Ovarian Cancer 4

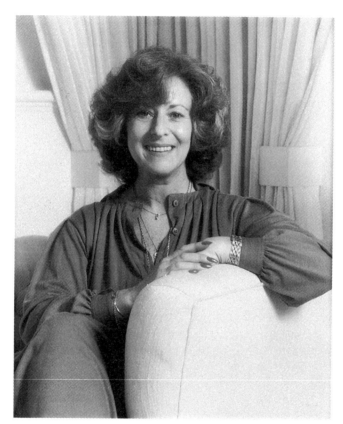
Helene Harris

Ovarian Cancer 4

Edited by

Frank Sharp

Department of Obstetrics and Gynaecology,
Northern General Hospital, Sheffield University, Sheffield, UK

Tony Blackett

Department of Obstetrics and Gynaecology,
Northern General Hospital, Sheffield University, Sheffield, UK

Robin Leake

Faculty of Medicine,
University of Glasgow, Glasgow, UK

Jonathan Berek

Division of Gynecologic Oncology,
UCLA School of Medicine, Los Angeles, USA

CHAPMAN & HALL MEDICAL
London · Glasgow · Weinheim · New York · Tokyo · Melbourne · Madras

Published by
Chapman & Hall, 2–6 Boundary Row, London SE1 8HN, UK

Chapman & Hall, 2–6 Boundary Row, London SE1 8HN, UK

Blackie Academic & Professional, Wester Cleddens Road, Bishopbriggs, Glasgow G64 2NZ, UK

Chapman & Hall GmbH, Pappelallee 3, 69469 Weinheim, Germany

Chapman & Hall USA, 115 Fifth Avenue, New York, NY 10003, USA

Chapman & Hall Japan, ITP-Japan, Kyowa Building, 3F, 2-2-1 Hirakawacho, Chiyoda-ku, Tokyo 102, Japan

Chapman & Hall Australia, 102 Dodds Street, South Melbourne, Victoria 3205, Australia

Chapman & Hall India, R. Seshadri, 32 Second Main Road, CIT East, Madras 600 035, India

First edition 1996

© 1996 Chapman & Hall

Printed in Great Britain by the University Press, Cambridge

ISBN 0 412 72370 0

Erratum

The images of figures 5.4 and 5.5, appearing on pages 55 and 56 respectively, have been transposed.

Ovarian Cancer 4. Edited by F. Sharp, T. Blackett, R. Leake and J. Berek. Published in 1996 by Chapman & Hall, London. ISBN 0 412 72370 0

Contents

Contents

Contributors

Nelly Auersperg
Department of Obstetrics and Gynaecology, University of British Columbia, BC Women's Hospital, 4490 Oak Street, Vancouver BC V6H 3V5, Canada

Nigel P Bailey
Division of Oncology, Newcastle General Hospital, Westgate Road, Newcastle-upon-Tyne NE4 6BE, UK

Rachael G Barton
University of Birmingham CRC Institute for Cancer Studies, Birmingham B15 2TJ, UK

Robert C Bast Jr.
University of Texas, MD Anderson Cancer Center, Houston, TX 77030, USA

Andrew Berchuck
Duke University Medical Center, Durham, North Carolina, 27710, USA

Jonathan S Berek
Division of Gynecologic Oncology, Department of Obstetrics and Gynecology, UCLA School of Medicine, Los Angeles, CA 90024-2740, USA

Alan P Boddy
University of Newcastle, Newcastle-upon-Tyne, UK

Michael A Bookman
Fox Chase Cancer Center, 7701 Burholme Avenue, Philadelphia, PA 19111, USA

Cinda M Boyer
Duke University Medical Center, Durham, North Carolina, 27710, USA

Peter Boyle
Division of Epidemiology and Biostatistics, European Institute of Oncology, Via Ripamonti 435, 20141 Milano, Italy

Robert Brown
CRC Department of Medical Oncology, CRC Beatson Laboratories, Garscube Estate, Switchback Road, Glasgow G61 1BD, UK

A Hilary Calvert
Division of Oncology, Newcastle General Hospital, Westgate Road, Newcastle-upon-Tyne NE4 6BE, UK

Lisa Cannon-Albright
Genetic Epidemiology Group, Department of Medical Informatics, University of Utah, Salt Lake City, UT, USA

K K Chan
Department of Obstetrics and Gynaecology, City Hospital Trust, Dudley Road, Birmingham B18 7QH, UK

Randolph D Christen
Department of Medicine and the Cancer Center, University of California San Diego, La Jolla, California 92093, USA

Brian B Cohen
School of Biological and Medical Sciences, University of St Andrews, UK

William P Collins
Department of Obstetrics and Gynaecology, King's College Hospital, Denmark Hill, London SE5 8RX, UK

Aileen E C Crosbie
Department of Clinical Genetics, Western General Hospital NHS Trust, Edinburgh, UK

Robert M Dable
Duke University Medical Center, Durham, North Carolina, 27710, USA

Elisabeth G E de Vries
Division of Medical Oncology, Department of Internal Medicine, University Hospital, Oostersingel 59, 9713 EZ Groningen, The Netherlands

Johannes Dietl
Department of Obstetrics and Gynaecology, University of Tübingen, Schleichstraße 4, 72076 Tübingen, Germany

Helen G Dyck
Department of Obstetrics and Gynaecology, University of British Columbia, BC Women's Hospital, 4490 Oak Street, Vancouver BC, V6H 3V5, Canada

Hani Gabra
ICRF Medical Oncology Unit, Western General Hospital NHS Trust, Edinburgh, UK

Lori A Getts
Department of Medical Oncology, Fox Chase Cancer Center, Philadelphia, PA 19111, USA

Moira G Gilligan
University of Birmingham, CRC Institute for Cancer Studies, Birmingham B15 2TJ, UK

Charles R Gillis
Beatson Oncology Centre, Western Infirmary, Dumbarton Road, Glasgow, UK

Andrew K Godwin
Department of Medical Oncology, Fox Chase Cancer Center, Philadelphia, PA 19111, USA

David E Goldgar
Genetic Epidemiology Group, Department of Medical Informatics, University of Utah, Salt Lake City, UT 84108, USA

Martin E Gore
Gynaecology Unit, Royal Marsden Hospital, Fulham Road, London SW3 6JJ, UK

Thomas C Hamilton
Department of Medical Oncology, Fox Chase Cancer Center, Philadelphia, PA 19111, USA

Ian R Hart
Richard Dimbleby Department of Cancer Research/ICRF Laboratory, St Thomas's Hospital, Lambeth Palace Road, London SE1 7EH, UK

David J Hole
Beatson Oncology Centre, Western Infirmary, Dumbarton Road, Glasgow, UK

Hans-Peter Horny
Institute of Pathology, University of Tübingen, Germany

Stephen B Howell
Department of Medicine 0812, University of California, San Diego, La Jolla, CA 92093, USA

Andrew Hughes
Division of Oncology, Newcastle General Hospital Westgate Road, Newcastle-upon-Tyne NE4 6BE, UK

Richard Hutson
Department of Obstetrics and Gynaecology, St James's University Hospital, Leeds LS9 7TF, UK

Elizabeth J Junor
Beatson Oncology Centre, Western Infirmary, Dumbarton Road, Glasgow, UK

Hilbert J Kappen
University of Nijmegen, Laboratory for Medical and Biophysics and Dutch Foundation for Neural Networks, Geert Grooteplein Noord 21, 6525 EZ Nijmegen, The Netherlands

Stanley B Kaye
CRC Department of Medical Oncology, University of Glasgow, CRC Beatson Laboratories, Alexander Stone Building, Garscube Estate, Switchback Road, Bearsden, Glasgow G61 1BD, UK

Sean Kehoe
Department of Obstetrics and Gynaecology, City Hospital Trust, Dudley Road, Birmingham B18 7QH, UK

Lloyd R Kelland
CRC Centre for Cancer Therapeutics, The Institute of Cancer Research, 15 Cotswold Road, Sutton, Surrey SM2 5NG, UK

David J Kerr
University of Birmingham, CRC Institute for Cancer Studies, Birmingham B15 2TJ, UK

Buran Kurdi-Haidar
Department of Medicine and Cancer Center, University of California, San Diego, La Jolla, CA 92093, USA

Robin E Leake
Department of Biochemistry, University of Glasgow, Glasgow G12 8QQ, UK

Alastair Lessels
Department of Pathology, Western General Hospital NHS Trust, Edinburgh, UK

Cathryn M Lewis
Genetic Epidemiology Group, Department of Medical Informatics, University of Utah, Salt Lake City, UT, USA

Michael J Lind
Division of Oncology, Newcastle General Hospital Westgate Road, Newcastle-upon-Tyne NE4 6BE, UK

Gerrit Los
Department of Medicine and Cancer Center, University of California San Diego, La Jolla, California 92093, USA

David Luesley
Department of Obstetrics and Gynaecology, City Hospital Trust, Dudley Road, Birmingham B18 7QH, UK

Patrick McClean
Department of Medical Oncology, Charing Cross Hospital, London W6 8RF, UK

James Mackay
ICRF Department of Medical Oncology, Western General Hospital NHS Trust, Edinburgh EH4 2XU, UK

Sarah L Maines-Bandiera
Department of Obstetrics and Gynaecology, University of British Columbia, BC Women's Hospital, 4490 Oak Street, Vancouver BC, V6H 3V5, Canada

Paul D Miller
Department of Medical Oncology, Fox Chase Cancer Center, Philadelphia, PA 19111, USA

John Monaghan
Regional Department of Gynaecological Oncology, Queen Elizabeth Hospital, Gateshead, Tyne and Wear NE9 6SX, UK

Jan P Neijt
Utrecht University Hospital, Department of Internal Medicine, Heidelberglaan 100, PO Box 85500, 3508 GA Utrecht, The Netherlands

Anne Nelstrop
Department of Medical Oncology, Charing Cross Hospital, London W6 8RF, UK

Susan Neuhausen
Genetic Epidemiology Group, Department of Medical Informatics, University of Utah, Salt Lake City, UT, USA

D R Herbie Newell
University of Newcastle, Newcastle-upon-Tyne NE4 6BE, UK

Franco Odicino
Department of Gynaecologic Oncology, University of Brescia and the European Institute of Oncology, Via Ripamonti 435, 20141 Milano, Italy

Robert F Ozols
Fox Chase Cancer Center, 7701 Burholme Avenue, Philadelphia, PA 19111, USA

Sergio Pecorelli
Department of Gynaecologic Oncology, University of Brescia and the European Institute of Oncology, Via Ripamonti 435, 20141 Milano, Italy

Martine J Piccart
Institut Jules Bordet, Rue Heger-Bordet 1, Brussels, Belgium

Bruce Ponder
CRC Human Cancer Genetics Research Group, Addenbrooke's Hospital, Hills Road, Cambridge CB2 2QQ, UK

Peter Ruck
Institute of Pathology, University of Tübingen, Germany

Gordon J S Rustin
Department of Medical Oncology, Charing Cross Hospital, London W6 8RF, UK

Udo Schumacher
Department of Human Morphology, University of Southampton, UK

Peter F Searle
University of Birmingham, CRC Institute for Cancer Studies, Birmingham B15 2TJ, UK

Jean Selleslags
Institut Jules Bordet, Rue Heger-Bordet 1, Brussels, Belgium

Anne P Shapter
Division of Gynecologic Oncology, Department of Obstetrics and Gynecology, UCLA School of Medicine, Los Angeles, CA 90024-1740, USA

Neelam Siddique
Division of Oncology, Newcastle General Hospital, Westgate Road, Newcastle-upon-Tyne NE4 6BE, UK

Mark Skolnick
Genetic Epidemiology Group, Department of Medical Informatics, University of Utah, Salt Lake City, UT, USA

George E Smart
Department of Obstetrics and Gynaecology, Royal Infirmary of Edinburgh NHS Trust, Edinburgh, UK

Stephen K Smith
Department of Obstetrics and Gynaecology, University of Cambridge, Rosie Maternity Hospital, Cambridge CB2 2SW, UK

John F Smyth
ICRF Department of Medical Oncology, Western General Hospital NHS Trust, Edinburgh, UK

C Michael Steel
Department of Biological and Medical Sciences, University of St Andrews, St Andrews, UK

Linda Steele
Genetic Epidemiology Group, Department of Medical Informatics, University of Utah, Salt Lake City, UT, USA

Wim ten Bokkel Huinink
The Netherlands Cancer Institute, Amsterdam, The Netherlands

Antonella Tessadrelli
Department of Gynaecologic Oncology, University of Brescia and the European Institute of Oncology, Via Ripamonti 435, 20141 Milano, Italy

Annet te Velde
The Netherlands Cancer Institute, Amsterdam, The Netherlands

Marc M H J Theeuwen
University of Nijmegen, Laboratory for Medical and Biophysics and Dutch Foundation for Neural Networks, Geert Grooteplein Noord 21, EZ Nojmegen, The Netherlands

Huw Thomas
University of Newcastle, Newcastle-upon-Tyne NE4 6BE, UK

Maria van der Burg
Daniel den Hoed Kliniek, Rotterdam, The Netherlands

Ate G J van der Zee
Division of Gynecologic Oncology, University Hospital, Oostersingel 59, 9713 EZ Groningen, The Netherlands

Peter van Geene
Department of Obstetrics and Gynaecology, City Hospital Trust, Dudley Road, Birmingham B18 7QH, UK

Allan van Oosterom
University Hospital, Antwerp, Belgium

Jantien Wanders
New Drug Development Office, Amsterdam, The Netherlands

Kim Ward
Department of Obstetrics and Gynaecology, City Hospital Trust, Dudley Road, Birmingham B18 7QH, UK

Michael Wells
Department of Pathology, St James's University Hospital, Leeds LS9 7TF, UK

John Welsh
Olav Kerr Professor of Palliative Medicine, Glasgow University, Hunters Hill Marie Curie Centre, 1 Belmont Road, Glasgow G21 3AY, UK

Alastair Williams
Department of Pathology, Medical School, University of Edinburgh, Edinburgh, UK

Feng-Ji Xu
University of Texas, MD Anderson Cancer Centre, Houston, Texas 77030, USA

Lawrence S Young
University of Birmingham CRC Institute for Cancer Studies, Birmingham B15 2TJ, UK

Yin-Hua Yu
University of Texas, MD Anderson Cancer Centre, Houston, Texas 77030, USA

Preface

With the publication of this volume, it has now been a decade since the Helene Harris Memorial Trust was born. An important decision was made by its benefactor, Mr John Harris, to establish a series of meetings to present the state of research and discuss the management of ovarian cancer. There have been now five biennial meetings and this outstanding programme has witnessed and promoted great progress in our understanding of the basic biology, genetics, mechanisms of resistance and the new therapeutic strategies of ovarian cancer. This international programme has brought together many capable and distinguished scientists and clinicians who are dedicated to the study of ovarian cancer, and has facilitated the interaction of many scholars, leading to an exchange of ideas and many collaborations.

The last decade has witnessed the discovery of specific genes that may control the development of ovarian cancer, a clearer understanding of the inherent biology of the disease process, and several leaps forward in our understanding of the treatment of the disease. Methods for screening have been refined and, although we do not yet have a suitable answer, the series of meetings has helped to produce a strategy that may very well ultimately lead to the early detection of ovarian cancer.

In the most recent meeting held in Glasgow, Scotland on 3–7 May 1995, the important question of whether or not there is an identifiable premalignant lesion was addressed. While the data on this issue are controversial, a clear summary of the problem was defined and is presented. One of the most exciting areas of progress in the past decade has been in the genetics of ovarian cancer and a prominent discussion was undertaken on the current situation of gene mutations associated with the disease. The discovery and cloning of the BRCA1 gene is clearly a milestone in the understanding of genetic predisposition of ovarian cancer and undoubtedly will be the first amongst several discoveries that will allow us to characterize its molecular epidemiology. Discussions were undertaken to summarize the optimal treatment of ovarian cancer, including the appropriate strategies for primary and intervention surgeries, better means of defining response and survival and new chemotherapeutic approaches that now incorporate the taxanes. Important new studies defined the use of CA125 for response, the impact of location and type of physician treating women with ovarian cancer, as well as the use of the innovative new technique of using neural networks to predict survival.

Many new treatment approaches, including biological therapies and methods of overcoming drug resistance, have developed over the past decade. A major session was devoted purely to evolving gene therapy strategies, because DNA-based therapy will undoubtedly become a reality. This symposium well summarizes the current status of this important new approach.

We are proud to dedicate this book to the 'decade of progress' that has taken place since the inception of the Helene Harris Memorial Trust. We continue to dedicate our efforts to the women and their families who are diagnosed and treated for ovarian cancer. To their great courage, we reaffirm our goal to detect and cure the disease.

Frank Sharp, Sheffield
Tony Blackett, Sheffield
Robin Leake, Glasgow
Jonathan Berek, Los Angeles

Helene Harris Memorial Trust Introduction

This latest book on ovarian cancer published for the Helene Harris Memorial Trust by Chapman & Hall covers the work of the 1995 HHMT Forum in Glasgow.

This fifth major international meeting was most significant covering, as it did, the new developments in gene therapy plus many other aspects in the treatment and management of ovarian cancer. I believe that research workers, clinicians and all others involved in probing the biology of ovarian cancer and developing improved treatment will find this work invaluable.

The HHMT owes a debt to many people. To the distinguished contributors go our sincere thanks, also to our fine administrators, Shirley Claff and Geraldine Presland, whose voluntary efforts organizing all aspects of the Forum have made everything run smoothly. Finally a very special acknowledgement to our editors, Frank Sharp, Tony Blackett, Robin Leake and Jonathan Berek for their most professional and efficient compilation of a very fine book.

John E. Harris

Part One

Is there an Identifiable Premalignant Lesion?

Chapter 1

Phenotypic plasticity of ovarian surface epithelium: possible implications for ovarian carcinogenesis

Nelly AUERSPERG, Sarah L. MAINES-BANDIERA and Helen G. DYCK

1.1 INTRODUCTION

A high proportion of the common epithelial ovarian carcinomas express complex phenotypic characteristics of Müllerian duct-derived epithelia, and a lesser but significant proportion resemble Wolffian duct derivatives, and even intestinal cells [1,2]. Such diverse characteristics take the form of epithelial specializations at the cellular level, such as apical microvilli, junctional complexes, epithelial membrane antigens and secretory products including mucins and CA125. They are also expressed at the level of multicellular morphogenesis or tissue formation, in the form of polarized epithelia, papillae, cysts and glandular structures. These complex, highly differentiated tumours arise in a simple squamous to cuboidal epithelium, the ovarian surface epithelium (OSE), which is the pelvic mesothelium covering the ovary. Like some other simple epithelia, OSE is characterized by low molecular weight keratins, simple desmosomes, apical microvilli and a basal lamina [3]. Importantly however, many of the more highly specialized epithelial characteristics found in ovarian carcinomas are lacking or are expressed weakly and inconsistently in normal OSE. These include high molecular weight keratins, E-cadherin, CA125, mucin and several epithelial antigens [1,4-6]. Thus, unlike carcinomas in most other organs, where epithelial cells become less differentiated in the course of neoplastic progression than the epithelium from which they arise, ovarian carcinomas are frequently more highly differentiated than OSE [2].

Embryologically, the OSE originates in coelomic epithelium which overlies the gonadal ridge. It is therefore of mesodermal origin, and closely related to the underlying stromal fibroblasts [7]. Coelomic epithelial cells penetrate into the fetal ovary and contribute to the development of granulosa cells; furthermore, the gonadal ridge lies near the region where invagination of the coelomic epithelium gives rise to the Müllerian (paramesonephric) ducts, *i.e.* the primordia for the epithelia of the oviduct, uterus and upper vagina. Thus, in the embryo, the coelomic epithelium in the gonadal region is competent to develop along many different pathways. The relatively simple phenotype of the adult OSE, and its capacity to differentiate into such striking variety of ovarian carcinomas, have led to the concept that adult OSE is relatively uncommitted and closer to a stem cell form than other coelomic epithelial derivatives such as the endometrium and the oviductal epithelium.

There are indications that even the differentiation of OSE into a simple epithelium is not as firmly determined as in most other adult epithelia. Evidence of its mesodermal origin and its developmental relationship to stromal fibroblasts persist in the adult: OSE *in vivo* and *in vitro* contains vimentin filaments, which are typical for mesenchymal cells, concurrently with keratin filaments [3,8]. In culture, it produces not only epithelial (laminin and collagen IV) but also mesenchymal (collagen types I and III) components of extracellular matrix [3], and it modulates from an epithelial to a mesenchymal morphology in response to a variety of environmental cues [9,10].

In this review, we discuss some of the possible implications of the limited deter-mination and persistent competence for phenotypic plasticity of adult OSE, with particular emphasis on its capacity to undergo epithelio-mesenchymal conversion, on the changes in plasticity and respon-siveness to environmental controls that occur with neoplastic progression, and on possible alterations in these characteristics that may occur in normal OSE from women with familial ovarian cancer.

1.2 NORMAL OVARIAN SURFACE EPITHELIUM (OSE)

Recent studies aimed at characterizing human OSE cells indicate that this epithelium is far more complicated and physiologically versatile than would be predicted from its inconspicuous appearance. The normal OSE has the capacity to remodel the ovarian cortex through synthetic, physical and proteolytic functions which may influence ovulation and the repair of ovulatory defects, as well as the ovarian shrinkage and cyst

formation which occur with age [10,11]. The discoveries that OSE cells secrete biologically active cytokines [12] and growth factors [13] and that they have oestrogen receptors [14,15] suggest that OSE plays an integral part in the network of hormones and short range-acting factors which regulate normal ovarian physiology.

In vitro studies have demonstrated that normal OSE is highly responsive to environmental influences. Under standard culture conditions, that is on a plastic substratum in serum-supplemented culture media, OSE cells retain their cobblestone epithelial appearance as long as they are maintained under confluent conditions in primary culture, that is as long as they are not disrupted and passaged. If the monolayer is disrupted, then the cells lose their characteristic cuboidal epithelial morphology in exchange for one resembling flattened extraovarian mesothelium and, subsequently, an atypical, fibroblast-like phenotype (Figure 1.1). Epithelio-mesen-chymal conversion is characterized by a switch from an apico-basal to an anterio-posterior polarity, loss of intercellular contacts, expression of the connective tissue type collagens types I and III, and prolyl-4-hydroxylase [16], and by the loss of epithelial markers [3]. Preliminary data indicate that OSE *in situ*, on the ovarian surface, does not produce collagen III, but that the secretion of this extracellular matrix component is triggered by explantation into culture [17]. Though most cells in primary culture retain vimentin, keratin and microvilli, the proportion of keratin-positive cells as well as the number of keratin subtypes decrease over several passages, while vimentin is retained. Microvilli disappear even more rapidly as there are only a few villi on less than 5% of cells by passage 1. CA125, an epithelial differen-tiation marker present in small proportions of OSE cells in primary culture

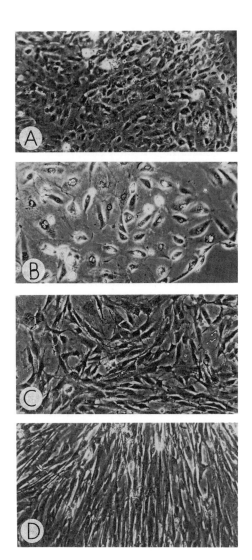

Figure 1.1 Morphological variation among cultures of human ovarian surface epithelium (OSE) in low passage. (a) compact, cobblestone epithelial monolayer in primary culture; (b) flat epithelial monolayer, frequently seen in passages 2-3; (c) atypical growth with cellular overlap and mesenchymal features, characteristic of cultures in passages 3 and beyond; (d) stromal fibroblasts, showing more parallel alignment and spindle shapes than the cells in (c). Phase contrast microscopy, x 250.

and passage 1, diminishes and disappears over subsequent passages. E-cadherin could not be demonstrated in primary cultures of OSE cells by either immunofluorescence or Western blotting, though it is expressed, albeit weakly and inconsistently, by OSE *in vivo* [18]. Similarly, desmoplakin I and II are present in the OSE of ovarian sections but could not be demonstrated once the cells are cultured. Among epithelial markers, only the epithelial basement membrane components laminin and collagen type IV persist with passaging in culture. It should be noted, however, that these forms of extracellular matrix are also found in association with certain cells that are classically considered components of connective tissue, such as smooth muscle cells and adipocytes. In contrast to the epithelial markers, vimentin, collagens I and III and prolyl-4-hydroxylase persist in prolonged culture [3].

Whether OSE cells remain epithelial or undergo conversion to a mesenchymal phenotype depends on the culture substratum [10]. Under two sets of conditions, some epithelial characteristics of OSE are maintained and in both instances the substratum resembles one that OSE cells normally encounter *in vivo*:

1. Cells grown on fibrin clots, which mimic the surface on which OSE cells migrate during the repair of the ovulatory defect, retain an epithelial morphology though they separate from one another and migrate actively.

2. Matrigel, a substratum consisting predominantly of the epithelial components of the basement membrane [19] supports the formation of nonproliferative clusters of epithelioid OSE cells [10].

In contrast, OSE cells cultured on collagen-, gelatin- or fibronectin-coated dishes, on collagen gel, and on a collagen-rich stroma produced by rat OSE [20] assume

5

mesenchymal characteristics. OSE cells also convert to the mesenchymal form if they are grown directly on plastic or in a three-dimensional sponge matrix which provides a rigid scaffolding of inert, denatured pig skin collagen (Health Designs Industries, Rochester, NY). The substitution of three-dimensional for two-dimensional culture conditions induces major changes in signal transduction and gene expression [21,22], and increases the resemblance to *in vivo* conditions [23]. In the three-dimensional collagenous sponge matrix, epithelial morphogenesis by OSE and its derivatives was defined by the capacity of the cells to form structures such as epithelial linings, papillae and cysts, whereas mesenchymal morphogenesis was defined by a dispersed, fibroblast-like cell distribution and secretion of extracellular matrix. Importantly, both on plastic and in the matrix, the normal OSE cells secrete connective tissue type collagens. In the three-dimensional matrix, in particular, OSE cells produce a copious, fibrillar extracellular matrix with the cells dispersed singly, in a manner indistinguishable from fibroblasts within loose connective tissue (Figure 1.2). Together, these variations in growth patterns suggest that extracellular matrix components contribute to the environmental signals which determine whether OSE will express epithelial or mesenchymal characteristics, and that these signals may take the form of either endogenous or exogenous matrix components.

Sponge contraction was examined as an additional indicator of the mesenchymal phenotype. Sponge contraction and collagen gel contraction in culture are functions which are characteristic of connective tissue fibroblasts and are thought to mimic the contraction of connective tissues that is carried out by fibroblasts *in vivo* during wound healing [17]. It is known that fibroblasts cultured within collagen gels contract the gels as a result of tractional forces exerted by the cells attached to the collagen fibres. This contraction requires a functional cytoskeleton, and the traction is transduced on the collagen matrix through integrins, specifically integrin a2b1. The force generated by such cultured fibroblasts resembles the force observed in contracting skin wounds [reviewed in 24]. When low passage OSE cells were cultured in the three-dimensional sponge matrix, they contracted it to approximately half its original size within a few weeks.

It has been known for a long time [25,26] that cells, in general, respond to explantation into culture as they would to wounding, and that they consequently undergo changes in phenotype and in gene expression that are seen in regenerative responses and wound healing [27]. Specific signals that elicit this response include the disruption of intercellular contacts and the exposure to serum which, *in vivo*, cells encounter only at sites of tissue damage. By analogy, the response of OSE to explantation into culture may mimic the responses that occur *in vivo* during postovulatory repair and, perhaps, when fragments of OSE are displaced from the ovarian surface by adhesions or become trapped in the stroma as a result of changes in the ovarian contours with pregnancies and ageing. Under such conditions, OSE cells disperse, migrate, proliferate and assume different shapes [28]. The modulation of cobblestone OSE to flat epithelial cells in culture may be analogous to the appearance of the flat 'B' type OSE cells that have been observed *in vivo* in regions on the ovarian surface where OSE overlies sites of previous ovulatory rupture [29]. The assumption of the mesenchymal phenotype occurs particularly consistently in association with endogenous and exogenous collagenous extracellular matrices. Therefore, the

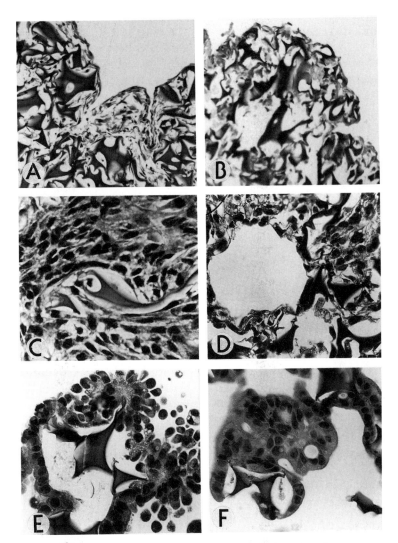

Figure 1.2. Morphology of cultures grown in a three-dimensional sponge matrix. (a) OSE from a woman with no family history (NFH) of ovarian cancer, p.5: growth resembles loose connective tissue with the cells dispersed in an abundant extracellular matrix. The tissue is thrown into folds as a result of sponge contraction; (b) OSE from a woman with a family history (FH) of ovarian cancer, p.4: the cells adhere to sponge spicules as small groups. There is no visible extracellular matrix and no sponge contraction; (c) Immortalized NFH-OSE p.7: the amount of extracellular matrix is reduced compared to (a). The cells retain a mesenchymal form and intercellular organization; (d) Immortalized FH-OSE p.8: round cells are interspersed in a network of extracellular matrix; (e,f) ovarian carcinoma cell lines OVCAR 3 (e) and OVCAR 5 (f) showing an epithelial morphology (rows of columnar cells, papillae, cyst-like structures).

Light microscopy, hematoxylin & eosin; (a,b) x 120; (c-f) x 350. p = passage number modulation to the mesenchymal form in culture may, perhaps, reflect an *in vivo* response of OSE cells to displacement from the ovarian surface into the ovarian stroma, which would allow them to assume the properties of connective tissue fibroblasts. In OSE-derived organoids in culture [11] cells that are trapped within the 'stroma' appear fibroblastic in morphology and growth pattern, but continue to express keratin. Similar modulations to a mesenchymal form have been observed in cultures from other types of mesodermally derived epithelia, including pleural mesothelium, endothelial cells and kidney cells [30-34]. Furthermore, similar epithelio-mesenchymal conversions occur normally *in vivo* in at least two cell types that are closely related to OSE anatomically and developmentally:

1. In reactive mesothelial cells engaged in repair in response to pleural injury, Davila and Crouch [35] found co-expression of keratin with vimentin and collagen I propeptide, both on the regenerating lining and in the submesothelial regions.

2. When the cells of the developing Müllerian duct regress in response to Müllerian inhibiting substance in male embryos, they dissociate from one another, assume a mesenchymal form and migrate into the surrounding stroma [36].

While there is at present no conclusive evidence for a similar phenomenon in human ovaries, we have observed occasional keratin positive spindle-shaped cells in corpora lutea and their surrounding stroma, and similar observations have been reported by others [1,8].

1.3 NEOPLASTIC PROGRESSION

In contrast to normal OSE, immortalized OSE and especially ovarian carcinomas maintain epithelial characteristics in prolonged culture [3,15,37]. As reported previously [38] we immortalized OSE cells in low passage by transfection with SV40 large T antigen. The characteristics of the immortalized lines reflected the morphology and differentiation markers of the low passage cells at the time of transfection. In lines derived from epithelial, keratin-positive OSE cells, an epithelial morphology, keratin, laminin and collagen type IV persisted in nearly 100% of cells after repeated subculturing. In addition, about 50% of cells in one of the lines retained abundant apical microvilli, though these structures disappear rapidly in nonimmortalized OSE cultures. Like normal OSE cells in low passage culture, the immortalized lines co-express the epithelial markers with mesenchymal characteristics, namely collagens type I and III and prolyl-4-hydroxylase. Immortalized OSE lines grow well in three-dimensional sponge matrix, filling the spaces with tightly packed cells (Figure 1.2). Like low passage OSE cells, the immortalized cells contract the sponge matrix to about half its original size within a few weeks. Interestingly, even though they form epithelial monolayers when grown in two dimensions, their growth patterns in the sponge matrix remain mesenchymal, sometimes resembling sarcomas. Therefore, the cues which induce epithelio-mesenchymal conversion in low passage OSE appear to be altered in the immortalized lines.

Ovarian carcinoma lines exhibited the most typically epithelial phenotypes of all the cell types examined. On plastic, all but one of eight lines analysed were epithelial. Six of the eight lines expressed keratin in 100% of cells, and several of them retained apical microvilli. In addition, and in contrast to both low passage and immortalized OSE cells, two carcinoma lines tested for E-cadherin and for CA125 expressed these markers of Müllerian epithelial differentiation in a high proportion of cells, while collagen III was expressed only by few cells in three lines. The carcinoma lines retained epithelial growth patterns in three-dimensional sponge matrix culture where they formed columnar epithelia, papillae, aggregates and cyst-like structures, sometimes closely resembling ovarian carcinomas *in vivo* (Figure 1.2). In contrast to low passage- and immortalized OSE, there was no sponge contraction by any of the cancer cell lines.

Immortalization by SV40 large T antigen interferes with the normal function of p53, a tumour suppressor gene which is frequently mutated in ovarian carcinomas [39,40]. Our results support other data which indicate that interference with p53 function is insufficient to shift the phenotype of OSE to that of ovarian carcinomas. They show further that such interference permits the continued expression of differentiation markers that characterize the OSE cells of origin, but does not induce a more complex epithelial phenotype with properties of Müllerian epithelial derivatives. Thus, although the SV40 early genes induce (pre)neoplastic changes in the form of reduced phenotypic plasticity and uncontrolled proliferation, the consequences of their expression are insufficient to completely mimic ovarian carcinogenesis.

In addition to the epithelial characteristics that were maintained in the immortalized lines, the carcinoma lines also expressed E-cadherin and CA125, formed complex epithelial structures in three-dimensional matrix, and lacked at least one of the connective tissue type collagens found in low passage- and immortalized OSE [17]. These results demonstrate that our culture conditions permit the expression of at least some of the Müllerian duct characteristics that are commonly acquired by OSE cells in the course of malignant transformation *in vivo*. They support the concept that the ovarian carcinoma cells have become firmly committed to differentiation along the lines of Müllerian duct epithelia and are no longer responsive to the signals which induce mesenchymal phenotypes in their non-malignant precursors. Our findings complement *in vivo* comparisons of epithelial differentiation markers in OSE and ovarian cancers. Ovarian cancers express an epithelial cell type 200-kDa glycoprotein, human milk fat globule antigen and high molecular weight keratins [1,5] and form complex epithelial histological structures [2], while OSE is negative for these epithelial markers; vimentin, in contrast, is uniformly present in OSE but more heterogeneously among carcinomas [1]. Interestingly, possession of a vimentin cytoskeleton seems to predispose certain epithelia to give rise to mesenchymal-shaped cells [41]. The similarities between our findings and the *in vivo* characteristics of OSE and of ovarian cancers, respectively, suggest that the differences in differentiation observed here may be significant in the process of ovarian carcinogenesis.

1.4 FAMILIAL OVARIAN CANCER

There has been little progress in the detection of preneoplastic changes in the OSE. This lack of information poses a particular problem for women with hereditary ovarian cancer syndromes, where there is a need to define criteria for prevention and surveillance [42]. Although most epithelial ovarian carcinomas arise without known predictive factors, recent progress in genetic analysis, and in particular the identification of the BRCA-1 gene, has identified some women who are at high risk of developing ovarian cancer [43]. However, not all women with BRCA-1 mutations develop ovarian cancer, and there are other individuals who are at increased risk of developing the disease because of a family history that may be linked through other loci, or where

9

linkage testing is not feasible. Studies of women with familial ovarian cancer [44] and with unilateral ovarian cancer [45,46] have revealed benign histological changes in the OSE and stroma of overtly normal ovaries. In view of these observations, it seemed possible that the OSE from women with family histories of ovarian cancer might express an altered phenotype in culture, and that such alterations might reveal early changes and, perhaps, predictive markers for ovarian carcinogenesis.

As discussed earlier in this review, it appears that, in the course of carcinogenesis, OSE cells become more firmly committed to an epithelial phenotype and less apt to undergo epithelio-mesenchymal conversion in response to the environmental signals encountered in culture. We therefore examined OSE cultures from women with family histories of ovarian cancer to test the hypothesis that their capacity for epithelio-mesenchymal conversion may be reduced. The parameters that were chosen for evaluation included the cellular morphology and growth patterns in two- and three-dimensional culture, the capacity for sponge contraction, and the expression of CA125, keratin and collagen type III. As described above, sponge contraction is a characteristic of fibroblasts thought to correspond to the contractile activity of connective tissue fibroblasts during wound healing *in vivo* [24]. CA125 is an epithelial differentiation antigen that is normally expressed by oviductal epithelium and endometrium [4,47] and is also secreted by a high proportion of ovarian serous adenocarcinomas [48]. Whereas CA125 expression by normal OSE on the ovarian surface is often weak or absent, the OSE in inclusion cysts, where carcinomas tend to arise, is more consistently CA125 positive. Changes in CA125 expression may therefore occur very early, or even precede, neoplastic progression in OSE

cells. The concurrent expression of keratin and collagen type III, as an epithelial and a mesenchymal marker respectively, were compared. Keratin is one of the most uniformly expressed epithelial markers for normal OSE *in vivo* and in primary culture, and it diminishes with passaging. Collagen type III is one of the connective tissue type collagens and is particularly abundant *in vivo* during wound repair [49]; it appears to be absent in intact OSE *in vivo* , and is induced in primary culture.

We compared the above markers in overtly normal OSE from patients with no family history (NFH, 27 cases), patients with strong family histories, defined as at least two first degree relatives with breast or ovarian cancer (FH, 7 cases), and patients with minor family histories (mFH, 6 cases). The FH cases were obtained through collaboration with Drs. Henry T. Lynch, Creighton University, and Dr. Thomas C. Hamilton, Fox Chase Cancer Center. Within the FH group, four patients were 17q linkage positive. There were no consistent differences between the phenotypes of OSE from these four patients and the phenotypes of the remaining FH cases.

In contrast to NFH-OSE cells which modulated from epithelial monolayers in primary culture to a mesenchymal form by passage 2-4, FH-OSE cells retained a predominantly flat epithelial phenotype throughout the study, that is up to passage 5. The morphological changes among the mFH-OSE cultures were intermediate between the other two groups [50]. In three-dimensional sponge culture, low passage NFH-OSE cells proliferated rapidly, filled the sponge with a loose extracellular matrix which was interspersed with single, spindle-shaped cells and contracted the sponge to approximately half its original size. In contrast, FH-OSE cells grew very slowly in a three-dimensional sponge and never filled it. They adhered to

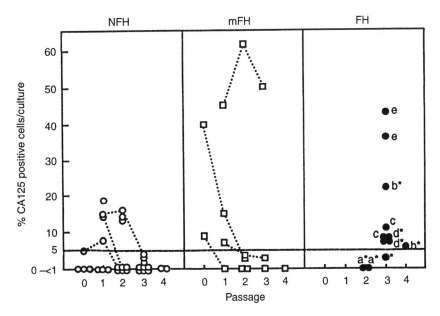

Figure 1.3 The proportion of cells expressing CA125 in cultures of OSE from women with no family history (NFH), with a minor family history (mFH) and with a strong family history (FH) of ovarian cancer. Most of the latter group were available for analysis only in passage 3. In cases where cells from the same patient were tested in more than one passage, the symbols are connected by lines. Asterisks indicate women with 17q linkage. The same letter next to two symbols in the FH group denotes the right and left ovary from the same indivdual. Note that the proportion of CA125-positive cells tends to drop with passaging to less than 5% in cultures from women in the NFH and mFH groups, but not in cultures from women in the FH group. (Reproduced, with permission, from *Am. J. Obstet. Gynecol.*)

the sponge spicules as single rounded cells, small aggregates and short rows of cuboidal cells, did not produce detectable extracellular matrix and did not contract the sponge matrix (Figure 1.2). Thus, compared to NFH-OSE, FH-OSE remained more epithelial when grown either in two or three dimensions [17].

Most primary NFH-OSE cultures contained very few CA125 positive cells (Figure 1.3). Upon subsequent passage, the proportion of cultures with five percent or more CA125 positive cells rose in passage 1 and diminished thereafter to very low levels in passage 4. With some exceptions, cultures derived from mFH patients followed a similar pattern. However, CA125 expression in the FH-OSE cultures was different: five percent or more of the cells retained CA125 in 9 of 12 cultures in passages 2-4, and in 9 of 10 cultures in passages 3-4. Thus, FH-OSE cultures retained subpopulations of CA125-expressing cells over longer time periods and more population doublings than did other cultures. In cultures with mixed cell morphologies, the CA125 positive cells were characteristically epithelial [50].

In contrast to NFH-OSE cultures, where the number of cells expressing keratin diminished with passages while collagen expression remained high, cultures of FH-

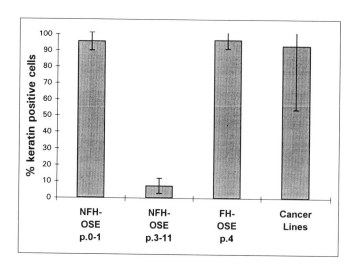

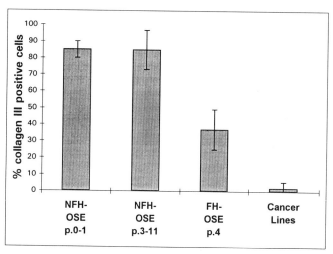

Figure 1.4 The percentage of OSE cells expressing keratin and collagen type III, based on counts of 1000 cells or more. NFH, no family history of ovarian cancer; FH, family history of ovarian cancer; p., passage; cancer lines, eight cell lines of ovarian carcinomas [17]. Keratin expression in the p. 3-11 NFH-OSE group is significantly lower (P<0.01) than in the other groups, which are statistically similar. The passage distribution in this group was: 1 x each of p.3, 5, 6, 11 and 2 x p.4. Collagen III expression is higher in both p. 0-1 and p. 3-11 NFH-OSE than in the FH-OSE (p<0.01). The cancer lines are significantly lower than all other groups (p<0.01).

12

OSE retained a high proportion of keratin positive cells throughout the study, while the proportion of collagen III positive cells was significantly reduced (Figure 1.4).

Cultures from seven FH patients were immortalized by transfection with SV40 early genes. All but one of the lines remained morphologically epithelial. In contrast to low passage FH-OSE, the immortalized FH-OSE proliferated rapidly in three-dimensional sponge, filling it within three weeks. They formed a lacy network of loosely packed cells within the sponge spaces, lined cavities with a squamous to cuboidal epithelium, and produced a small amount of ECM (Figure 1.2). However, like FH-OSE and unlike the immortalized NFH-OSE, they did not contract the sponge.

Although there were exceptions and inconsistencies in these studies as a result of uncontrolled variables among patients, differences between cultures, and the small number of observations, the results suggest that overtly normal OSE from women with family histories of ovarian cancer may differ from the OSE of women with no family histories not only at the genetic level, but also phenotypically. The increased stability of the epithelial phenotype observed in the FH-OSE might be related to the increased propensity of these cells to undergo neoplastic transformation, since OSE cells become more firmly committed to an epithelial phenotype with neoplastic progression. Importantly, the differences between the NFH-OSE and FH-OSE phenotypes described here may not be detectable in the intact epithelium, because they are differences in the responses of the NFH-OSE and FH-OSE cells to particular environmental signals, encountered upon explantation into culture. One of the most interesting changes observed in the OSE from patients with familial ovarian cancer was its inability to contract the three-dimensional sponge matrix, both in low passage and after immortalization. This change suggests that FH-OSE may differ from NFH-OSE in its response to wound healing signals.

1.5 CONCLUSIONS

Compared to most other adult epithelia, the ovarian surface epithelium (OSE) appears relatively uncommitted and retains a considerable phenotypic plasticity, reminiscent of stem cells. This phenotypic plasticity allows normal OSE cells to respond appropriately to extracellular signals and to adapt to varying conditions and changing environments. OSE cells respond to explantation into culture by conversion to a mesenchymal phenotype, which includes a fibroblast-like shape, reduced intercellular adhesion, the ability to contract collagen substrata, the expression of stromal extracellular matrix components, and loss of epithelial markers such as keratin and desmoplakin [3,51]. By analogy with the behaviour of other cell types, this conversion may mimic a regenerative or repair response of OSE cells *in vivo*. Such responses occur following ovulation, and perhaps also when fragments of OSE are displaced from the ovarian surface by adhesions, or become trapped in the stroma through changes in the ovarian contours.

In contrast to normal OSE, immortalized OSE and especially ovarian carcinoma cells maintain their epithelial characteristics in prolonged culture. Immortalization with SV40 large T antigen results in improved preservation of the epithelial characteristics of the OSE, but does not appear to induce any of the inappropriate differentiation markers that characterize ovarian carcinomas, such as the characteristics of Müllerian duct-derived epithelia. While in normal OSE phenotypic plasticity is a means to adapt to variable conditions, in ovarian carcinomas the phenotypic plasticity of OSE is shown by a capacity to re-express the developmental potential and differentiation pathways of the embryonic coelomic epithelium: most commonly, neoplastic OSE assumes the complex epithelial phenotypes of Müllerian duct-derived epithelia. It is not known what factors are responsible for this inappropriate differentiation of OSE. It seems clear, however, that the differentiation of ovarian carcinomas along Müllerian lines is accompanied by a loss of the adaptability to changing environments that exists in normal OSE. In culture, the differentiation of ovarian carcinomas seems irreversible and is maintained under conditions that induce epithelio-mesenchymal modulation in low passage and in immortalized OSE. One of the most fundamental characteristics of neoplasia in general is a change in phenotypic plasticity, as neoplastic cells substitute autoregulatory mechanisms for responses to external cues. The lack of responsiveness of the ovarian carcinomas to the environmental influences which determine the characteristics of normal OSE reflects this autonomy.

Overtly normal OSE cells from patients with family histories of ovarian cancer were also found to maintain more epithelial characteristics in culture than did OSE from the general population. These results suggest that the normal OSE of women with family histories of ovarian cancer might differ from other OSE not only genetically but also phenotypically.

The observations summarized in this review indicate that, with neoplastic progression, OSE cells become more firmly committed to an epithelial phenotype and less apt to undergo epithelio-mesenchymal conversion in response to environmental signals. In analogy with the behaviour in culture of other cell types, this change may reflect an altered or defective capacity to take part in repair processes. The changes in OSE from women with familial ovarian cancer suggest further that an increased commitment to an epithelial phenotype and/or reduced responsiveness to the environmental signals encountered in culture may be among the earliest changes in the process of ovarian carcinogenesis.

ACKNOWLEDGEMENTS

The work described in this review was supported by grants to N.A. from the Medical Research Council of Canada and the National Cancer Institute of Canada. N.A. is a Terry Fox Research Scientist of the National Cancer Institute of Canada, and H.G.D. received a Studentship from the B.C. Foundation for Non-Animal Research.

REFERENCES

1. Van Niekerk, C.C., Ramaekers, F.C.S., Hanselaar, A.G.J.M. *et al.* (1993) Changes in expression of differentiation markers between normal ovarian cells and derived tumors. *Am. J. Pathol.* **142**, 157-77.
2. Young, R.H., Clement, P.B. and Scully, R.E. (1989) The ovary. In *Diagnostic Surgical Pathology* (ed. S.S.Sternberg), Raven Press, New York, pp.1655-734.
3. Auersperg, N., Maines-Bandiera, S.L., Dyck H.G. *et al.* (1994) Characterization of cultured human ovarian surface epithelial cells: phenotypic plasticity and premalignant changes. *Lab. Invest.* **71**, 510-18.
4. Jacobs I. and Bast R.C. (1989) The CA 125 tumour-associated antigen: A review of the literature. *Hum. Reprod.* **4**, 1-12.
5. Moll, R., Pitz, S., Weikel, W. *et al.* (1991) Complexity of expression of intermediate filament proteins, including glial filament protein, in endometrial and ovarian adenocarcinomas. *Hum. Pathol.* **22**, 989-1001.
6. Viale, G., Gambacorta, M., Dell'Orto, P.

14

and Coggi, G. (1988) Coexpression of cytokeratins and vimentin in common epithelial tumours of the ovary: an immunocytochemical study of eighty-three cases. *Virchows Arch. A Pathol.* **413**, 91-101.

7. Nicosia, S.V. (1983) Morphological changes in the human ovary throughout life. In *The Ovary* (ed G.B. Serra), Raven Press, New York, pp. 57-81.

8. Czernobilsky, B., Moll, R., Levy, R. *et al.* (1985) Co-expression of cytokeratin and vimentin filaments in mesothelial, granulosa, and rete ovarii cells of the human ovary. *Eur. J. Cell Biol.* **37**, 175-90.

9. Siemens, C.H. and Auersperg, N. (1988) Serial propagation of human ovarian surface epithelium in tissue culture. *J. Cell. Physiol.* **134**, 347-56.

10. Kruk, P.A., Uitto, V.J., Firth, J.D. *et al.* (1994) Reciprocal interactions between human ovarian surface epithelial cells and adjacent extracellular matrix. *Exp. Cell Res.* **215**, 97-108.

11. Kruk, P.A. and Auersperg, N. (1992) Human ovarian surface epithelial cells are capable of physically restructuring extracellular matrix. *Am. J. Obstet. Gynecol.* **167**, 1437-43.

12. Ziltener, H.J., Maines-Bandiera, S., Schrader, J.W. and Auersperg, N. (1993) Secretion of bioactive IL-1, IL-6 and colony stimulating factors by human ovarian surface epithelium. *Biol. Reprod.* **49**, 635-41.

13. Berchuck, A., Kohler, F.M., Boente, M.P. *et al.* (1993) Growth regulation and transformation of ovarian epithelium. *Cancer* **71**, 545-51.

14. Adams, A.T. and Auersperg, N. (1983) Autoradiographic investigation of estrogen binding in cultured rat ovarian surface epithelial cells. *J. Histochem. Cytochem.* **31**, 1321-25.

15. Hamilton, T.C., Young, R.C., McKoy, W.M. *et al.* (1983) Characterization of a human ovarian carcinoma cell line (NIH:OVCAR-3) with androgen and estrogen receptors. *Cancer Res.* **43**, 5379-89.

16. Hoyhtya, M., Myllyla, A., Siuva, J. *et al.* (1984) Monoclonal antibodies to human prolyl 4-hydroxylase. *Eur. J. Biochem.* **141**, 477-82.

17. Dyck, H.G., Hamilton, T.C., Lynch, H.T. and Auersperg, N. (1995) Expression of epithelial and mesenchymal characteristics in human ovarian surface epithelium: changes associated with a family history of ovarian cancer and with neoplastic progression. *Submitted.*

18. Auersperg, N. and Maines-Bandiera, S.L. (1995) E-cadherin expression by ovarian surface epithelium: changes in culture and with neoplastic progression. *Submitted.*

19. Kleinman, H.K., McGarvey, M.L., Liotta, L.A. *et al.* (1982) Isolation and characterization of type IV procollagen, laminin, and heparin sulfate proteoglycan from the EHS sarcoma. *Biochemistry* **21**, 6188-93.

20. Kruk, P.A. and Auersperg, N. (1994) A line of rat ovarian surface epithelium (ROSE) provides a continuous source of complex extracellular matrix. *In Vitro Cell Develop. Biol.* **30A**, 217-25.

21. Mauch, C., Hatamochi, A., Scharffetter, K. and Krieg, T. (1988) Regulation of collagen synthesis in fibroblasts within a three-dimensional collagen gel. *Exp. Cell Res.* **178**, 493-503.

22. Mansbridge, J.N., Ausserer, W.A., Knapp, M.A. and Sutherland, R.M. (1994) Adaptation of EGF receptor signal transduction to three-dimensional culture conditions: changes in surface receptor expression and protein tyrosine phosphorylation. *J. Cell Physiol.* **161**, 374-82.

23. Leighton, J. (1994) Exploring processes of

organization of normal and neoplastic epithelial tissues in gradient culture. *J. Cell. Biochem.* **56**, 29-36.

24. Chiquet-Ehrismann, R., Tannheimer, M., Koch, M. *et al.* (1994) Tenascin-C expression by fibroblasts is elevated in stressed collagen gels. *J. Cell Biol.* **127**, 2093-101.

25. Auersperg, N. and Finnegan, C.V. (1974) The differentiation and organization of tumors *in vitro*. In *Neoplasia and cell differentiation* (ed. G.V. Sherbet), S. Karger, Basel, pp. 279-318.

26. Bissell, M.J. (1981) The differentiated state of normal and malignant cells or how to define a 'normal' cell in culture. *Int. Rev. Cytol.* **70**, 27-100.

27. Desmouliere, A. and Gabbiani, G. (1994) Modulation of fibroblastic cytoskeletal features during pathological situations: the role of extracellular matrix and cytokines. *Cell Motil. Cytoskel.* **29**, 195-203.

28. Nicosia, S.V., Saunders, B.O., Acevedo-Duncan, M.E. *et al.* (1991) Biopathology of ovarian mesothelium. In *Ultrastructure of the ovary* (eds. G. Familiari, S. Makabe and P.M. Motta), Kluwer, Boston, pp.288-307.

29. Gillett, W.R., Mitchell, A. and Hurst, P.R. (1991) A scanning electron microscopic study of the human ovarian surface epithelium: characterization of two cell types. *Hum. Reprod.* **6**, 645-50.

30. Connell, N.D. and Rheinwald, J.G. (1983) Regulation of the cytoskeleton in mesothelial cells: reversible loss of keratin and increase in vimentin during rapid growth in culture. *Cell* **34**, 245-53.

31. Lipton, B.H., Bensch, K.G. and Karasek, M. A. (1991) Histamine-modulated trans-differentiation of dermal microvascular endothelial cells. *Differentiation* **46**, 117-33.

32. Mackay, A.M., Tracy, R.P. and Craighead, J.E. (1990) Cytokeratin expression in rat mesothelial cells *in vitro* is controlled by the extracellular matrix. *J. Cell Sci.* **95**, 97-107.

33. Augustin, H.G., Kozian, D.H. and Johnson, R.C (1994) Differentiation of endothelial cells: analysis of the constitutive and activated endothelial cell phenotypes. *BioEssays* **16**, 901-6.

34. Zuk, A., Matlin, K. and Hay, E.D. (1989) Type 1 collagen gel induces Madin-Darby canine kidney cells to become fusiform in shape and lose apical-basal polarity. *J. Cell Biol.* **108**, 903-20.

35. Davila, R.M. and Crouch, E.C. (1993) Role of mesothelial and submesothelial stromal cells in matrix remodeling following pleural injury. *Am. J. Pathol.* **142**, 547-55.

36. Trelstad, R.L., Hayashi, A., Hayashi, K., and Donahoe, P.K. (1982) The epithelial-mesenchymal interface of the male rat Müllerian duct: loss of basement membrane integrity and ductal regression. *Dev. Biol.* **92**, 27-40.

37. Fogh, J. and Tremple, G. (1975) New human tumor cell lines. In *Human Tumor Cells in Vitro*, (ed J.Fogh), Plenum, New York, pp. 115-160.

38. Maines-Bandiera, S.L., Kruk, P.A. and Auersperg, N. (1992) Simian virus 40–transformed human ovarian surface epithelial cells escape normal growth controls but retain morphogenetic responses to extracellular matrix. *Am. J. Obstet. Gynecol.* **167**, 729-35.

39. Marks, J.R., Davidoff, A.M., Kerns, B.J. *et al.* (1991) Overexpression and mutation of p53 in epithelial ovarian cancer. *Cancer Res.* **51**, 2979-84.

40. Kupryjanczyk, J., Thor, A.D., Beauchamp, R. *et al.* (1993) p53 gene mutations and protein accumulation in human ovarian cancer. *Proc. Natl. Acad. Sci. USA* **90**, 4961-5.

41. Hay, E.D. (1989) Extracellular matrix, cell skeletons, and embryonic development. *Am. J. Med. Genet.* **4**, 14-29.

42. Lynch, H.T. and Lynch, J.F. (1992) Hereditary ovarian carcinoma. *Hemat. Oncol. Clin. N. Am.* **6**, 783-811.

43. Ford, D., Easton, D.F., Bishop, D.T. *et al.* (1994) Risks of cancer in BRCA1-mutation carriers. *Lancet* **343**, 692-5.

44. Hamilton, T.C., Godwin, A.K., Salazar, H *et al.* (1994) Premalignant and early malignant ovarian neoplasms in prophylactic oophorectomy specimens from women with a strong family history of ovarian cancer. *Proc. Am. Soc. Clin. Oncol.* **13**, 836.

45. Resta, L., Russo, S., Colucci, G.A. and Prat, J. (1993) Morphological precursors of ovarian epithelial tumors. *Obstet. Gynecol.* **82**, 181-6.

46. Mittal, K.R., Zeleniuch-Jacquotte, A., Cooper, J.L. and Demopoulos, R.I. (1993) Contralateral ovary in unilateral ovarian carcinoma: A search for preneoplastic lesions. *Int. J. Gynecol. Pathol.* **12**, 59-63.

47. Nouwen, E.J., Dauwe, S. and De Broe M.E. (1990) Occurrence of the mucinous differentiation antigen CA125 in genital tract and conductive airway epithelia of diverse mammalian species (rabbit, dog, monkey). *Differentiation* **45**, 192-8.

48. Leake, J., Woolas, R.P., Oram, J.D. *et al.* (1994) Immunocytochemical and serological expression of CA 125: a clinicopathological study of 40 malignant ovarian epithelial tumours. *Histopathology* **24**, 57-64.

49. Risteli, L., Risteli, J., Puistola, U. *et al.* (1992) Aminoterminal propeptide of type III procollagen in ovarian cancer. *Acta Obstet. Gynecol. Scand.* **71** Suppl. 155, 99-103.

50. Auersperg, N., Maines-Bandiera, S., Booth, J.H. *et al.* (1995) Expression of two mucin antigens in cultured human ovarian surface epithelium: influence of a family history of ovarian cancer. *Am. J. Obstet. Gynecol.* **173**, 558-65.

51. Auersperg, N., Maines-Bandiera, S.L. and Kruk, P.A. (1994) Human ovarian surface epithelium: Growth patterns and differentiation. In *Ovarian Cancer 3* (eds. F.Sharp, P. Mason, A.D.Blackett and J.S.Berek), Chapman & Hall, London, pp. 157-69.

Chapter 2

Cystadenocarcinoma of the ovary: an immunohistochemical investigation

Johannes DIETL, Hans-Peter HORNY, Peter RUCK and Udo SCHUMACHER

2.1 INTRODUCTION

The majority of human ovarian cancers arise as a result of malignant transformation of the epithelial cells covering the surface of the ovary [1]. The morphology of the surface epithelium changes constantly throughout life [2]. It is a dynamic tissue with considerable morphological variation and is capable of rapid mitotic activity to accommodate the changes in size of the ovary during the different phases of the menstrual cycle. The uniqueness of ovarian surface changes and their rather abrupt disappearance in immediately adjacent mesothelia suggest that local factors may play an important role in modulating the growth and morphogenesis of the ovarian mesothelium. This study demonstrates some immunohistochemical features of the ovarian surface epithelium and cystadenocarcinoma of the ovary, with special reference to mucinous cystadenocarcinoma.

2.2 TRANSITION BETWEEN BENIGN AND MALIGNANT EPITHELIUM

Normal ovarian surface epithelium and cystadenocarcinoma of the ovary exhibit differences in proliferative activity and oncogene expression. Figure 2.1a shows ovarian surface epithelium below a serous surface papillary adenocarcinoma. The

tissue has been stained by the antibody DC10, which detects the proliferating cell nuclear antigen (PCNA). PCNA is a nuclear protein that is an absolute prerequisite for DNA synthesis [3] and is a marker of proliferative activity. MIB-1 is another antibody that reacts with proliferating cells. It detects the Ki-67 antigen [4]. Figure 2.1b shows normal surface epithelium and a serous surface papillary adenocarcinoma stained with MIB-1. The flat surface epithelium exhibits very few stained nuclei, but a greater proportion of cells in the transition zone of the surface epithelium are stained, and the tumour is strongly reactive. The same case, stained for p53 protein, is illustrated in Figure 2.1c. The tumour is strongly reactive, but the normal surface epithelium is nonreactive.

It seems that the surface epithelium does not become malignant in its entirety in all cases. There are probably distinct foci of surface cells that become malignant. Although we found areas of transition between normal surface epithelium and tumour in 5 out of 6 serous borderline tumours, it is still not clear whether the presence of multiple tumour foci on the surface represents metastatic spread or simultaneous multifocality. On the other hand, a single tumour is often found to contain both benign and malignant

19

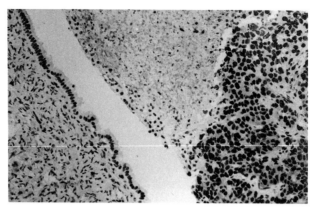

Figure 2.1a Many cell nuclei in the normal ovarian surface epithelium on the left exhibit immunoreactivity for PCNA. Virtually all the tumour cells of the serous cystadenocarcinoma on the right are also stained. x 120

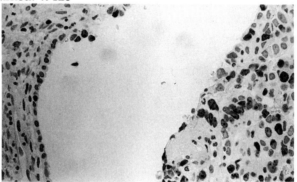

Figure 2.1b MIB-1 stains only very few cells in the normal flat surface epithelium seen on the left. Continuous with this, at the top of the illustration, is an area with increased nuclear pleomorphism that represents the transition zone, in which a larger proportion of cell nuclei are stained. Many cell nuclei are stained in the serous cystadenocarcinoma seen on the right. x 120

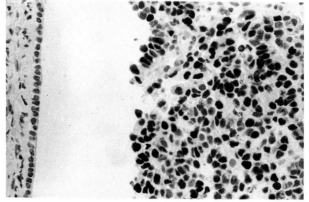

Figure 2.1c Immunoreactivity for p53 protein is seen in this serous cystadenocarcinoma of the ovary (right), but the ovarian surface epithelium (left) remains unstained. x 120

Table 2.1 Frequency of adjacent benign epithelium in serous and mucinous cystadenocarcinoma

Tumour type	No. of cases with adjacent benign epithelium
Mucinous (n = 32)	
Borderline (n = 6)	6
Carcinoma (n = 26)	23
Serous (n = 42)	
Borderline (n = 8)	8
Carcinoma (n = 34)	21

components. Table 2.1 gives the frequency of adjacent benign epithelium in serous and mucinous cystadenocarcinoma of the ovary. Benign epithelium was noted adjacent to borderline epithelium in all tumours of low malignant potential. It was found adjacent to malignant epithelium in 23 out of 26 mucinous cystadenocarcinomas and 21 out of 34 serous cystadenocarcinomas. Puls and colleagues [5] demonstrated an inverse relationship between the presence of benign epithelium and tumour grade. Their observations confirm a continuum in the epithelial lining of certain serous ovarian tumours from benign to borderline to malignant.

Abnormalities of c-erbB2 and p53 expression are common in epithelial ovarian cancer [6,7]. The proportion of tumour cells positive for c-erbB2 and p53 protein is of interest. We found only about 10 % of tumour cells to be stained in most cases of mucinous cystadenocarcinoma (Figure 2.2). Cells with a c-erbB2 or p53 mutation therefore do not appear to have a clear growth advantage and do not represent the predominant tumour cell population in mucinous cystadenocarcinoma. Although Berchuck and colleagues [7] and Rubin and colleagues [6] demonstrated that over-

expression of p53 and c-erbB2 is not a feature of benign and borderline epithelial ovarian tumours, it is still not clear whether activation of c-erbB2 and p53 is an early causative event in tumourigenesis or a late event that confers metastatic potential.

2.3 IMMUNOPHENOTYPE OF MUCINOUS CYSTADENOCARCINOMA

2.3.1 INTERMEDIATE FILAMENTS

The main intermediate filaments expressed by ovarian epithelial tumours are cytokeratins, but vimentin is also found [8]. Table 2.2 shows the cytokeratin profile of mucinous cystadenocarcinoma. Cytokeratins number 7, 18, 19 and 20 are expressed by most examples of this tumour, but 10 and 13 are absent. Cytokeratin-7 expression is restricted to a subtype of glandular epithelium and has recently been reported to be present in primary ovarian adenocarcinomas but not in colonic adenocarcinomas or their ovarian metastases [9-11], a finding that could be of diagnostic value. Cytokeratin 20 is not expressed by non-mucinous Müllerian duct tumours but is commonly found in colonic adenocarcinomas [12]. The cytokeratin profile of the ovarian surface epithelium is identical to that of normal mesothelial cells and Müllerian

Table 2.2 Cytokeratin profile of mucinous cystadenocarcinoma (n = 15)

Cytokeratin	No. of cases reactive
CK 19	15
CK 7	13
CK 20	9
CK 18	3
CK 10	0
CK 13	0

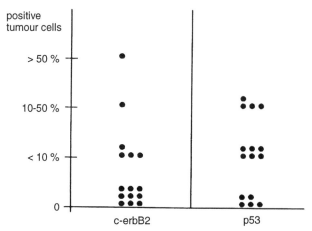

Figure 2.2 Pattern of immunoreactivity for c-erbB2 and p53 protein in 15 cases of mucinous cystadenocarcinoma of the ovary.

epithelium, including the epithelium of the endometrium, endocervix and upper part of the vagina [13]. We found coexpression of cytokeratins and vimentin in 3 out of 15 mucinous cystadenocarcinomas. In a recent study, de Nictolis and colleagues [14] found 31 out of 47 mucinous cystadenocarcinomas of intestinal-type epithelium to exhibit varying degrees of vimentin expression. The coexpression of cytokeratins and vimentin is also seen in the ovarian surface epithelium [13] and in the epithelium of the Fallopian tube and endometrium, but not in that of the endocervix. It has also been described in certain other normal tissues [15] and both mesenchymal [16] and epithelial [15] tumours.

2.3.2 OTHER MARKERS

Fifteen mucinous cystadenocarcinomas were immunostained with a broad panel of antibodies against various non-haemopoietic antigens (Table 2.3). Only the antibodies against CEA, CA19-9, E-cadherin, TGF-α, and PDGF-R stained the majority of cases. Most of the other antibodies stained only a few cases or none at all.

The classical marker for ovarian carcinoma is CA125, but very few tumour cells in mucinous cystadenocarcinoma of the ovary were found to be reactive. The antibody against CEA stained the largest number of tumours, most of which were stained very strongly. Most investigators have found CEA expression to be absent in serous carcinomas, but present in mucinous tumours [17]. It is usually seen in invasive mucinous tumours but is very rare in benign mucinous cystadenomas [18]. Although PLAP is not a typical marker for mucinous cystadenocarcinoma, it was found in 3 out of 15 cases. PLAP is expressed by serous and endometrioid carcinomas but is not usually found in mucinous tumours [17].

On average, 50% of ovarian carcinomas express oestrogen receptors (OR) [19]. However, only 4 of our 15 cases were OR-positive, and progesterone receptor (PR) expression was found in only 2 cases. No correlation between OR and PR expression and histological grade, tumour type, age or stage has been found in ovarian carcinoma [19, 20].

Chromogranin A is widely distributed in

Table 2.3 Immunohistochemical profile of mucinous cystadenocarcinoma (n = 15)

	Proportion of cells stained	
	0-10%	>10%
CEA	3	12
CA 19-9	4	11
E-cadherin	5	10
TGF-α	6	9
PDGF-R	6	9
Leu-M1 (CD15)	10	5
Oestrogen receptor	11	4
DC 10 (PCNA)	11	4
PLAP	12	3
Chromogranin A	12	3
MIB-1	10	2
Progesterone receptor	13	2
CD44	13	2
MIC 2 (CD99)	14	1
α-amylase	15	0
β-HCG	15	0
AFP	15	0
BMA 120	15	0
QBEND 10 (CD 34)	15	0
NSE	15	0
PSAP	15	0
SM-actin	15	0
S100 protein	15	0
CA-125	15	0

Abbreviations:

TGF-α = transforming growth factor-α,
PDGF-R = platelet-derived growth factor receptor,
PCNA = proliferating cell nuclear antigen,
PLAP = placental alkaline phosphatase,
NSE = neuron specific enolase,
PSAP = prostate specific acid phosphatase,
SM = smooth muscle

human polypeptide hormone-producing tissues and can be a useful marker for tumours derived from them. In this study, we found cells immunoreactive for chromogranin A in 3 of the 15 mucinous cystadenocarcinomas. The immunoreactive cells resembled intestinal enterochromaffin cells. Thus some mucinous cystadeno-carcinomas of the ovary exhibit neuroendocrine differentiation [21]. The origin of endocrine cells in mucinous ovarian tumours, however, has not been established with certainty.

The proliferative activity of mucinous cystadenocarcinoma was investigated with the antibodies MIB-1 and DC10 (PCNA). In most cases, fewer than 10% of tumour cells were reactive.

The peptide growth factors TGF-α and the receptor for PDGF were detected in 9 of the 15 cases. Peptide growth factors are glycoproteins that stimulate proliferation or differentiation by binding to specific cell-membrane receptors. They usually act locally via autocrine, paracrine, or juxtacrine mechanisms. Jindal *et al.* [22] found that surface cells and ovarian cancers produce TGF-α. This was interpreted as suggestive of the presence of an autocrine growth stimulatory pathway.

2.4 TUMOUR-INFILTRATING LYMPHORETICULAR CELLS IN MUCINOUS CYSTADENOCARCINOMA

In all the cases, the majority of the reactive tumour-infiltrating lymphoreticular cells (TIL) were found to be T cells or macrophages. B cells and natural killer cells were generally found in only small numbers (Table 2.4). This is in keeping with findings reported by other investigators [23] and suggests that the *in situ* host response to ovarian mucinous cystadenocarcinoma is predominantly cell-mediated. Although TIL are commonly found in human tumours, the significance of their presence is poorly understood. They may represent a true anti-tumour response or, on the other hand, promote tumour progression.

The aberrant expression of certain lymphoid and macrophage-associated anti-

Table 2.4 Tumour-infiltrating lympho-reticular cells (TIL) in mucinous cystadeno-carcinoma (n = 15)

Antibody	Proportion of TIL stained	
	0-10 %	>10 %
PG-M1 (CD 68)	0	15
UCHL1 (CD45R0)	1	14
KP1 (CD 68)	2	13
HAM (CD 68)	4	11
OPD 4	6	9
DF-T1 (CD 43)	9	6
L26 (CD 20)	13	2
Leu-7 (CD 57)	13	2

gens, such as the T-cell associated antigen CD45R0 (UCHL1) and the macrophage associated antigen CD68 (HAM, KP1), by a small proportion of the tumour cells may play a role in facilitating infiltration and subsequent tumour dissemination.

2.5 IMMUNOPHENOTYPE OF TRANSPLANTED OVARIAN CANCER CELLS

Little is known about the mechanisms that enable ovarian cancer cells to form peritoneal metastases with such frequency. Recent reports, however, indicate that changes in cell adhesion molecule expression may be involved in the spread of ovarian cancers [24, 25]. We have studied the immunophenotype of primary human ovarian cystadeno-carcinoma and its metastasizing explants in an established SCID-mouse model [26]. When SCID-mouse ascites-derived cells were transplanted subcutaneously into SCID mice, they formed solid cystic tumours that metastasized to the lungs. The tumour cells were found to have a stable immuno-phenotype in all settings, and it is particularly interesting that E-cadherin and CD44v6 expression did not vary between the

primary tumour, SCID-mice ascites and solid SCID-mice tumour. Immunostaining for p53 protein was more intense in the ascites-derived cells and solid tumours in the SCID-mice than in the human primary tumour. Cellular proliferation, as measured by MIB-1 and PCNA immunostaining, was the same in the ascites-derived cells, the human primary tumour and the solid tumour that developed in the SCID mice after subcutaneous implantation.

Our findings strongly suggest that the expression of adhesion molecules such as E-cadherin and CD44v6 is not influenced by environmental factors. Cannistra and co-workers [24] recently reported that CD44 is responsible for the binding of ovarian cancer cells to peritoneal mesothelial cells. The mechanism of adhesion to other tissues is probably similar.

2.6 CONCLUSION

Our findings support data which suggest that benign ovarian tumours may undergo malignant transformation. Bourne and co-workers [27] reported a significant increase in the frequency of benign epithelial ovarian tumours in primary and secondary relatives of patients with ovarian cancer.

Immunohistochemical studies are useful in the investigation of cases of ovarian carcinoma, but there are inherent limitations because of heterogeneity of antigen expression by different examples of the same tumour type and variations in the specificities of available markers.

We have demonstrated that the immunophenotype of growing human ovarian cystadenocarcinoma cells in the peritoneal cavity of SCID mice does not differ from that of the human primary tumour. The ovarian surface and the peritoneum probably represent the same field of tumour growth.

Recent advances in the molecular genetics

and molecular biology of carcinogenesis suggest a very complex sequential process involving oncogenes, suppressor genes, growth factors and cytokines in tumour development. Further molecular studies will be needed to determine where and how these biological factors are active during carcinogenesis in the ovary.

REFERENCES

1. Scully, R.E. (1977) Ovarian tumors. A review. *Am. J. Pathol.* **87**, 686-720.
2. Nicosia, S.V. (1983) Morphological changes of the human ovary throughout life. In *The Ovary* (ed. G.B. Serra), Raven Press, New York, pp. 57-81.
3. Bravo, R., Frank, R., Blundell, P.A. and Macdonald-Bravo, H. (1987) Cyclin /PCNA is the auxilliary protein of DNA-polymerase-δ. *Nature* **326**, 515-17.
4. Key, G., Becker, M.H., Baron, B. *et al.* (1993) New Ki-67 equivalent murine monoclonal antibodies (MiB 1-3) generated against bacterially expressed parts of the Ki-67 c-DNA containing three 62 base pair repetitive elements encoding for the Ki-67 epitope. *Lab. Invest.* **68**, 629-36.
5. Puls, L.E., Powell, D.E., De-Priest, P.D. *et al.* (1992) Transition from benign to malignant epithelium in mucinous and serous ovarian cystadenocarcinoma. *Gynecol. Oncol.* **47**, 53-7.
6. Rubin, S.C., Finstad, C.L., Federici, M.G. *et al.* (1994) Prevalence and significance of HER-2/*neu*-expression in early epithelial ovarian cancer. *Cancer* **73**, 1456-59.
7. Berchuck, A., Kohler, M.F., Hopkins, M.P. *et al.* (1994) Overexpression of p53 is not a feature of benign and early-stage borderline epithelial ovarian tumors. *Gynecol. Oncol.* **52**, 232-6.
8. Dabbs, D.J. and Geissinger, K.R. (1988) Common epithelial ovarian tumors. Immunohistochemical intermediate filament profiles. *Cancer* **62**, 368-74.
9. Ramaekers, F., van Niekerk, C., Poels, L. *et al.* (1990) Use of monoclonal antibodies to keratin 7 in the differential diagnosis of adenocarcinomas. *Am. J. Pathol.* **136**, 641-55.
10. van Niekerk, C.C. (1993) Changes in expression of differentiation markers between normal ovarian cells and derived tumors. *Am. J. Pathol.* **142**, 157-77
11. Ueda, G., Sawada, M., Ogawa, H. *et al.* (1993) Immunohistochemical study of cytokeratin 7 for the differential diagnosis of adenocarcinomas in the ovary. *Gynecol. Oncol.* **51**, 219-23.
12. Moll, R., Löwe, A., Laufer, J. and Frank, W.W. (1992) Cytokeratin 20 in human carcinoma. *Am. J. Pathol.* **140**, 1-2.
13. Moll, R., Levy, R., Czernobilsky, B. *et al.* (1983) Cytokeratins of normal epithelia and some neoplasms of the female genital tract. *Lab. Invest.* **49**, 599-610.
14. de Nictolis, M., Montironi, R., Tommasoni, S. *et al.* (1994) Benign, borderline, and well-differentiated malignant intestinal mucinous tumors of the ovary: A clinico-pathologic, histochemical, immunohistochemical, and nuclear quantitative study of 57 cases. *Int. J. Gynecol. Pathol.* **13**, 19-21.
15. Mc Nutt, M.A. *et al.* (1985) Coexpression of intermediate filaments in human epithelial neoplasms. *Ultrastruct. Pathol.* **9**, 31-43.
16. Manivel, J.C., Wick, M.R., Dehner, L.P. and Sibley, R.K. (1987) Epitheloid sarcoma. An immunohistochemical study. *Am. J. Clin. Pathol.* **87**, 319-326.
17. Nouwen, E.J., Hendrix, P.G., Dauwe, S. *et al.* (1987) Tumor markers in the human ovary and its neoplasms. *Am. J. Pathol.* **126**, 230-42.
18. Benjamin, E. (1992) Immunohistochemical markers in gynaecological pathology. In

Advances in Gynaecological Pathology (eds. D. Lowe and H. Fox), Churchill Livingstone, Edinburgh, pp. 35-62.

19. Bizzi, A., Cadegoni, A.M., Landoni, F. *et al.* (1988) Steroid receptors in epithelial ovarian carcinoma: relation to clinical parameters and survival. *Cancer Res.* **48**, 6222-6.

20. Palmer, D.C., Muir, I.M., Alexander, A.I. *et al.* (1988) The prognostic importance of steroid receptors in endometrial carcinoma. *Obstet. Gynecol.* **72**, 388-93.

21. Sasaki, E., Sasano, N., Kimura, N. *et al.* (1989) Demonstration of neuroendocrine cells in ovarian mucinous tumors. *Int. J. Gynecol. Pathol.* **8**, 189-200.

22. Jindal, S.K., Snoey, D.M., Lobb, D.K. and Dorrington, J.H. (1994) Transforming growth factor α localization and role in surface epithelium of normal human ovaries and in ovarian carcinoma cells. *Gynecol. Oncol.* **53**, 17-23.

23. Kabawat, S.E., Bast, R.C.Jnr., Welch, W.R. *et al.* (1983) Expression of major histocompatibility antigens and nature of inflammatory cellular infiltrate in ovarian neoplams. *Int. J. Cancer* **32**, 547-54.

24. Cannistra, S.A, Kansa, G.S., Niloff, J. *et al.* (1993) Binding of ovarian cancer cells to peritoneal mesothelium *in vitro* is partly mediated by CD 44 H. *Cancer Res.* **53**, 3830-8.

25. Risinger, J.I., Berchuck, A., Kohler, M.F. and Boyd, J. (1994) Mutations of the E-cadherin gene in human gynecologic cancers. *Nat. Genet.* **7**, 98-102.

26. Schumacher, U., Adam, E., Horny, H.-P. and Dietl, J. (1995) Transplantation of a human ovarian cystadenocarcinoma into severe combined immunodeficient (SCID) mice alterations of the tumor phenotype and metastases in the SCID mice. *Submitted for publication*

27. Bourne, T.H., Whitehead, M.I., Campbell, S. *et al.* (1991) Ultrasound screening for familial ovarian cancer. *Gynecol. Oncol.* **43**, 92-7.

Chapter 3

Candidate precursor lesions

Michael WELLS and Richard HUTSON

3.1 INTRODUCTION

The recognition of a precursor lesion for epithelial ovarian cancer would have important implications for our understanding of its pathogenesis. Early-stage ovarian cancer produces no symptoms with the majority of patients presenting with advanced disease where the prognosis is poor. As a result there has been little change in the overall survival rate of ovarian cancer patients during the past thirty years. The duration of the pre-clinical phase in epithelial ovarian cancer is unknown. Recent advances in molecular biology are leading to an understanding of the genetic basis of ovarian cancer though it is not yet possible to formulate a multistep pathway of ovarian carcinogenesis analogous to that described for colorectal cancer. Given the histological diversity of these tumours it would not be surprising if more than one oncogenic route could operate. The disruption and proliferation of ovarian surface epithelium that occurs in association with ovulation and the formation of epithelial inclusion cysts, may provide an important initiating stimulus for somatic mutation leading to oncogene activation and loss of normal tumour suppressor gene function. Such events, combined with the inherent ability of ovarian epithelial cells to respond to and produce cytokines and growth factors, could explain, in part, the aetiology of ovarian cancer and its association with ovulation.

3.2 PRESENT EVIDENCE FOR A PRECURSOR LESION

It is believed that most epithelial ovarian cancer arises from surface epithelium or from epithelial inclusion cysts resulting from invagination of surface epithelium and entrapment of the surface epithelium within the ovarian stroma associated with the trauma of ovulation. The evidence for this includes the following observations:

1. Atypia (dysplasia or ovarian intraepithelial neoplasia) involving the surface epithelium of the ovary has been reported adjacent to invasive areas of stage I epithelial ovarian cancer [1].

2. There is an increased frequency of inclusion cysts (Figure 3.1) in apparently normal ovaries contralateral to ovarian cancer compared to ovaries from age matched women without ovarian cancer [2].

3. The surface epithelium of ovaries adjacent to epithelial ovarian cancer has a higher incidence of metaplastic and hyperplastic change than ovaries from healthy women [3].

One of the principal hypotheses of the pathogenesis of ovarian cancer states that a woman's risk of ovarian cancer increases with the number of ovulations she experiences. After each ovulation, the ovary undergoes a process of repair of the surface epithelium. It has been suggested that this repair process leads to the formation of epithelial inclusion cysts. If the formation of these cysts is indeed the

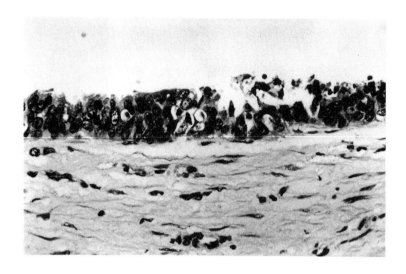

Figure 3.1 Wall of epithelial inclusion cyst showing atypia.

mechanism by which frequent ovulation leads to increased risk of ovarian cancer, then women with ovarian cancer should have more epithelial inclusion cysts. This theory has been supported by work carried out by Mittal *et al.* [2] but refuted by Westhoff *et al.* [4]. The former studied contralateral ovaries of women with stage I ovarian adenocarcinoma. Epithelial inclusion cysts also showed tubal metaplasia more frequently than inclusion cysts in patients without ovarian cancer.

Nuclear pleomorphism, irregular nuclear chromatin pattern, stratification, and loss of nuclear polarity have been described as characteristic features of ovarian intraepithelial neoplasia [1,5]. Inclusion cysts are seen with considerable frequency in the ovary; however in the experience of most pathologists, detection of atypia within the lining of inclusion cysts is extremely rare. Certainly there has been no systematic documentation of *in situ* neoplastic change within such cysts. An early immuno-histochemical study showed the presence of 'tumour markers' such as carcinoembryonic antigen and the beta subunit of human chorionic

gonadotrophin in some but not all epithelial inclusion cysts; a feature shared with some adenocarcinomas [6].

It has been suggested that benign or borderline epithelial changes may be the precursor of ovarian cancer. In many cases of ovarian cancer adjacent areas of benign, serous or mucinous epithelium may be seen and in 40% of cases a direct transition from benign or borderline to invasive epithelium is visible [7,8].

74–90% of mucinous carcinomas contain benign epithelium compared to 15–56% of serous carcinomas [7,8]. The great majority of serous carcinomas probably arise *de novo* from the surface epithelium and its inclusions but a sizeable proportion of mucinous carcinomas probably arise from mucinous cystadenomas. Mucinous metaplasia of the surface epithelium and mucinous epithelial inclusions are rare. Focal evolution into an obvious adenocarcinoma occurs much more commonly in mucinous tumours of borderline malignancy than in serous borderline tumours. However foci of early invasion have recently been described in serous tumours of borderline malignancy [9,10].

The very high reported association of endometriosis with endometrioid carcinoma and clear cell carcinoma (28% and 49% respectively) in contrast with its very low frequency in association with serous and mucinous carcinomas of the ovary (3% and 4% respectively) furnishes strong evidence that endometriosis of the ovary is a precancerous lesion [8,11]. Most interestingly, using a recombinant DNA X-chromosome inactivation technique, Nilbert and colleagues have recently shown that 3 of 5 endometriotic cysts exhibited a monoclonal X-chromosome inactivation pattern indicating that the cell populations of these cysts were each derived from a single cell and thus represent neoplastic cell growth. Identification of endometriotic cysts of monoclonal origin may be of clinical value in order to estimate the neoplastic potential of the cysts [12].

Our present knowledge of the genetic events in ovarian cancer now allows a molecular approach to studying candidate precursor lesions and their relationship to invasive disease. The main molecular genetic findings in sporadic and epithelial ovarian cancer may be summarized as follows:

1. Linkage to chromosome 17q in familial breast/ovarian cancer
A rare dominant gene BRCA1 which has recently been identified increases the risk of breast and ovarian cancer [13,14]. Analysis of loss of heterozygosity in tumours from familial breast/ovarian cancer families suggests that the BRCA1 gene is a tumour suppressor gene [15]. 95% of cases of ovarian cancer, however, are sporadic rather than familial.

2. Growth factors
Loss of the inhibitory function of transforming growth factor beta (TGF-β) may represent a step in ovarian carcinogenesis [16]. Macrophage colony stimulating factor (M-CSF) is a ligand for a cell surface receptor encoded by the c-fms proto-oncogene. Normal ovarian surface epithelium does not express c-fms whereas the majority of ovarian cancer cells do express the receptor [17].

3. Growth factor receptors
The c-erbB2 (HER-2/neu) oncogene encodes a protein kinase transmembrane receptor which binds a ligand similar to epidermal growth factor. The c-erbB2 gene product is expressed by the ovarian surface epithelium of normal adult ovaries, although fetal expression has not been demonstrated. Amplification of the c-erbB2 gene is found in about 30% of ovarian cancers [18]. Epidermal growth factor receptor also shows increased expression in ovarian cancer cells [19].

4. Oncogenes
Amplification of c-myc is seen in approximately one-third of ovarian cancers [20]. k-ras mutation may be an important and relatively early event in mucinous ovarian tumours [21] and has been reported in borderline tumours [22].

5. Tumour suppressor genes
It is known that p53 is definitely implicated in ovarian neoplasia with at least 50% of advanced stage ovarian cancers demonstrating point mutations. Most occur within the highly conserved exons 5–8 of the gene [23–29]. Overexpression of protein in ovarian cancer has generally been assumed to reflect p53 mutation, since wild-type protein is not usually demonstrable by immunohistochemistry [30,31]. p53 mutation is a clonal event with the same point mutation occurring in both the primary tumour and metastatic deposits [32].

6. Loss of heterozygosity
A high frequency of allelic loss has been shown in ovarian cancer for 6p, 6q, 13q, 17p, 17q, 18q, 22q and Xp. The most important of these is 17q since BRCA1 is located here. BRCA1 may play a role in sporadic disease but other (as yet unidentified) tumour suppressor genes may also be involved [33].

3.3 P53 PROTEIN EXPRESSION IN PUTATIVE PRECURSOR LESIONS

p53 is a nuclear phosphoprotein weighing 53kDa which accumulates in cells following DNA damage [34]. In its turn p53 activates another gene encoding a protein (p21) which causes the affected cell to arrest in G1 of the cell cycle [35]. p53 plays an important part in conserving genomic stability and is a major biochemical regulator of growth control as cells with inactivation of p53 have a growth advantage over their neighbours [36]. The gene coding for p53 protein is located on chromosome 17p13, a common site for allelic deletions in human tumours.

We have studied p53 protein expression in epithelial inclusion cysts adjacent to and contralateral to serous carcinoma of the ovary and compared them to epithelial inclusion cysts associated with borderline tumours and in normal ovaries [37]. Serous adenocarcinomas were chosen as they have been shown to have a significantly higher incidence of p53 mutations than mucinous and endometrioid type tumours.

Normal ovaries and cases of ovarian serous borderline tumours and serous adeno-carcinomas were selected from the surgical pathology files of St James's University Hospital, Leeds. A total of 13 advanced stage (FIGO stage III) serous ovarian adenocarcinomas, 5 serous borderline tumours and 13 normal ovaries were studied. The median age was 50 years (range 26–72 years). The distribution of epithelial inclusion cysts with and without cytological atypia was assessed in the normal ovaries, serous borderline tumours and serous carcinomas.

Three micron thick sections were cut from the paraffin blocks, mounted on 3-aminoproplytriethoxysilane (APES) coated slides and air dried. They were stained with haematoxylin and eosin and immuno-histochemistry was performed as follows. The sections were deparaffinized in xylene and

rinsed in absolute alcohol (100%), before being rehydrated in tap water. Endogenous peroxidase activity was then blocked by incubating in 98ml methanol and 2ml 30% hydrogen peroxide for ten minutes. The slides were then placed in citrate buffer (pH6.0) and microwaved at 100°C for one minute. This procedure was repeated four more times at five minute intervals. The solution was then allowed to cool for twenty minutes before the slides were washed in Tris buffered saline for five minutes. The slides were then assembled in a Sequenza (Shandon), and incubated in 1:20 rabbit serum for three minutes. The primary monoclonal antibody (Ab-2 to human wild-type and mutant p53, Oncogene Science) was applied at a dilution of 1:50 in 5% rabbit serum in PBS for ninety minutes. Sections were then incubated for thirty minutes in a biotinylated monoclonal conjugate of rabbit anti-mouse 1gG (dilution 1:200) and then for a further thirty minutes with peroxidase conjugated Streptavidin:Biotin complex (Dako). The slides were then removed from the Sequenza and incubated with 2,3-diaminobenzidine (DAB) for ten minutes. The sections were then rinsed in water before being counterstained in Mayer's haematoxylin for thirty seconds and blued in Scott's tap water substitute. This was followed by routine dehydration, clearing and mounting. Sections of colonic cancer were used as a positive control. In preliminary experiments the primary monoclonal antibody was omitted as a negative control.

The total number of cases (11) having epithelial inclusion cysts was the same for both serous adenocarcinomas and normal ovaries. In their study, Mittal *et al.* showed that the number of inclusion cysts was increased in ovaries from patients with ovarian carcinoma compared to normal controls [2]. We were unable to show this difference between normal ovaries and serous epithelial tumours in this small series but 8/13 serous carcinomas had epithelial inclusion cysts with atypia whereas no atypia were seen in epithelial inclusion cysts in normal ovaries.

Immunohistochemical reactivity was assessed and graded as strong staining (+++), moderate (++), weak (+) or negative (-). A positive immunohistochemical reaction was found in all 13 serous ovarian carcinomas and

all five of the borderline tumours, though weaker staining was apparent in the borderline tumours (Table 3.1). In 10/13 serous adenocarcinomas and 4/5 borderline tumours, the surface epithelium showed strong immunoreactivity for p53 but this was seen in

Table 3.1 p53 immunoreactivity in serous carcinomas and borderline tumours and normal ovaries

	Strong	*Moderate*	*Weak*	*Negative*
		p53 immunoreactivity		
Serous carcinomas	7	2	4	0
Serous borderline tumours	0	1	4	0
Normal ovaries (epithelial inclusion cysts)	0	0	2	11

Table 3.2 p53 immunoreactivity found in surface epithelium and epithelial inclusion cysts (IC) of serous carcinomas and borderline tumours and normal ovaries

	Serous carcinoma	*Serous borderline tumours*	*Norma ovary*
Total Number	13	5	13
Surface epithelium negative	3	1	12
Surface epithelium positive	10	4	1
Total number having inclusion cysts (IC)	11	2	11
Number of cases with some IC positive for p53 *	7	1	2
Number of cases with some IC negative for p53 *	7	2	11

Note that some cases contain both positively- and negatively-staining inclusion cysts

Table 3.3 Number of cases with inclusion cysts showing immunoreactivity for p53

	No atypia	*With atypia*
Serous (n=7)	2	5
Borderline (n=1)	1	0
Normal (n=2)	2	0
(weak immunoreactivity)		

only 1/13 normal ovaries (Table 3.2). In eight of the tumour cases (7 carcinomas, 1 borderline) epithelial inclusion cysts were positive but only two cases of normal ovaries had epithelial inclusion cysts which were weakly positive for p53. In five cases of advanced serous carcinomas, positive immunoreactivity for p53 protein was seen only in those epithelial inclusion cysts showing atypia (Table 3.3). No atypia of epithelial inclusion cysts was seen in borderline tumours or normal ovaries.

p53 overexpression in epithelial ovarian cancer has been reported by several authors; the level of expression ranging from 33 to 80% [25,27,29-31]. We found the level of expression to be 100% in both advanced (stage III) serous ovarian cancer and borderline tumours. One possible explanation for this is that our specimens were microwaved which has been shown to enhance immunohistochemical reactivity [38,39].

Some workers have found no p53 protein expression in borderline tumours of the ovary in contrast to the findings in the present study [31,32]. In one case of borderline tumour in our study immunoreactivity for p53 was detected in an epithelial inclusion cyst showing no atypia. Our findings, therefore, do not support the suggestion that aberrant expression of the p53 protein is an event that frequently occurs in the development of ovarian cancer but not in borderline tumours of the ovary. We therefore cannot conclude that p53 expression occurs at the step when the tumour 'progresses' from borderline neoplasia to cancer. Kupryjanczyk *et al.* have recently reported p53 immunoreactivity in 8 out of 12 borderline tumours but in none of these were they able to show genetic alterations in the p53 gene using single-stranded conformational polymorphism analysis [40]. In contrast they found mutation of the p53 gene in 40% (4/10) of stage I carcinomas and conclude that p53 mutations may not be commonly associated with the borderline phenotype of ovarian epithelial tumours but may occur

during malignant transformation. In another recent paper Mittal *et al.* studied immunoreactivity of epithelial inclusion cysts in ovaries contralateral to stage I ovarian carcinoma or borderline tumours [41]. No immunoreactivity for p53 protein was seen in any of the cases. No comment was made on the presence or absence of cytological atypia, but in their earlier paper the authors reported that changes of ovarian intraepithelial neoplasia were not seen in epithelial inclusion cysts contralateral to ovarian cancer [2].

3.4 CONCLUSIONS AND FUTURE DIRECTIONS

From our own study we conclude that p53 expression is seen more frequently in surface epithelium and epithelial inclusion cysts associated with ovarian serous neoplasia than in normal ovaries. It is likely therefore that loss of normal p53 tumour suppressor gene function is a key event in ovarian carcinogenesis. Ovarian intraepithelial neoplasia may be the precursor of ovarian malignancy and in some cases, at least, p53 protein expression may precede overt cytological abnormalities.

In p53 studies DNA sequencing ideally should be combined with immunohistochemical approaches. Microdissection techniques should be explored further when comparing phenotypically normal ovarian surface epithelium adjacent to the neoplastic lesion. Molecular genetic analysis of tissue can be made after selective ultraviolet radiation fractionation and the polymerase chain reaction. Cells in histological sections from archival tissues can be selected for DNA amplification by painting the glass slide with black ink to cover the area of tissue of interest. The sections can then be irradiated with ultra-violet light which will result in degradation of all DNA except in the areas protected by black ink [42,43]. Molecular analysis can include the study of loss of heterozygosity by PCR-based microsatellite polymorphisms [44], single stranded conformational polymorphism analysis for p53 mutation [40] and molecular analysis by *in situ* hybridization.

It is likely also, that further immuno-histochemical studies will contribute to our understanding of putative precursor lesions of epithelial ovarian cancer. For example, the monoclonal antibody MAb12C3 appears to be useful in identifying early histological malignant transformation of ovarian tumours, especially in cases of borderline malignancy. In 56% (14/25) of the specimens of borderline malignancy, MAb12C3 reacted exclusively with the cells of suspected malignant foci, which were composed of papillary projections into the lumen lined by cells exhibiting moderate nuclear atypia [45]. It would be interesting to determine the status of atypical and non-atypical epithelial inclusion cysts with this antibody.

REFERENCES

1. Plaxe, S.C., Deligdisch, L., Dottino, P.R. and Cohen CJ. (1990) Ovarian intraepithelial neoplasia demonstrated in patients with stage I ovarian carcinoma. *Gynecol. Oncol.* **38**, 367-72.
2. Mittal, K.R.,, Zeleniuch-Jacquotte, A. Cooper, J.L. and Demopoulos, R.I. (1993) Contralateral ovary in unilateral ovarian carcinoma, A search for preneoplastic lesion. *Int. J. Gynecol. Pathol.* **12**, 59-63.
3. Resta, L., Russo, S., Colucci, G.A. and Prat, J. (1993) Morphologic precursors of ovarian epithelial tumors. *Obstet. Gynecol.* **82**, 181-6.
4. Westhoff, C., Murphy, P., Heller, D. and Halim, A. (1993) Is ovarian cancer associated with an increased frequency of germinal inclusion cysts? *Am. J. Epidemiol.* **138**, 90-3.
5. Deligdisch, L. and Gil, J. (1989) Characterization of ovarian dysplasia by interactive morphometry. *Cancer* **63**, 748-55.
6. Blaustein, A. Kaganowicz, A. and Wells J. (1982) Tumor markers in inclusion cysts of the ovary. *Cancer* **49**, 722-726.
7. Puls, L.E., Powell, D.E., DePriest, P.D. *et al.* (1992) Transition from benign to malignant epithelium in mucinous and serous ovarian cystadenocarcinoma. *Gynecol. Oncol.* **47**, 53-7.
8. Scully, R.E., Bell, D.A. and Abu-Jawdeh, G.M. (1994) Update on early ovarian cancer and cancer developing in benign ovarian tumors, in *Ovarian Cancer 3* (eds F. Sharp, P. Mason, T. Blackett and J. Berek) Chapman & Hall, London, pp. 139-44.
9. Bell, D.A. and Scully, R.E. (1990) Ovarian serous borderline tumors with stromal microinvasion. A report of 21 cases. *Hum. Pathol.* **21**, 397-403.
10. Tavassoli, F.A. (1988) Serous tumors of low malignant potential with early stromal invasion (serous LMP with microinvasion). *Mod. Pathol.* **1**, 407-14.
11. Fox, H. (1993) Pathology of early malignant change in the ovary. *Int. J. Gynecol. Pathol.* **12**, 153-5.
12. Nilbert, M., Pejovic, T., Mandahl, N. *et al.* (1995) Monoclonal origin of endometriotic cysts. *Int. J. Gynecol. Cancer* **5**, 61-3.
13. Miki, Y., Swensen, J., Shattuck-Eidens, D. *et al.* (1994) A strong candidate for the breast and ovarian cancer susceptibility gene BRCA1. *Science* **266**, 66-71.
14. Futreal, P.A., Liu, Q.Y., Shattuck-Eidens, D. *et al.* (1994) BRCA 1 mutations in primary breast and ovarian carcinomas. *Science* **266**, 120-2.
15. Smith, S.A., Easton, D.F., Ford, D. *et al.* (1993) Genetic heterogeneity and localization of a familial breast-ovarian cancer gene on chromosome 17q12-q21. *Am. J. Hum. Genet.* **52**, 767-76.
16. Berchuck, A., Rodriguez, G., Olt, G. *et al.* (1992) Regulation of growth of normal ovarian epithelial cells and ovarian cancer cell lines by transforming growth factor-beta. *Am. J. Obstet. Gynecol.* **166**, 676-84.
17. Kacinski, B.M., Carter, D., Mittal, K. *et al.* (1990) Ovarian adenocarcinomas express fms-complementary transcripts and fms

antigen, often with coexpression of CSF-1. *Am. J. Pathol.* **137**, 135-47.

18. Rubin, S.C., Finstad, C.L., Federici, M.G. *et al.* (1994) Prevalence and significance of HER-2/*neu* expression in early epithelial ovarian cancer. *Cancer* **73**, 1456-9.

19. Berchuck, A., Rodriguez, G.C., Kamel, A. *et al.* (1991) Epidermal growth factor receptor expression in normal ovarian epithelium and ovarian cancer.I. Correlation of receptor expression with prognostic factors in patients with ovarian cancer. *Am. J. Obstet. Gynecol.* **164**, 669-74.

20. Tashiro, H., Miyazaki, K., Okamura, H. *et al.* (1992) c-myc over-expression in human primary ovarian tumours,its relevance to tumour progression. *Int. J. Cancer.* **50**, 828-33.

21. Ichikawa, Y., Nishida, M., Suzuki, H. *et al.* (1994) Mutation of K-ras protooncogene is associated with histological subtypes in human mucinous ovarian tumors (published erratum appears in *Cancer Res.* 1994 **54**, 1391). *Cancer Res.* **54**, 33-5.

22. Teneriello, M.G., Ebina, M., Linnoila, R.I. *et al.* (1993) p53 and Ki-*ras* mutations in epithelial ovarian neoplasms. *Cancer Res.* **53**, 3103-8.

23. Kohler, M.F., Marks, J.R., Wiseman, R.W. *et al.* (1993) Spectrum of mutation and frequency of allelic deletion of the p53 gene in ovarian cancer. *J. Nat. Cancer Inst.* **85**, 1513-9.

24. Milner, B.J., Allan, L.A., Eccles, D.M. *et al.* (1993) p53 mutation is a common genetic event in ovarian carcinoma. *Cancer Res.* **53**, 2128-32.

25. Marks, J.R., Davidoff, A.M., Kerns, B.J. *et al.* (1991) Overexpression and mutation of p53 in epithelial ovarian cancer. *Cancer Res.* **51**, 2979-84.

26. Mazars, R., Pujol, P., Maudelonde, T. *et al.* (1991) p53 mutations in ovarian cancer: a late event? *Oncogene* **6**, 1685-90.

27. Kohler, M.F., Kerns, B.M., Humphrey, P.A. *et al.* (1993) Mutation and overexpression of p53 in early stage epithelial ovarian cancer. *Obstet. Gynecol.* **81**, 643-50.

28. Okamoto, A., Sameshima, Y., Yokoyama, S. *et al.* (1991) Frequent allelic losses and mutations of the p53 gene in human ovarian cancer. *Cancer Res.* **51**, 5171-6.

29. Eccles, D.M., Brett, L., Lessells, A. *et al.* (1992) Overexpression of the p53 protein and allele loss at 17p13 in ovarian carcinoma. *Br. J. Cancer* **65**, 40-4.

30. McManus, D.T., Yap, E.P.H., Maxwell, P. *et al.* (1994) p53 expression, mutation and allelic deletion in ovarian cancer. *J. Pathol.* **174**, 159-68.

31. Klemi, P.J., Takahashi, S., Joensuu, H. *et al.* (1994) Immunohistochemical detection of p53 protein in borderline and malignant serous ovarian tumours. *Int. J. Gynecol. Pathol.* **13**, 228-33.

32. Kiyokawa, T. (1994) Alteration of p53 in ovarian cancer; Its occurrence and maintenance in tumour progression. *Int. J. Gynecol. Pathol.* **13**, 311-18.

33. Jacobs, I.J., Smith, S.A., Wiseman, R.W. *et al.* (1993) A deletion unit on chromosome 17q in epithelial ovarian tumors distal to the familial breast/ovarian cancer locus. *Cancer Res.* **53**, 1218-21.

34. Kuerbitz, S.J., Plunket, B.S., Walsh, W.V. *et al.* (1992) Wild-type p53 is a cell cycle check point determinant following irradiation. *Proc. Natl. Acad. Sci. USA* **89**, 7491-5.

35. Pines, J. (1994) Arresting developments in cell-cycle control. *T.I.B.S.* **19**, 143-5.

36. Pietenpol, J.A. and Vogelstein, B. (1993) Tumour Suppressor Genes, No room at the p53 inn. *Nature* **365**, 17-8.

37. Hutson, R., Ramsdale, J. and Wells, M. (1995) p53 protein expression in putative precursor lesions of epithelial ovarian cancer. *Histopathology - in press*

38. Shi, S.R., Kay, M.E. and Kalra, K.L. (1991) Antigen retrieval in formalin-fixed, paraffin-embedded tissues,An enhancement method for immunohistochemical staining based on

microwave oven heating of tissue sections. *J. Histochem. Cytochem.* **39**, 741-8.

39. Resnick, J.M., Cherwitz, D., Knapp, D. *et al.* (1995) A microwave method that enhances detection of aberrant p53 expression in formalin-fixed paraffin-embedded tissues. *Arch. Pathol. Lab. Med.* **119**, 360-6.

40. Kupryjanczyk, J., Bell, D.A., Dimeo, D. *et al.* (1995) p53 gene analysis of ovarian borderline tumours and stage I carcinomas. *Hum. Pathol.* **26**, 387-92.

41. Mittal, K.R., Goswami, S. and Demopoulos, R.I. (1995) Immunohistochemical profile of ovarian inclusion cysts in patients with and without ovarian carcinoma. *Histochem. J.* **27**, 119-22.

42. Shibata, D., Hawes, D., Li, Z-H. *et al.* (1992) Specific genetic analysis of microscopic tissue after selective ultraviolet radiation fractionation and the polymerase chain reaction. *Am. J. Pathol.* **141**, 539-41.

43. Zheng, J., Wan, M., Zweizig, S. *et al.* (1993) Histologically benign or low-grade malignant tumours adjacent to high-grade ovarian carcinomas contain molecular characteristics of high-grade carcinomas. *Cancer Res.* **53**, 4138-42.

44. Gruis, N.A., Abeln, E.C.A., Bardoel, A.F.J. *et al.* (1992) PCR-based microsatellite polymorphisms in the detection of loss of heterozygosity in fresh and archival tumour tissue. *Br. J. Cancer* **68**, 308-13.

45. Yamada, K., Ohkawa, K. and Joh, K. (1995) Monoclonal antibody, MAb 12C3, is a sensitive immunohistochemical marker of early malignant change in epithelial ovarian tumours. *Am. J. Clin. Pathol.* **103**, 288-94.

Chapter 4

Ovary-specific retroviral-like genomic elements

Thomas C. HAMILTON, Paul D. MILLER, Lori A. GETTS and

Andrew K. GODWIN

4.1 INTRODUCTION

The inconsistent symptoms which result in the detection of ovarian cancer, most often only after it has metastasized beyond the ovaries, not only lead to frequent mortality but also have hampered our ability to gain insights into the genes which cause this disease. An understanding of the rationale for this view is aided by a brief summary of differences in strategies being used to determine the genetic basis of colon cancer (where substantial progress is being made) compared to those required for similar efforts to directly study clinical ovarian cancer. These observations have suggested to us that animal models of ovarian cancer could provide an alternative means to detect important ovarian cancer genes. The frequency of colon cancer compared to ovarian cancer is an asset yielding more independent specimens for study. Two additional characteristics of colon cancer are substantial assets:

1. Colonoscopy is a cost-effective means to screen for early disease and has acceptable morbidity. Such cannot be said for laparoscopy and ovarian cancer, except perhaps for individuals with a substantial family history of the disease (see below for limitations of the study of such cases) [1].

Hence, the majority of ovarian cancer specimens available for study are from late stage patients [2,3] where the complexity of genetic changes present [4-10] suggests that they likely are a combination of causal and random. It should also be noted that many of the limited number of stage one lesions which are available are large tumours since detection must await the occurrence of the vague symptoms typical of the disease. In such large stage one tumours (many centimetres in diameter) compared to small ones (<1cm in diameter), the difference in tumour cell population doublings is substantial and could result in the addition of random genetic events to those causally involved in tumour initiation.

2. Polyps are accepted precursor lesions in colon cancer. In the case of ovarian cancer, there is failure among pathologists to agree as to whether precursor lesions exist. For example, there is discussion [11], but no general agreement, as to whether inclusion cysts are precursors of benign ovarian cystadenomas and whether these, in turn, are precursors of ovarian cancers [12,13]. There is even substantial speculation that tumours of low malignant potential and inherited disease have different routes of causation than sporadic ovarian cancer [14]. This is in contrast to colon cancer where there is

37

substantial evidence that the study of familial disease has markedly aided in the apparent understanding of the genetic causation of sporadic disease [15,16].

In summary, the frequency, the ability to obtain early malignant lesions and normal progenitor cells (in many cases all from the same individual), the recognition of accepted precursor lesions, and the relationship between the genesis of familial and sporadic colon cancer are in marked contrast to the situation in ovarian cancer.

4.2 THE INHERITED COMPONENT

It is clear that a portion of ovarian cancers occur at high frequency within individual families and often in combination with breast cancer [17]. The majority of these familial cancers (only 5-10% of all ovarian cancers) can be attributed to inheritance of a gene conferring high risk [17]. In 1994, the breast cancer susceptibility gene, known as BRCA1, was cloned [18]. It has been determined that alterations within both alleles of the gene (which presumably inactivate or result in abnormal function) occur in the majority of ovarian and breast cancers that develop in these families [19-23]. Among the many reasons for great excitement prior to the cloning of BRCA1 was the expectation that somatic mutations in the gene would be found to contribute to the aetiology of the far more frequent sporadic forms of ovarian and breast carcinoma. This hypothesis was predicted based on the observation that loss of heterogeneity (LOH), the hallmark of tumour suppressor gene inactivation, was common in sporadic ovarian cancer in the region of chromosome 17 known to include BRCA1 [2,4,8-10]. Interestingly, initial studies indicate that the gene appears to play only a very limited role in non-inherited ovarian cancer [24,25]. The simplest explanation (with certain caveats) is that hereditary and sporadic forms of ovarian

cancer have different routes to causation as has been speculated by pathologists and gynaecological oncologists. Indeed, the exact role of BRCA1 in inherited breast and ovarian cancer is far from defined based on the recent discovery of an individual that inherited a mutant allele of BRCA1 from each parent. At the age of 32 years, the only malady in this clinical knockout so far is unilateral breast cancer [26]. What is evident is that the genetic basis for more than 80% of ovarian cancer is still unknown, indicating the need to identify additional genes involved in the initiation and clinical manifestation of this disease.

4.3 MODEL SYSTEMS

An alternative to the study of inherited cancer or late stage sporadic ovarian cancer specimens is the use of model systems which may be genetically simpler than clinical cancer. This may make it easier to identify candidate genes separated from the morass of genetic changes characteristic of late stage cancer [2,4-10]. At present, the only well characterized model of ovarian cancer is the system of growth-associated transformation of rat ovarian surface epithelial cells developed by us [27-29]. Briefly, rat ovarian surface epithelial cells were isolated and placed in tissue culture. These cells were found to grow rapidly to cover the culture surface as if repairing a wound in the ovarian surface [27]. When the cells covered the surface, mitotic activity stopped and the cells could be maintained as a quiescent viable culture for long periods of time. Under these conditions, the cells developed no features characteristic of malignancy. Alternatively, the cells could be harvested with trypsin, diluted, and returned to a new culture flask. These cells would again grow to cover the culture vessel's surface. By repeating the process multiple times, the repetitious wound repair as occurs with incessant ovulation was mimicked in a simple way. Rat ovarian surface epithelial cells subjected to such growth stress frequently acquire features characteristic of malignant cells [27,29]. These changes include loss of the contact inhibited phenotype, acquisition of the capacity for substrate independent growth which was modulated by epidermal growth factor and transforming growth factor beta, and the ability to form tumours in xenogeneic hosts [29,30]. The histological features of the tumours produced by the transformed rat ovarian surface epithelial cells supported the relevance of the model in that they recapitulated clinical ovarian cancer. All of the tumours had features which were consistent with designation as adenocarcinomas. They varied from poorly differentiated to well-differentiated tumours [29-31]. In summary, this model provides some of the first experimental data suggestive that repetitious mitotic activity of the surface epithelium, as occurs in the absence of pregnancy or other means of inhibition of ovulation, may contribute to the initiation of ovarian cancer. Furthermore, the features of the tumours produced by transformed rat surface epithelial cells provide some experimental support to the dogma that ovarian cancer arises from the surface epithelium.

We believe that the ability to produce many independent transformants and have the normal progenitor cells from which they were derived will facilitate the identification of genetic differences between the normal and malignant cells. Furthermore, some indication that the genetic changes that accompany malignant transformation in our system are less complex than is typical of the majority of late stage clinical cancers [5-7] has been provided by cytogenetic analysis [29]. Cells of individual undifferentiated tumours have as few as three, but average only five to eight clonal abnormalities, whereas the more

differentiated tumours have just one or two changes. These numbers are far lower than is typical of clinical specimens. Thus, the majority of the genes which may be identified using this model could be causally involved in the disease process. There is no guarantee, however, that this will be true in every case. Hence, it is important to note that the availability of an experimental system will markedly facilitate testing the functional role of candidate genes.

One approach that we are currently using to detect genetic differences between normal and malignantly transformed rat ovarian surface epithelial cells is genome scanning. This method is related to DNA fingerprinting but uses a much more abundant repetitive DNA sequence (~500–1000 copies per genome) to detect DNA fragments on a Southern blot [32]. The technique favours detection of relatively large duplications or deletions with less likelihood of detecting small differences such as point mutations [32]. The goal is to resolve large numbers of individual bands on a Southern blot. Hence, detection of a genetic difference requires the presence of the repetitive sequence in a restriction fragment associated with the alteration. The technique allows a significant portion of the genome to be examined for sequence differences related to a mutant locus. The sensitivity of the method is related to copy number and dispersion of the repetitive sequence, the number of distinct repetitive sequence probes used, the number of restriction endonucleases individually used on each related group of DNA samples, and the type and extent of mutations.

4.4 EXPERIMENTAL FINDINGS

We have chosen to use a retroviral-like element identified by us as our genome scanning probe. This sequence has many features which make it well-suited to the purpose. It is present as ~1000–3000 copies

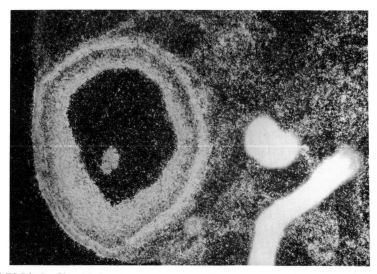

Figure 4.1 OST RNA *In Situ* Hybridization. A section of an adult rat ovary was hybridized with ^{35}S-labelled OST cDNA probes. The photographs were taken with epiluminescence, resulting in the silver grains appearing as white dots. Shown is expression of OST in the granulosa cells and theca cells of a large pre-ovulatory follicles. Note its abundant expression in the surface epithelial cells directly above the follicle. Magnification x50.

in the rat genome and is widely distributed as demonstrated by fluorescence *in situ* hybridization [30]. These characteristics alone make it appropriate to detect alterations in DNA between phenotypically different populations of rat ovarian surface epithelial cells. It, however, has additional features which are of interest. It is well known that retrovirus-like sequences are endogenous to the genomes of most if not all species. These sequences may be divided into families based on sequence and structure. They vary in abundance from single members to >1000 copies per genome [33]. In the human as well as rodents, they may occur as solitary long terminal repeats (LTRs), but often are characterized by 3' and 5' LTRs and intervening sequence with homology to viral *gag, pol* and/or *env* genes [33, 34]. This latter arrangement is characteristic of the element we have discovered. The features of such sequences

confer upon them much potential to influence evolution and oncogenesis [33, 35]. Their interspersed repetitive nature allows for homologous recombination which may yield increased copy number of intervening genes. Their mobility on an evolutionary time scale, also, creates the potential for gene disruption and hence inactivation of gene function. For example, it has recently been found that the inactivation of the TSC2 gene by a full-length retroviral-like element is the basis for inherited renal cancer in the Eker rat [36]. Furthermore, the promoter characteristics of LTRs, evidenced by the fact that retrovirus-like sequences are often transcribed suggests their potential to regulate adjacent gene expression [37]. Of great interest, is the fact that in some instances there is tissue specificity to retrovirus-like element expression, and such is the case with the family of sequences we discovered. Examination of Northern blots

Table 4.1. DNA alterations detected by genome scanning between normal and transformed rat ovarian surface epithelial cells*

Restriction enzyme	Cell line							
	8	9	10	12	14	19	23	26
	9S, 44S, T	17S, 44S T	9S, 44S, T	9S, 44S T	7S, 44S, T	9S, 44S, T	9S, 44S, T	9S, 44S,T
Hae III		No diff.	No diff.				No diff.	- - +
Hpa II			- + + + - -					+
Msp I		No diff.	No diff.			No diff.		- - +
Rsa I	No diff.	No diff.	- + + + - -	No diff.	No diff.	No diff.	- + +	No diff.
Taq I		No diff.	No diff.					- - +
Hinf I		No diff.	No diff.			No diff.	- + +	No diff.
Apa I	+ + -	+ + -	No diff.	No diff.	- + +	No diff.	- + +	No diff.
Bam HI	No diff.	No diff.			No diff.			- +
Bgl II		No diff.						- +
Bmy I	No diff.	No diff.		No diff.	No diff.			- +
Eco RI	No diff.	No diff.		No diff.	No diff.	No diff.	- + +	- +
Eco RV	No diff.	+ + -		No diff.	- + +	No diff.	- + +	- +
Hind III	No diff.	No diff.					No diff.	- +
Hpa I								- +
Pst I	No diff.	No diff.				No diff.		- +
Pvu II	No diff.	No diff.						- +
Sst I	No diff.	No diff.		No diff.	No diff.			- +

* DNA was isolated and subjected to genome scanning analysis as previously described [30,32]
- = loss of band; + = gain (amplification) of a band, S = subculture, T = tumour cell line

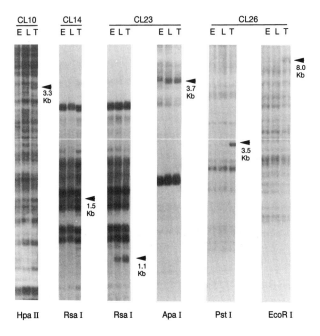

Figure 4.2 Autoradiographs of Southern transfer of genome scanning gels. Blot was probed with the 1.6 kbp OST fragment. Arrows indicate bands gained or lost along with their approximate size. The restriction endonuclease used is indicated under each cell line (CL) triplet: early passage (E), late passage transformed (L), and cells from the tumours produced by transformed cells (T).

prepared with RNA from mature rat ovary, brain, muscle, heart, kidney, lung, spleen, liver, Fallopian tube and uterus revealed the presence of an abundant family of transcripts only in the ovarian RNA [30]. Hence, we refer to this family as Ovarian Specific Transcripts (OSTs). We have examined the expression of OST in more detail within the ovary using *in situ* hybridization on histological sections [30 and Figure 4.1]. We found that expression followed follicular growth in a similar but distinct pattern from leutinizing and follicle stimulating hormones [30, 38]. Of great interest, was the finding of abundant expression in surface epithelial cells adjacent to large antral follicles (Figure 4.1). Such information on expression

increases the utility of the OST sequence as a tool for the identification of alterations including amplification and deletion of genetic material associated with transformation using genome scanning technology.

We have used the OST probe and genome scanning to examine the DNA from eight cell line triplets for alterations. A cell line triplet consisted of early passage cells (phenotypically and cytogenetically normal), late passage malignantly transformed cells derived from the same early passage cells and cells derived from the tumour which the transformed cells produced when injected into nude mice. Southern blots were prepared from the DNA of triplets after

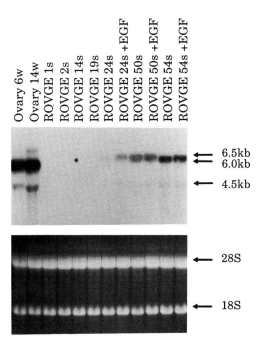

Figure 4.3 Northern blot analysis of normal and malignantly transformed rat ovarian surface epithelial cells (with and without exposure to exogenous epidermal growth factor). The top panel shows examination with OST 30-1 [30]. Loading equivalency is demonstrated in the lower panel by ethidium staining of total RNA (15µg per lane). Size is shown in kilobases (kb); w= weeks of age; s=subculture; EGF=epidermal growth factor. Cells at late passage >50S are malignantly transformed.

treatment with 3 to 15 individual restriction endonucleases. As summarized in Table 4.1, six of the eight cell lines showed banding alterations including both the appearance and disappearance of bands in the transformed and tumour cells, and increased band intensity in these cells compared to normal cells. The group showing the most frequent changes was from cell line 26 whereas no changes were seen in cell lines 12 and 19, which is consistent with the limited karyotypic abnormalities seen in these latter two tumour cell lines [29]. Representative data are pictorially presented in Figure 4.2. An additional finding of interest was related to the expression of OSTs in rat ovarian surface epithelial cells in culture. As shown in Figure 4.3, OSTs were not expressed in early passage normal cells subjected to routine *in vitro* growth conditions. However, transformation in some cases was associated with activation of transcription of genomic ovarian specific transcription units. Furthermore, limited data show that the transcriptional activity of these units is modulated by epidermal growth factor at intermediate *in vitro* passage, *i.e.* at an early step in transformation (Figure 4.3).

4.5 CONCLUSIONS

Frequent findings on genome scanning blots were bands of increased intensity in transformed cells. This is consistent with amplification of genetic material and this possibility is supported by analysis of the karyotypes of transformed cells. We observed evidence for gene amplification in three of the tumour cell lines (lines 8, 9 and 26) in the form of double minute chromosomes (line 9) and homogeneously staining chromosomal regions (lines 8 and 26) [29]. Based on these data, we have initiated efforts to clone the apparent amplicon in one of the transformed cell lines, cell line 26. This is the first step necessary to determine whether a gene of significance to the malignant transformation process is embedded within the amplicon. In summary, we have identified a new family of retroviral-like elements. These elements are widely distributed in the rat genome and are expressed only in the rat ovary. Furthermore, we have shown the utility of an OST probe to detect genetic differences between normal and malignantly transformed rat ovarian surface epithelial cells by genome scanning and transformation associated transcriptional activation of the genomic units which serve as templates for OSTs.

ACKNOWLEDGEMENTS

The authors are supported by the following grants from the National Cancer Institute: CA56916 (TCH), CA51228 (TCH), and CA60643 (AKG).

REFERENCES

1. Puls L., Powell D., DePriest P. *et al.* (1992) Transition from benign to malignant epithelium in mucinous and serous ovarian cystadenocarcinoma. *Gynecol. Oncol.* **47**, 53-7.
2. Godwin A., Vanderveer L., Schultz D. *et al.* (1994) A common region of deletion on chromosome 17q in both sporadic and familial epithelial ovarian tumors distal to BRCA1. *Am. J. Hum. Genet.* **55**, 666-77.
3. Schultz D., Vanderveer L., Buetow K. *et al.* (1995) Characterization of chromosome 9 in human ovarian neoplasia identifies frequent genetic imbalance on 9q are rare alterations involving 9p, including CDKN2. *Cancer Res.* **55**, 2150-7.
4. Yang-Feng T., Han H., Chen K. *et al.* (1993) Allelic loss in ovarian cancer. *Int. J. Cancer* **54**, 546-51.
5. Testa J. (1995) Chromosome alterations in human lung cancer. *In*, H. Pass, J. Mitchell, D. Johnson and A. Turrisi (eds.), *Lung Cancer, Principles and Practice*, JB Lippincott, Philadelphia.
6. Tenaka K., Boice C. and Testa J. (1989) Chromosome aberrations in nine patients with ovarian cancer. *Cancer Genet. Cytogenet.* **43**, 1-14.
7. Lukeis R., Ball D., Irving L. *et al.* (1993) Chromosome abnormalities in non-small cell lung cancer pleural effusions. *Genes Chrom. Cancer* **8**, 262-9.
8. Sato T., Saito H., Morita R. *et al.* (1991) Allelotype of human ovarian cancer. *Cancer Res.* **51**, 5118-22.
9. Osborne R. J. and Leech V. (1994) Polymerase chain reaction allelotyping of human ovarian cancers. *Br. J. Cancer*, **69** 429-38.
10. Cliby W., Ritland S., Hartmann L. *et al.* (1993) Human epithelial cancer allelotype. *Cancer Res.* **53**, 2393-8.
11. Radisavljevic S. (1976) The pathogenesis of ovarian inclusion cysts and cystomas. *Obstet. Gynecol.* **49**, 424-9.
12. Fox H. (1993) Pathology of early malignant change in the ovary. *Int. J. Gynecol. Pathol.* **12**, 153-5.
13. Zheng J., Benedict W., Xu H.-J. *et al.* (1995) Genetic disparity between morphologically benign cysts contiguous to ovarian carcinomas and solitary cystadenomas. *J. Nat. Cancer Inst.* **87**, 1146-53.
14. Powell D., Puls L., and van Nagell J.J.

(1992) Current concepts in ovarian epithelial tumors, Does benign to malignant transformation occur? *Hum. Pathol.* 23, 846-7.

15. Fearon E. and Vogelstein B. (1990) A genetic model for colorectal tumorgenesis. *Cell*, 61, 759-767

16. Parsons R., Li G., Longley M. *et al.* (1993) Hypermutability and mismatch repair deficiency in RER+ tumor cells. *Cell* 75, 1227-36.

17. Narod S., Feunteun J., Lynch H. *et al.* (1991) Familial breast-ovarian cancer locus on 17q12-q23. *Lancet* 338, 82-3.

18. Miki Y., Swensen J., Shattuck-Eldens D. *et al.* (1994) A strong candidate for the breast and ovarian cancer susceptibility gene BRCA1. *Science* 266, 66-71.

19. Castilla L., Couch F., Erdos M. *et al.* (1994) Mutations in the BRCA1 gene in families with early-onset breast and ovarian cancer. *Nat. Genet.* 8, 387-91.

20. Friedman L., Ostermeyer E., Szabo C. *et al.* (1994) Confirmation of BRCA1 by analysis of germline mutations linked to breast and ovarian cancer in ten families. *Nat. Genet.* 8, 399-404.

21. Simard J., Tonin P., Durocher F. *et al.* (1994) Common origins of BRCA1 mutations in Canadian breast and ovarian cancer families. *Nat. Genet.* 8,392-8.

22. Shattuck-Eidens D., McClure M., Simard J. *et al.* (1995) A collaborative survey of 80 mutations in the BRCA1 breast and ovarian cancer susceptibility gene. *JAMA* 273, 535-41.

23. Takahashi H. (1995) Mutation analysis of the BRCA1 gene in ovarian cancers. *Cancer Res.* 55, 2998-3002.

24. Futreal P., Liu Q., Shattuck-Eldens D. *et al.* (1994) BRCA1 mutations in primary breast and ovarian carcinomas. *Science* 266, 120-2.

25. Hosking L., Trowsdale J., Nicolai H. *et al.* (1995) A somatic BRCA1 mutation in an ovarian tumor. *Nat. Genet.*, 9, 343-4.

26. Boyd M., Harris F., McFarlane R., Davidson H., and Black D. (1995) A human BRCA1 gene knockout. *Nature* 375, 541-2.

27. Godwin A., Testa J., Handel L. *et al.* (1992) Spontaneous transformation of rat ovarian surface epithelial cells implicates repeated ovulation in ovarian cancer etiology and is associated with clonal cytogenetic changes. *J. Nat. Cancer Inst.* 84, 592-601.

28. Hamilton T. (1992) Ovarian cancer. Part I, Biology. *Curr. Prob. Cancer* 16, 1-57.

29. Testa J., Getts L., Salazar H. *et al.* (1994) Spontaneous transformation of rat ovarian surface epithelial cells results in well to poorly differentiated tumors with a parallel range of cytogenetic complexity. *Cancer Res.* 54, 2778-84.

30. Godwin A., Miller P., Getts L. *et al.* (1995) Retroviral-like sequences specifically expressed in the rat ovary detect genetic differences between normal and transformed rat ovarian surface epithelial cells. *Endocrinology* 136, 4640-9.

31. Salazar H., Godwin A., Getts L. *et al.* (1995) Spontaneous transformation of the ovarian surface epithelium and the biology of ovarian cancer. *In*, F. Sharp, P. Mason, T. Blackett and J. Berek (eds.), *Ovarian Cancer 3.* Chapman & Hall Medical, London, pp. 145-56.

32. Brilliant M., Gondo Y. and Eicher E. (1991) Direct molecular identification of the mouse pink-eyed unstable mutation by genome scanning. *Science* 252, 566-9.

33. Stoye J. and Coffin J. (1985) Endogenous Retroviruses. *In*, R. Weiss, N. Teich, H. Varmus and J. Coffin (eds.), *Molecular Biology of Tumor Viruses, Part III. RNA Tumor Viruses,*. Cold Spring Harbor Laboratory, Cold Spring Harbor, NY, pp. 357-404.

34. Leib-Mosch C., Brack-Werner R., Werner

T. *et al.* (1990) Endogenous retroviral elements in human DNA. *Cancer Res.* **50**, 5636-42.

35. Keshet E., Schiff R., and Itin A. (1991) Mouse retrotransposons, a cellular reservior of long terminal repeat (LTR) elements with diverse transcriptional specificities. *Adv. Cancer Res.* **56**, 215-51.

36. Xiao G.-H., Jin F., and Yeung R. (1995) Germ-line *Tsc2* mutation in a dominantly inherited cancer model defines a novel family of rat intracisternal-A particle elements. *Oncogene* **11**, 81-7.

37. Feuchter-Murthy A., Freeman J., and Mager D. (1993) Splicing of a human endogenous retrovirus to a novel phospholipase A2 related gene. *Nucleic Acids Res.* **21**, 135-45.

38. Vanderveer L., Jackson K., Hamilton T. and Godwin A. (1992) Identification of a novel ovarian specific transcript that is expressed in spontaneously transformed rat ovarian surface epithelial cells. *Proc. Am. Assoc. Cancer Res.* **33**, 357.

Part Two

Genetics and Epidemiology

Chapter 5

Breast and ovarian cancer in Utah kindreds with three BRCA1 mutations

David E. GOLDGAR, Linda STEELE, Susan NEUHAUSEN,

Lisa CANNON-ALBRIGHT, Cathryn M. LEWIS and Mark SKOLNICK

5.1 INTRODUCTION

Ovarian cancer has been recognized as having a significant familial component with estimates ranging between a two- and a three-and-a-half-fold increased risk of ovarian cancer among first-degree relatives of women with ovarian cancer [1,2]. In addition, some population-based studies have shown familial associations between ovarian cancer, early-onset breast cancer and early-onset colon cancer [3,4]. These associations are believed to be largely due to two familial cancer syndromes, the Breast/Ovarian [5-7] and Hereditary Non-Polyposis Colorectal Cancer (HNPCC) [8], respectively. It is now known that the former syndrome is due in large part to the BRCA1 gene on chromosome 17q [9] and to a lesser extent, to the BRCA2 locus on chromosome 13q [10], while the latter syndrome is due to mutations in at least four genes involved in DNA repair [11-13]. It is likely that the overwhelming majority of the excess familial risk in ovarian cancer is due to these specific, high-penetrant, autosomal dominant genes [14]. It is also noteworthy that most site-specific ovarian cancer appears to be due to the BRCA1 locus as well as those with early-onset breast cancer [15]. Based on

linkage analyses of 214 breast cancer families collected as part of the international Breast Cancer Linkage Consortium (BCLC), it was estimated that 80% of families with the breast-ovarian syndrome were due to the BRCA1 locus [5,16] and that the risk of developing ovarian cancer for female carriers of a BRCA1 mutation was 0.63 by age 60 [17].

Of perhaps greater interest was the finding that there was statistically significant evidence of heterogeneity of ovarian cancer risk among these families with the vast majority (89%) of families having a relatively low, but still highly elevated over general population rates, risk (0.23), while the remaining families had a very high lifetime risk of developing ovarian cancer (0.84) [17]. At the time when this study was performed, the BRCA1 gene had not yet been isolated, and it was assumed that this difference would very likely be due to differences in the specific BRCA1 mutation segregating in high and low risk ovarian cancer families.

With the recent isolation of BRCA1 [9] and the subsequent identification of large numbers of families with BRCA1 mutations [18,19], it is now possible to examine the ovarian cancer risk in families with specific, known, BRCA1 mutations. Somewhat surprisingly, there was not a striking

49

association of ovarian cancer risk with specific BRCA1 mutations, although there was some slight evidence that mutations in the 3' end of the gene were associated with a lower ovarian cancer risk [19]. However, even among diverse families with identical mutations on the same haplotypic background, one finds a great diversity in the proportion of affected individuals who develop ovarian cancer [18]. It is therefore important to examine other potential factors which may modify the risk of ovarian cancer among BRCA1 mutation carriers.

The obvious candidates for these factors are environmental factors which are known to be associated with sporadic ovarian cancer risk in large epidemiological studies. For example, a number of reproductive and hormonally-related factors convey increased risk for ovarian cancer. Nulliparity as well as having relatively few pregnancies have been very consistently related to a higher risk for developing ovarian cancer. A clear dose-response relationship exists where increasing numbers of pregnancies decrease the risk for ovarian cancer [20]. In contrast to breast cancer, age at first pregnancy does not appear to have a large effect on ovarian cancer.

It is unlikely, however, that these factors can explain all the observed variation in ovarian cancer risk among BRCA1 carriers. In this paper we examine the pattern of inheritance of breast and ovarian cancer in four large Utah kindreds in which a specific BRCA1 mutation has been identified. These four families contain a total of 47 cases of breast cancer and 29 cases of ovarian cancer in known carriers of BRCA1 mutations (or in a few cases in first degree relatives of known carriers on whom testing was not possible). We have collected preliminary risk factor information on carriers of these mutations in an effort to explain the observed variation in

ovarian cancer incidence in these families. The largest such family, K2082, has been studied in detail previously [21] but has been updated for the present study.

5.2 METHODS

5.2.1 ASCERTAINMENT OF FAMILIES

Three of the four families reported in this paper (K2082, K2301 and K2305) were ascertained from the Utah Population Database (UPDB) [22] on the basis of a cluster of early onset breast cancers and ovarian cancers among related individuals (K2082) or for multiple cases of ovarian cancer (K2301,K2305). The fourth family (K1001) was ascertained in 1980 from physician referral as a result of diagnosis of two early-onset breast cancer cases. The ascertainment of these families has been described in more detail previously [21, 23]. Permission to contact eligible proband cases was elicited from their physicians, an introductory letter was sent, followed by a phone call from a clinic coordinator. Once permission was obtained, each kindred was extended through all available connecting relatives, and to all informative first degree relatives of each proband or cancer case. All ovarian or breast cancer cases reported in the kindred which were not confirmed in the Utah Cancer Registry were researched by the clinic coordinator and, where possible, medical records or death certificates were obtained for confirmation of all cancers. Risk factor data was gathered via a telephone interview on living subjects. Surrogate data was obtained for parity and age at first and last pregnancy through both genealogical records and interview with living relatives. All subjects gave informed consent for blood sampling and interviewing and all research was approved by the Institutional Review Board of the University of Utah.

5.2.2 DETECTION OF MUTATIONS AND IDENTIFICATION OF CARRIERS

Initially, linkage analysis was performed using short tandem repeat markers located in the BRCA1 region of chromosome 17. Convincing linkage evidence was found for K2082, but the other three families had initially either negative or uninformative lod scores with these markers, largely due to the presence of sporadic cases within the family. With the isolation of the BRCA1 gene it became possible to test patient samples from these families directly for mutations by direct sequencing of the entire coding region and intron:exon boundaries of the BRCA1 gene. When mutations were identified in a given family, allele-specific oligonucleotide hybridization was used to identify mutation carrier status of at-risk individuals.

5.2.3 STATISTICAL ANALYSIS

Risks of breast and ovarian cancer were calculated using survival analysis (life table) methods of women who were (a) known to carry the BRCA1 gene by mutation testing or by pedigree relationship to other known carriers; or (b) who were affected first degree relatives of a known gene carrier, but whose carrier status could not be inferred. A non-parametric Kaplan-Meier analysis was used to estimate the probability of developing cancer as a function of age. Unaffected women were classified as censored at their current age or age at death, if deceased. In the penetrance analysis, age-specific risks of developing breast and ovarian cancers were estimated separately, assuming in each case that women with the other cancer were unaffected for the one being considered.

Table 5.1 Relationship of reproductive risk factors to phenotype.

(a) Comparison of risk factors among the three phenotypic groups.

	Breast		Ovarian		Unaffected[1]		P_{AU} [2]	P_{BO} [3]
	n=43		n=29		n=26			
	Mean	SD	Mean	SD	Mean	SD		
Parity	4.2	2.6	4.2	2.4	5.0	2.9	0.18	0.94
Age first pregnancy	23.5	3.6	24.0	4.0	21.8	4.2	0.03	0.59
Age last pregnancy	33.2	6.7	33.2	6.0	33.4	7.3	0.89	0.99
Age/Age at death	45.1	12.3	50.6	10.3	48.2	10.3	0.88	0.05

[1] Only includes unaffected gene carriers 40 years or older
[2] Significance level for testing differences between affected and unaffected gene carriers.
[3] Significance level for testing differences between breast and ovarian cases.

(b) Correlations with age at diagnosis

	Breast	Ovarian	Unaffected
Parity	0.40**	0.31	0.33
Age first pregnancy	0.12	0.32	0.21
Age last pregnancy	0.44**	0.54**	0.32

** p<0.01

Women who underwent prophylactic surgery were censored at the age at which surgery was performed.

Factors of interest which may influence age specific risk such as mutation, parity, and age at first/last pregnancy were tested using the log-rank test to see if they affected the risks of cancer for BRCA1 mutation carriers. Because of the possible confounding effect of temporal changes in reproductive patterns, year of birth was included in all tests of the reproductive cohorts on cancer risk. The computer program Lifetest (SAS Inc., Cary, NC) was used to estimate the penetrance curves and test for covariate effects and for differences in risks for pre-defined strata.

Comparisons between affected and unaffected subjects for the various risk factors of parity, age at first pregnancy, and age of last pregnancy was done adjusting for year of birth using the SAS GLM program. To examine the effects of these known risk factors for breast and ovarian cancer, two sets of analyses were performed. The first analysis compared three groups of BRCA1 gene carriers in these four families: unaffected women over 40 years of age; women affected with breast cancer; and women affected with ovarian cancer. Women with both breast and ovarian cancer were included in the ovarian category. The comparison between the two cancer-affected groups was subdivided into two orthogonal single degree of freedom contrasts: affected vs. unaffected; and breast vs. ovarian. The results of these analyses are shown in Table 5.1.

5.3 RESULTS

The mutations found in these four families have been described elsewhere [19]. Families 2301 and 1001 had identical mutations which have also been found in three additional families from other centres; moreover these families shared an identical haplotype at markers within and surrounding the BRCA1 locus [18], indicating a common ancestral origin of the mutation found in these families. The data from these two families were pooled in the analysis of mutational heterogeneity. The mutations found in the other two families have not, to our knowledge, been found in any other families. The characteristics of the four families are summarized in Table 5.2 and abbreviated pedigree drawings for three of the kindreds are shown in Figures 5.1–5.3. The pedigree drawing of the largest kindred, K2082, has been published previously [21]. As shown in Table 5.2, the kindreds appear to have quite diverse phenotypic expression. Kindred 1001 contains 11 cases of breast cancer due likely to the BRCA1 mutation in the family, the majority of which were diagnosed before age 40. Thus far, there have been no cases of ovarian cancer diagnosed in K1001. Kindred 2305, on the other hand, contains seven cases of ovarian cancer and six cases of breast, only one of which was diagnosed before age 40.

A summary of the mean values for the three reproductive risk factors and age/age at diagnosis as a function of phenotype are shown in Table 5.1(a). The differences between the three phenotypic subgroups were subdivided into those between affected (with breast or ovarian) women and unaffected gene carriers over age 40 and those differences between women affected with breast cancer compared to those with ovarian cancer. Of the three risk factors examined, age at first pregnancy and parity differed significantly between those women who developed breast or ovarian cancer and those women over age 40 who were carriers of BRCA1 mutations but remained unaffected. There was no difference in age/age at diagnosis between affected and unaffected women. No risk factor differences were found between women with breast cancer and those with ovarian cancer.

Affected women had, on average, one less child than unaffected women. Interestingly, while age at last birth did not differ significantly between affected and unaffected women, nor between women with breast and ovarian cancer, this factor was most highly correlated with age at diagnosis of the disease; women who had their last child at a later age tended to have later age at diagnosis of their disease. This was true for both breast (r=0.44, p<0.01) and ovarian cancer (r=0.54, p<0.01).

5.3.1 RESULTS OF SURVIVAL ANALYSES

The results of the survival analyses described above in the methods section are given in Tables 5.3 and 5.4 and shown graphically in Figures 5.4 and 5.5. Table 5.3 shows the cumulative risks of breast, ovarian, or either cancer for the combined data set as a function of age. Table 5.4 assesses the impact of the reproductive covariates on these risks. Age at last pregnancy seems to have had the greatest impact on cumulative risk. For overall risk of cancer, this was highly significant and in a stepwize multivariate model, when age at last birth was included into the model, no other risk factors were significant. Figure 5.4 shows the estimated cumulative risk of ovarian cancer as a function of parity (<4 live births vs. 4 or more, panel a) and specific BRCA1 mutation (panel b), while Figure 5.5 shows similar data for breast cancer risk. While risk of ovarian cancer did not differ between the low and high parity groups, significant heterogeneity in risk was observed between the three distinct mutations. For breast cancer risk there were both differences according to parity, with the lower parity group of carriers having a lower risk of breast cancer, and mutation heterogeneity as well.

Table 5.2 Characteristics of the four BRCA1 families included in the study. For breast and ovarian cancer, both known carriers and first degree relatives of carriers are tabulated; in the unaffected category, only those women certain to be BRCA1 carriers are included.

Kindred			*Age /*	*age at*	*diagnosis*	
		Total	*<40*	*40-49*	*50-59*	*60+*
1001	Breast	11	7	3	0	1
	Ovarian	0	-	-	-	-
	Unaffected	4	1	3	0	0
2082	Breast	20	5	7	5	3
	Ovarian	18	1	7	6	3
	Unaffected.	33	14	11	3	5
2301	Breast	10	4	1	3	2
	Ovarian	3	0	0	3	0
	Unaffected	6	3	1	1	1
2305	Breast	6	1	2	1	2
	Ovarian	7	3	1	2	1
	Unaffected	2	1	0	1	0
Total	Breast	47	17	13	10	7
	Ovarian	28	4	9	11	4
	Unaffected	45	19	15	5	6

Kindred 1001

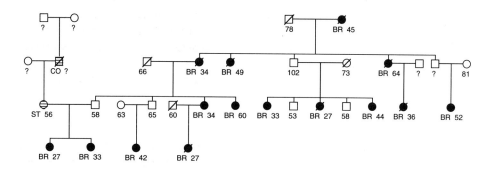

Kindred 2301

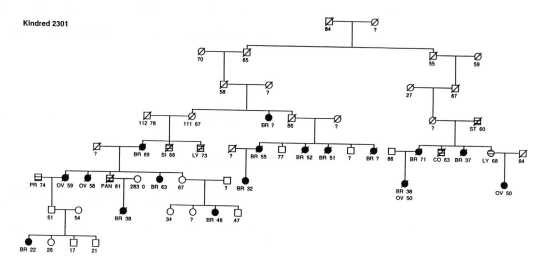

Kindred 2305

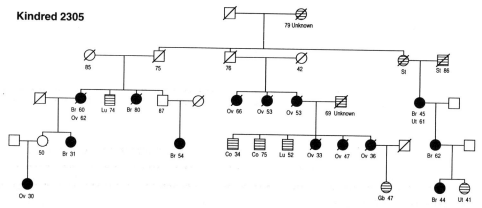

Figures 5.1-5.3 Pedigree drawings of families 1001, 2301, and 2305. Filled symbols indicate cases of breast or ovarian cancer. Horizontally striped symbols indicate cancers other than breast or ovarian:

Co = colon; Gb = gallbladder; Mela = malignant melanoma; Ut = Uterine; Pr = prostate; Lu = lung; St = stomach.

Table 5.3 Estimated risks of breast and ovarian cancer for all families pooled

Risks by Age	Breast Cancer	Ovarian Cancer	Either Cancer
40	0.16 (0.04)	0.05 (0.02)	0.20 (0.04)
50	0.33 (0.05)	0.18 (0.05)	0.46 (0.05)
60	0.50 (0.06)	0.40 (0.07)	0.74 (0.05)
70	0.77 (0.08)	0.52 (0.08)	0.95 (0.03)

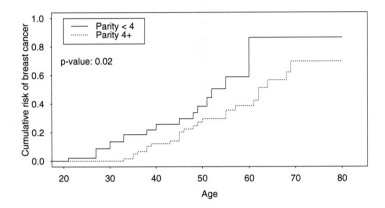

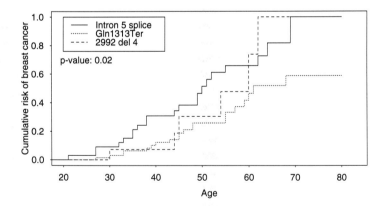

Figure 5.4 Kaplan-Meier plots of cumulative risk of ovarian cancer. Upper panel displays plots for two groups of women defined on parity <4 vs parity = 4 or more. The lower panel shows separate plots for the three mutations represented in the sample of four families.

Table 5.4. Test of reproductive risk factors as modifiers of BRCA1 cancer risk in Kaplan-Meier analysis

	Breast Cancer		Ovarian Cancer		Either Cancer	
	Univ[1]	Mult[2]	Univ	Mult	Univ	Mult
Age last pregnancy	0.06	0.06	0.10	NS	0.002	0.002
Birth Year	NS	NS	0.07	0.07	0.006	NS
Parity	0.18	NS	0.11	NS	0.01	NS
Age first pregnancy	NS	NS	NS	NS	NS	NS

[1] Test of each variable independently without including others in the model.

[2] Results of stepwize inclusion of risk factors; subsequent effects are adjusted for those already in the model.

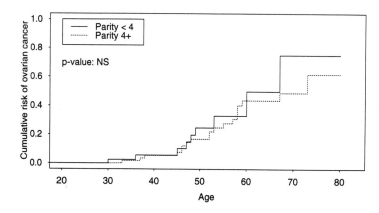

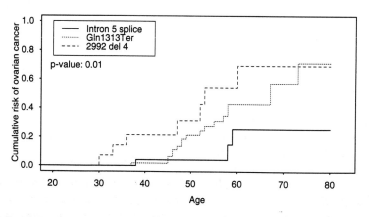

Figure 5.5 Kaplan-Meier plots of cumulative risk for breast cancer risk. Upper panel displays plots for two groups of women defined on parity <4 vs. parity = 4 or more. The lower panel shows separate plots for the three mutations represented in the sample of four families.

5.4 DISCUSSION

Beginning with the original linkage of early onset breast cancer to chromosome 17q [24] and the recognition that families with ovarian cancer as well as breast were also linked to the same region [15], there has since been recognition of the fact that the BRCA1 gene could be quite variable in expression. More recently, Narod *et al.* [25] analysed 145 families with breast and ovarian cancer and found statistical evidence for heterogeneity of ovarian cancer risk and Smith *al.* [26] demonstrated that families with largely site-specific ovarian cancer were also likely to be due to the BRCA1 gene. Previously, there was a presumption that these differences would largely be explained by mutational differences within the BRCA1 gene. Now that the BRCA1 gene has been isolated this question can be answered directly. Preliminary evidence shows some differences in the proportion of affected individuals within ovarian cancer families according to the position of the mutation in the gene. Families with mutations located in the 3' portion of the gene are generally found to have a lower incidence of ovarian cancer. That being said, it is also clear that when multiple families with the same mutation have been examined, there is still substantial variation observed in the proportions of breast and ovarian cancer, and also in the age at diagnosis of those cancers.

In this chapter, we have used four extended Utah kindreds to examine differences in age-specific risks of breast and ovarian cancer as a function of both mutional differences between families and in established reproductive risk factors within families. The results of our study indicate that for breast cancer, parity was associated with statistically significant differences in risk, with the direction of the effect consistent with the effect of parity in sporadic breast cancer. There were also mutation specific differences primarily due to a much lower risk of breast cancer in kindred 2082.

For ovarian cancer, the picture was somewhat less clear. There was no significant effect of any of the three risk factors on the cumulative ovarian cancer risk. However, if the ovarian cancer cases are considered separately, there was a significant correlation between age at diagnosis of those cancers and the age at last birth of the BRCA1 carrier. On the other hand, those women who went on to have ovarian or breast cancer were significantly older when they had their first child (24 *vs.* 22 years) than female gene carriers over age 40 who have not yet developed breast or ovarian cancer. This was true even after adjusting for the associated factor year of birth. There were no differences in age at last birth among the three groups.

Eventually, the goal will be to partition the observed phenotypic effects to genetic background (haplotype), specific genetic, and specific environmental effects and residual unexplained variation. These studies will require a larger sample size and complete pedigree data with detailed information on each individual who carries an altered BRCA1 susceptibility allele. The determination of predictors of phenotypic expression, not only in terms of type of cancer, but also in modulating age at onset, has great implications for screening and prevention strategies for women at dramatically increased risk of these cancers due to the BRCA1 gene.

ACKNOWLEDGEMENTS

The authors would like to express their thanks to the many family members who so kindly participated in this research. This work was supported by grants CA-55914, CA-48711, CN-05222, and RR-00064 from the National Institutes of Health.

REFERENCES

1. Hildreth, N.G., Kelsey, J.L., Li, V.A. *et al.* (1991) An epidemiologic study of epithelial carcinoma of the ovary. *Am. J. Epidemiol.* **114**, 398-405.

2. Schildkraut, J.M. and Thompson, W.D. (1988) Familial ovarian cancer: a population-based case-control study. *Am. J. Epidemiol.* **128**, 456-66.

3. Lynch, H.T., Guirgis, H.A., Albert, S. *et al.* (1974) Familial association of carcinoma of the breast and ovary. *Surgery* **38**, 717-24.

4. Watson, P. and Lynch, H.T. (1993) Extracolonic cancer in hereditary nonpolyposis colorectal cancer. *Cancer* **71**, 677-85.

5. Feunteun, J., Narod, S.A., Lynch H.T. *et al.* (1993) A breast-ovarian susceptibility gene maps to chromosome 17q21. *Am. J. Hum. Genet.* **52**, 736-42.

6. Go, R.C.P., King, M.C., Bailey-Wilson, J. *et al.* (1983) Genetic epidemiology of breast cancer and associated cancer in high risk families I. Segregation analysis. *J. Nat. Cancer Inst.* **71**, 455-61.

7. Lynch, H.T. (1981) *Genetics and Breast Cancer*, Van Nostrand Reinhold, New York.

8. Lynch, H.T., Kimberling, W., Albana, W. *et al.* (1985) Hereditary non polyposis colorectal cancer. *Cancer* **56**, 934-8.

9. Miki, Y., Swensen, J., Shattuck-Eidens, D. *et al.* (1994) A strong candidate for the 17q-linked breast and ovarian cancer susceptibility gene BRCA1. *Science* **266**, 66-71.

10. Wooster, R., Neuhausen, S., Mangion, J. *et al.* (1994) Localization of a breast cancer susceptibility gene, BRCA2 to chromosome 13q 12-13. *Science* **265**, 2088-90.

11. Leach, F.S., Nicolaides, N.C. and Papadopoulos, N., (1993) Mutations of a mutS homolog in hereditary non polyposis colorectal cancer. *Cell* **75**, 1215-25.

12. Papadopoulos, N., Nicolaides, N.C. and Wei, Y-F. (1994) Mutation of a mutL homolog in hereditary colon cancer. *Science* **263**, 1625-9.

13. Nicolaides, N.C., Papadopoulos, N. and Liu, B. (1994) Mutations of two PMS homologues in hereditary nonpolyposis colon cancer. *Nature* **371**, 75-80.

14. Newman, B., Austin, M.A., Lee, M. and King, M-C. (1988) Inheritance of human breast cancer: evidence for autosomal dominant transmission in high risk families. *Proc. Nat. Acad. Sci. USA* **85**, 3044-8.

15. Narod, S.A., Feunteun, J., Lynch, H.T. *et al.* (1991) Familial breast-ovarian cancer locus on chromosome 17q12-q23. *Lancet* **338**, 82-3.

16. Easton, D.F., Bishop, D.T., Ford, D. *et al.* (1993) Genetic linkage analysis in familial breast and ovarian cancer - results from 214 families. *Am. J. Hum. Genet.* **52**, 678-701.

17. Easton, D.F., Ford, D., Bishop, T.D. and the Breast Cancer Linkage Consortium (1995) Breast and ovarian cancer incidence in BRCA1 mutation carriers. *Am. J. Hum. Genet.* **56**, 265-71.

18. Simard, J., Tonin, P., Durocher, F. *et al.* (1994) Common origins of BRCA1 mutations in Canadian breast and ovarian cancer families. *Nat. Genet.* **8**, 392-8.

19. Shattuck-Eidens, D., McClure, M., Simard, J. *et al.* (1995) A collaborative survey of 80 mutations in the BRCA1 breast and ovarian cancer susceptibility gene. *JAMA* **273**, 535-41.

20. Daly, M.B. (1992) The epidemiology of ovarian cancer. *Hematol. Oncol. Clin. N. Am.* **6**, 729-38.

21. Goldgar, D.E., Fields, P., Lewis, C.M. *et al.* (1993) A large kindred with 17q-linked

breast and ovarian cancer: genetic, phenotypic and genealogical analysis. *J. Nat. Cancer Inst.* **86**, 200-9.

22. Skolnick, M. (1980) The Utah genealogical data base: a resource for genetic epidemiology. In *Banbury Report No 4: Cancer Incidence in Defined Populations* (eds. J Cairns, JL Lyon and M Skolnick). Cold Spring Harbor Laboratory, New York, pp. 285-97.

23. Goldgar, D.E., Cannon-Albright, L.A., Oliphant, A.R. *et al.* (1993) Chromosome 17q linkage studies of 18 Utah breast cancer kindreds. *Am. J. Hum. Genet.* **52**, 743-8.

24. Hall J.M., Lee, M.K., Newman, B. *et al.* (1990) Linkage of early-onset familial breast cancer to chromosome 17q21. *Science* **250**: 1684-9.

25. Narod, S.A., Ford, D., Devilee P. *et al.* (1995) An evaluation of genetic heterogeneity in 145 breast-ovarian cancer families. *Am. J. Hum. Genet.* **56**, 254-64.

26. Smith, S.A., Easton, D.F., Ford, D. *et al.* (1993) Genetic heterogeneity and localization of a familial breast-ovarian cancer gene on Chromosome 17q12-q21. *Am. J. Hum. Genet.* **52**, 767-76.

Chapter 6

Gene aberrations

C. Michael STEEL, Brian B. COHEN, Alastair LESSELS, Alastair WILLIAMS

and Hani GABRA

6.1 INTRODUCTION

It has to be admitted that progress in identifying specific molecular lesions (other than BRCA1 mutations) contributing to ovarian carcinogenesis has been disappointing, particularly in relation to the effort that has been expended by very many groups around the world. The reasons probably have as much to do with our lack of understanding of the fundamental biology of the disease as with limitations on experimental techniques in times past. As technological restraints are overcome, opportunities also arise for fresh analysis in the light of changing concepts of ovarian cancer evolution. There is therefore reason to hope that new findings – as well as the re-interpretation of accumulated data from older studies – will ultimately prove fruitful.

6.2 CYTOGENETICS AND TUMOUR CELL PLOIDY

Chromosome analysis of solid tumours is notoriously difficult and many of the studies of ovarian cancer have relied upon cells recovered from malignant ascites. Hence the published data probably display some bias towards more advanced tumours. Not surprisingly, chromo-some aberrations abound and consistency between reports is rather limited, discrepancies being particularly evident in relation to the scoring of double minutes or homogeneous staining regions. Rearrangements and deletions involving chromosomes 1, 3p, 6q, 9, 10, 11,12 and 14 are among the most frequently reported [1–16].

Overall, rates of aneuploidy (usually measured by integrated DNA densitometry in a flow cytometer) are high and there is generally a correlation between aneuploidy and adverse prognostic features [17,18] – though not all studies agree [19,20]. Aneuploidy occurs rarely in well differentiated, early stage tumours, which would otherwise be expected to have a high cure rate and, in that setting, may be an indication for adjuvant chemotherapy [21]. Similarly, aneuploidy may be a marker for a subset of borderline or 'low malignant potential' (LMP) lesions with a propensity to behave aggressively [22-24]. Nevertheless, it is important to recognize that completely benign tumours can be chromosomally abnormal; trisomy 12 in particular being a feature of some ovarian adenomas and fibromas [25,26].

6.3 ALLELOTYPING

There have been more than twenty-five major studies of 'allelic imbalance' or 'loss of heterozygosity' (LOH) in epithelial ovarian cancer, collectively covering every chromosome. Individually they have almost all suffered from inadequate numbers of tumours for analysis (specifically of the less common histological types) and from inadequate numbers of informative loci examined. This is not intended as a criticism of those responsible for the various publications (it applies equally to the work in which our own group has been involved!), rather, it reflects the sheer scale of operation required to generate a detailed map of chromosomal regions involved in major deletions, amplifications or mitotic exchanges. There appear to be both consistencies and inconsistencies among the various reports. For example, chromosomes 17p and q, 6q and 11p figure regularly among the regions with high rates of allelic imbalance, while, for 11q, the quoted rates of LOH have ranged from 0% to 52% [27–30]. Direct comparisons between published studies are difficult because different markers have been used and the findings have not always been broken down by histological type or FIGO stage of the tumours examined. We therefore do not propose to undertake an exhaustive meta-analysis of the data but rather to offer some interpretations of the material, following on the discussions by Foulkes and Trowsdale [29] and by Zweizig and colleagues [32] at the previous HHMT meeting in Toronto, and supplemented by more recent work, including some of our own data.

The first point to emphasize is that not all chromosomes are equal in terms of allelic imbalance. In our own series of epithelial ovarian cancers, LOH at all informative chromosome 17 loci has occurred in about half the cases, suggesting loss of one complete chromosome. Others find comparable, or even higher rates of whole chromosome loss [27]. Conversely, of 47 cases analysed for allele imbalance on chromosome 11, forty were positive at one or

more loci but only a single tumour gave a pattern consistent with whole chromosome loss [33]. This suggests that almost any chromosome 17 marker will yield an appreciable frequency of allele imbalance but the rates obtained with markers on other chromosomes may depend crucially on their precise map locations. That seems to be borne out, for example, in the cases of chromosomes 6q and 18q, both of which have now been studied intensively [34,35]. The use of multiple markers, even on chromosome 17, can reveal localized peaks and troughs of allele imbalance, implying, perhaps, the presence of several distinct loci of importance in ovarian carcinogenesis [30,31,36,37]. However, where the appropriate information is available, it appears that the frequency of allele imbalance at most loci correlates positively with histological grade and/or FIGO stage and much of the recorded data derives from advanced tumours [29,32,34,37]. Thus there may be over-representation of 'random noise' or of redundant chromosomal regions that can be deleted without compromising tumour cell growth potential.

A few loci, including regions of 11p, Xq and 17 can be implicated in allele imbalance in benign, borderline or LMP tumours, findings which may shed light on the relationship between these lesions and overt cancers [32,33,38].

In an attempt to circumvent the problem of limited numbers by combining comparable data from several sources for chromosomes 11 and 17 [28,29,33,36,37,39,40], we have compared the percentage of all informative loci on each chromosome arm showing allele imbalance, subdividing the tumours by histological type (Figure 6.1). The differences between the observed patterns on these chromosomes are immediately obvious. On chromosome 11 allele imbalance appears fairly uniformly distributed between the two

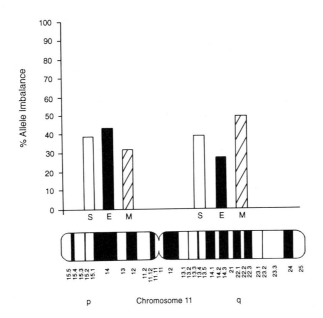

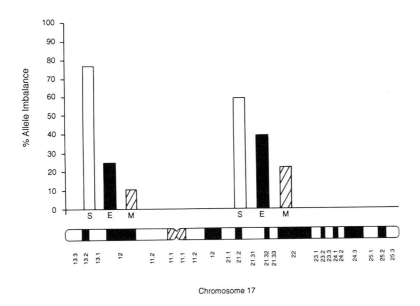

Figure 6.1 Allele imbalance on the long and short arms of chromosomes 11 and 17 in epithelial ovarian cancers. From published reports, for each chromosome arm, the aggregate proportion of all informative markers showing allele imbalance is shown as a vertical bar. Results are recorded separately for serous (S), mucinous (M) and endometrioid (E) carcinomas.

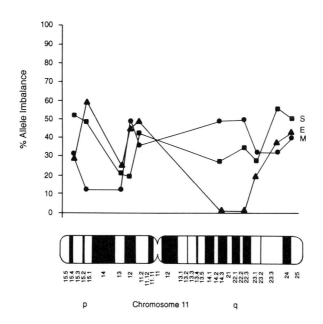

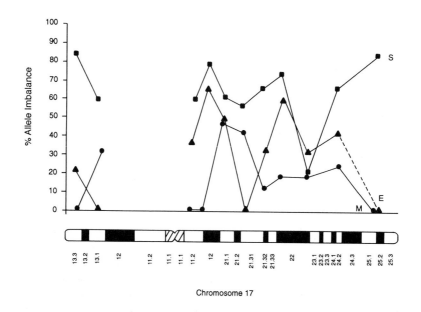

Figure 6.2 From Refs 33 and 37, proportional allele imbalance at ten loci on chromosome 11 and eleven loci on chromosome 17 plotted separately for serous (■), mucinous (●) and endometrioid (▲) ovarian cancers.

arms and among the three commonest histological types but on chromosome 17, imbalance, particularly on the short arm, is much more frequent in serous than in endometrioid or mucinous carcinomas.

When the patterns at individual loci are analysed (Figure 6.2), although the numbers are now smaller, several interesting additional features emerge. The complete absence of allele imbalance at 11q14-22, for ten endometrial carcinomas informative at one or both loci tested is striking and may be related to preservation of the progesterone receptor gene [41], as discussed later. The relative excess of serous carcinomas among tumours showing subtelomeric allele imbalance (on both arms of chromosome 11) may be important since, on follow-up, this pattern is associated with poor prognosis while the opposite distribution of allele imbalance (mainly peri-centromeric) is found predominantly in well-differentiated, lower grade tumours with a correspondingly better outlook [33].

The picture for chromosome 17 is, in some respects, similar. Allele imbalance on the short arm is strongly correlated with imbalance on the long arm, particularly in the distal region (q24-25) and with serous histology, advanced stage and bad prognosis [37]. These findings are in broad agreement with others already published [27,36,38].

There is additional data lending strong support to the view that allelotyping of ovarian cancer may have much to offer in the mapping of genes that are important in the initiation and progression of the disease and, hence, in defining distinct routes of tumour evolution. An example is the evidence that allele imbalance on chromosome 6q is both highly localized and correlated with histological type and differentiation grade [30,35]. Valuable information may, however, be obscured if adequate attention is not paid to sub-classification of the tumours included

in any series and if only a few loci are examined on any chromosome. There would be considerable merit in seeking agreement on a common set of polymorphic markers that could be applied by any group active in this field so that future results can be pooled.

6.4 CANDIDATE GENES

Three principal routes have led to the definition of candidate genes for ovarian carcinogenesis. The first is extrapolation from other types of cancer. A number of 'archetypal' oncogenes or tumour suppressors have been studied with positive results in varying proportions of cases. Activated and/or amplified ras (particularly Ki-ras, though occasionally Ha- or N-ras) has been demonstrated in around 15% of (mainly) advanced tumours [42-54]. In some instances, overexpression of ras product has been found without amplification of the gene [43]. Of particular interest is the finding of an activating Ki-ras mutation in a borderline ovarian tumour [44] though whether this may be a specific feature of the subset of aneuploid LMP tumours which can behave aggressively is currently unknown.

A somewhat higher proportion of tumours show overexpression of c-myc, usually accompanied by amplification of the gene [49,53–59]. The finding correlates well with high nuclear grade, serous histology and adverse clinical outcome [60-63].

C-erbB2 has been widely investigated in ovarian cancer and in up to 35% of cases overexpression of protein or of mRNA (which are very closely correlated) has been noted, again mainly in tumours with adverse prognostic features [64-68], though, as in the case of breast cancer, there is still debate over the prognostic significance of c-erbB2 over-expression [69,70]. The gene itself is amplified in only a proportion of these cases. By contrast, the homologue c-erbB3 appears to be more strongly expressed in borderline and early invasive ovarian tumours [71].

Other oncogenes have received less attention to date. One provocative report suggests that ovarian cancers may express the c-fms product (a homologue of the CSF-receptor) together with CSF-1 itself, thus generating an autocrine growth factor circuit [72]. There is also interest in the 11q13 amplicon that includes cyclin D, FGF3 and the high affinity folate receptor FOLR1 [61,73-75]. Foulkes and colleagues [28] found that this region was amplified in 4 of 28 ovarian cancers but did not detect correlations with overexpression of any of the putative oncogenes it carries. Aberrant expression of the nuclear oncogenes c-myb and c-jun have also been recorded in ovarian cancers but whether as causal events or as consequences of abnormal cellular proliferation is unclear [76,77].

In the case of TP53 and its product, p53, there is little doubt about its significance, which is discussed in more detail by several other contributors to this volume (see chapters 3,14,22,23). Mutations, allele loss and altered protein expression are detected in 30–50% of ovarian tumours, particularly in those with serous histology and of advanced stage, which carry a bad prognosis [78–81]. The role of the retinoblastoma gene is much more equivocal [61,82,83]. Reports of frequent allele imbalance on chromosome 13q [30,31] which raised the possibility of Rb involvement may be reinterpreted now that BRCA2 has been mapped to a contiguous region [84].

The second major route to ovarian cancer candidate genes is the study of familial cancers and here, of course, BRCA1 is pre-eminent, though it remains to be seen how relevant that particular locus may be to the high rate of allele imbalance at 17q12-21 in sporadic tumours [85,86]. BRCA2 is also associated with an excess of ovarian cancers in members of affected families [87] and the

characterization of that gene is awaited with very great interest. Few other cancer family syndromes include epithelial ovarian tumours in the clinical spectrum though cases have been recorded in association with constitutional p53 mutations [88,89] and in Lynch Type II families [90]. The latter category can be recognized by microsatellite instability in the tumours (due to defects in replication error repair) and it may be worth noting that such instability is rarely found in sporadic ovarian cancers [41,91].

Ataxia-telangiectasia, an autosomal recessive condition with an underlying DNA repair defect manifested (*inter alia*) by extreme radiosensitivity, is believed to be associated with an excess of epithelial cancers (particularly, but not exclusively, of the breast) in otherwise asymptomatic heterozygotes. There is considerable interest in the possibility that this gene (or genes) may make a significant contribution to the overall incidence of common cancers [92]. The locus maps to a region (11q23) that shows a high rate of allele imbalance in ovarian cancer but whether this is of any relevance at all may only emerge when the gene itself has been cloned and characterized.

The third route to ovarian cancer genes is the biological one. Recognizing that the sex hormones play a fundamental part in ovarian carcinogenesis [93,94] it is logical to examine the loci that regulate responses to the sex hormones. In fact, although chromosomes 6q25, 11q 22 and Xq – the sites of the oestrogen receptor (ER), progesterone receptor (PR) and androgen receptor respectively – are commonly implicated in allele imbalance, specific interpretation of the findings in terms of ER or PR expression has been attempted only recently [32,41]. These studies have found intriguing evidence that allele imbalance at the PR locus is associated with reduced PR expression that this, in turn, has a pronounced adverse influence on patient survival and that the effect is compounded in the presence of ER overexpression. Whether there is a comparable relationship between 6q25 allele imbalance and disturbed hormonal control of ovarian epithelial cell growth remains to be explored.

6.5 MODIFYING OR MINOR SUSCEPTIBILITY GENES

Finally, some comment should be made about possible 'modifying' genes that may not underlie familial clusters of ovarian cancer but could have a significant effect at the population level. The ataxia gene perhaps belongs to this category and the distinction between a low-penetrance predisposing gene and a modifying gene is almost a question of semantics. However, we are restricting the latter term to those genes (strictly alleles) that are relatively common in the general population and which might therefore provide the basis for a screening test. For breast cancer, certain alleles at the Ha-ras locus have been proposed [95] but there is insufficient data to suggest that they provide useful information on ovarian cancer risk. Very recently a polymorphism in the p53 gene (a 16 base pair insertion in intron 3) has been reported to be over-represented (almost two-fold) among patients with sporadic ovarian cancer and homozygotes for the less common allele had about an eight-fold increase in relative risk for ovarian cancer [96]. No such relationship had been found for breast cancer [97]. Our own preliminary data (Table 6.1) unfortunately do not support this promising observation which may reflect differences in the distribution of the polymorphism between the German and the Scottish populations.

Similarly, a Taq1 restriction site polymorph-ism in an intron of the progesterone receptor gene is reported to

Table 6.1 Distribution of p53PIN3 alleles [96,97)] in constitutional DNA of 25 epithelial ovarian cancer patients and 38 control subjects from the Scottish population

	p53'PIN3' alleles	
	A1	*A2*
Controls (n=38)	68 (89.5%)	8 (10.5%)
EOC (n=25)	47 (94%)	3 (6%)

There is no significant difference between the groups in the frequency of the A2 allele and no individual in either group was homozygous A2.

associate with ovarian cancer susceptibility in Germans but the finding was not confirmed in an Irish population [98].

In both cases, it will be worth exploring the claims further because the definition of the polymorphic markers is not technically demanding. Even if these initial reports are not upheld, relatively common determinants of cancer susceptibility may exist and their identification could have considerable clinical impact as well as making an important contribution to our understanding of the biology of the group of disorders that constitute ovarian cancer

6.6 FUTURE PROSPECTS

The availability of very large numbers of mapped, highly informative, microsatellite markers that can be applied to fixed archival tissues and which require only a few cells for comprehensive analysis, opens up the prospect of definitive allele imbalance studies. It will be particularly important to extend our knowledge of microscopic lesions that may represent early cancers, including any that can be detected in ovaries removed prophylactically from women who carry constitutional mutations at BRCA1, BRCA2 or other loci predisposing to ovarian cancer. Powerful new techniques for localizing amplifications and deletions in tumour DNA [99,100] such as comparative genomic hybridization (CGH) or representational difference analysis (RDA) have yet to be applied very widely in ovarian cancer but have the potential to carry the field forward very rapidly. Simply listing the sites of genomic alteration in a given tumour is, of course, of limited value. The object must be first, to characterize the genes involved and, second, to identify combinations and permutations of specific molecular changes that interact functionally to generate a tumour with particular histological characteristics and biological properties. Studies of tumour gene expression, for example by differential display analysis [101], will almost certainly make further significant contributions towards this end.

Much of our current activity in the molecular characterization of ovarian cancer represents the tedious but necessary phase of picking through the pieces of a jigsaw to put them the right way up and perhaps to identify edges and corners. The next decade should see the emergence of a complete picture.

REFERENCES

1. Atkin, N.B. and Baker, M.C. (1987) Abnormal chromosomes, including small metacentrics in 14 ovarian cancers. *Cancer Genet. Cytogenet.* **26**, 355-61.
2. Augustus, M., Bruderlein, S. and Gebhart. (1986). Cytogenetic and cell cycle studies in metastatic cells from ovarian carcinomas. *Anticancer Res.* **6**, 283-90.
3. Bello, M.J., Moreno, S. and Rey, J.A. (1990). Involvement of 9p in metastatic ovarian adenocarcinomas. *Cancer Genet. Cytogenet.* **45**, 223-9.
4. Bello, M.J. and Rey, J.A. (1990). Chromosome aberrations in metastatic ovarian cancer, relatioship with abnormalities in primary tumours. *Int. J. Cancer.* **45**, 50-4.
5. Gallion, H.H., Powell, D.E., Smith, L.W. *et al.* (1990). Chromosome abnormalities in human epithelial ovarian malignancies. *Gynecol. Oncol.* **38**, 473-7.
6. Kovacs, G. (1978). Abnormalities of chromosome no. 1 in human solid malignant tumours. *Int. J. Cancer* **21**, 688-94.
7. Mrozek, K., Limon, J., Nedoszytko, B. *et al.* (1989). Cytogenetical findings in human ovarian tumours. *Cancer Genet.* **38**, 182.
8. Nielsen, K., Andersen, J., Bertelsen, K. and Hansen, M.K. (1989). A cytogenetic study of 50 tumor samples from a consecutive series of 40 patients with ovarian cancer. *Cancer Genet.* **38**, 181.
9. Panani, A. and Ferti-Passantanopoulou, A. (1985). Common marker chromosomes in ovarian cancer. *Cancer Genet. Cytogenet.* **16**, 65-71.
10. Roberts, C.G. and Tattersall, M.H.N. (1990). Cytogenetic study of solid ovarian tumors. *Cancer Genet. Cytogenet.* **48**, 243-53.
11. Tanaka, K., Boice, C.R. and Testa, J.R. (1989). Chromosome aberrations in nine patients with ovarian cancer. *Cancer Genet. Cytogenet.* **43**, 1-14.
12. Tiepolo, L. and Zuffardi, O. (1973). Identification of normal and abnormal chromosomes in tumor cells. *Cytogenet. Cell Genet.* **12**, 8-16.
13. Trent, J.M. and Salmon, S.E. (1981). Karyotypic analysis of human ovarian carcinoma cells cloned in short term agar culture. *Cancer Genet. Cytogenet.* **3**, 279-91.
14. van-der Reit-Fox, M.F., Retief, A.E. and van Niekerk, W.A. (1979). Chromosome changes in 17 human neoplasms studied with banding. *Cancer* **44**, 2108-19.
15. Wake, N., Hreshchyshyn, M.W., Piver,

S.M. *et al.* (1980). Specific chromosome change in ovarian cancer. *Cancer Genet. Cytogenet.* **2**, 87-8.

16. Whang-Peng, J., Knutsen, T., Douglass, E.C. *et al.* (1984). Cytogenetic studies in ovarian cancer. *Cancer Genet. Cytogenet.* **11**, 91-106.

17. Brescia, R.J., Barakat, R.A., Beller, U. *et al.* (1990). The prognostic significance of nuclear DNA content in malignant epithelial tumours of the ovary. *Cancer* **65**, 141-7.

18. Friedlander, M.L., Hedley, D.H., Taylor, I. *et al.* (1984). Influence of cellular DNA content on survival in advanced ovarian cancer. *Cancer Res.* **44**, 397-400.

19. Sahni, K., Tribukait, B. and Einhorn, N. (1989). Flow cytometric measurement of ploidy and proliferation in effusions of ovarian carcinoma and their possible prognostic significance. *Gynecol. Oncol.* **35**, 240-5.

20. Schneider, J., Edler, L., Kleine, W. and Volm, M. (1990). DNA analysis, chemoresistance testing and hormone receptor levels as prognostic factors in advanced ovarian carcinoma. *Arch. Gynecol. Obstet.* **248**, 45-52.

21. Schueler, J.A., Cornelisse, C.J., Hermans, J. *et al.* (1993). Prognostic factors in well-differentiated early-stage epithelial ovarian cancer. *Cancer* **71**, 787-95.

22. Kaern, J., Trope, C., Kjorstad, K.E *et al.* (1990) Cellular DNA content as a new prognostic tool in patients with borderline tumors of the ovary. *Gynecol. Oncol.* **38**, 452-7.

23. Padberg, B.-C., Arps, H., Franke, U. *et al.* (1992). DNA cytophotometry and prognosis in ovarian tumors of borderline malignancy. *Cancer* **69**, 2510-4.

24. Kaern, J., Trope, C.G., Abeler, V. and Pettersen, E.O. (1995). Cellular DNA content, the most important prognostic factor in patients with borderline tumors

of the ovary. Can it prevent overtreatment ? In *Ovarian Cancer 3* (eds. F. Sharp, P. Mason, T. Blackett and J. Berek). Chapman & Hall, London. pp181-8.

25. Pejovic, T., Heim, S., Mandahl, M. *et al.* (1990). Trisomy 12 is a consistent chromosomal aberration in benign ovarian tumors. *Genes Chrom. Cancer* **2**, 48-52.

26. Leung, W.-Y., Schwartz, P., Ng, H.-T. and Yang-Feng, T.L. (1990). Trisomy 12 in benign fibroma and granulosa cell tumor of the ovary. *Gynecol. Oncol.* **38**, 28-31.

27. Foulkes, W.D., Black, D.M., Stamp, G.W.H. *et al.* (1993). Very frequent loss of heterozygosity throughout chromosome 17 in sporadic ovarian carcinoma. *Int. J. Cancer* **54**, 220-5.

28. Foulkes, W.D., Campbell, I.G., Stamp, G.W.H. and Trowsdale, J. (1993). Loss of heterozygosity and amplification on chromosome 11q in human ovarian cancer. *Br. J. Cancer* **67**, 268-73.

29. Foulkes, W.D. and Trowsdale, J.(1995). Isolating tumour suppressor genes relevant to ovarian carcinoma- the role of loss of heterozygosity. In *Ovarian Cancer 3.* (eds. F. Sharp, P. Mason, A. Blackett and J. Berek). Chapman & Hall. London. pp23-38.

30. Sato, T., Saito, H., Morita, R. *et al.* (1991). Allelotype of human ovarian cancer. *Cancer Res.* **51**, 5118-22.

31. Yang-Feng, T.L., Han, H., Chen, K.-C. *et al.* (1993). Allelic loss in ovarian cancer. *Int. J. Cancer* **54**, 546-51.

32. Zweizig, S., Zheng, J., Wan, M. *et al.* (1995). New insights into the genetics of ovarian epithelial tumor development. In *Ovarian Cancer 3.* (eds. F. Sharp, P. Mason, T. Blackett and J. Berek). Chapman & Hall, London. pp 61-73.

33. Gabra, H., Taylor, L., Cohen, B.B. *et al.* (1995). Chromosome 11 allele imbalance and clinicopathological correlates in

ovarian tumours. *Br. J. Cancer* **72**, 367-75.

34. Chenevix-Trench, G., Leary, G., Kerr, J. *et al.* (1992). Frequent loss of heterozygosity on chromosome 18 in ovarian carcinoma which does not always include the DCC locus. *Oncogene* **7**, 1059-65.

35. Orphanos, V., McGown, G., Hey, Y. *et al.* (1995). Allelic imbalance of chromosome 6q in ovarian tumours. *Br. J. Cancer* **71**, 666-9.

36. Saito, H., Inazawa, J., Saito, S. *et al.* (1993). Detailed deletion mapping of chromosome 17q in ovarian and breast cancers, 2-cM region on 17q21.3 often and commonly deleted in tumors. *Cancer Res.* **53**, 3382-5.

37. Steel, C.M., Eccles, D.M., Gruber, L. *et al.* (1995). Allele losses on chromosome 17 in ovarian tumours. In *Ovarian Cancer 3.* (eds. F. Sharp, P. Mason, T. Blackett and J. Berek). Chapman & Hall. London. pp 45-52.

38. Eccles, D.M., Russell, S.E.H., Haites, N.E. and the ABE Ovarian Cancer Genetics Group. (1992). Early loss of heterozygosity on 17q in ovarian cancer. *Oncogene* **7**, 2069-72.

39. Ehlen, T. and Dubeau, L. (1990). Loss of heterozygosity on chromosomal segments 3p, 6q and 11p in human ovarian carcinomas. *Oncogene* **5**, 219-23.

40. Viel, A., Giannani, F., Tumiotto, L. *et al.* (1992). Chromosomal localisation of two putative 11p oncosuppressor genes involved in human ovarian tumours. *Br. J. Cancer* **66**, 1030-6.

41. Gabra, H., Langdon, S.P., Watson, J.V. (1995) Allele loss at 11q22 correlates with low progesterone receptor content in epithelial ovarian cancer. *Submitted*

42. Bolz, E.M., Kefford, R.F., Leary, J.A. *et al.* (1989). Amplification of c-*ras*-Ki oncogene in human ovarian tumors. *Int. J. Cancer* **43**, 428-30.

43. Chien, C.-H., Chang, K.-T. and Chow, S.-

N. (1990). Amplification and expression of c-Ki-*ras* oncogene in human ovarian cancer. *Proc Natl. Science Council, Republic of China* **14**, 27-32.

44. Enomoto, T., Inoue, M., Perantoni, A.O. *et al.* (1990). K-*ras* activation in neoplasms of the human femal reproductive tract. *Cancer Res.* **50**, 6139-45.

45. Feig, L.A., Bast, R.C., Knapp, R.C. and Cooper, G.M. (1984). Somatic activation of *ras*^{K} gene in a human ovarian carcinoma. *Science* **223**, 698-700.

46. Filmus, J.E. and Buick, R.N. (1985). Stability of c-Ki-*ras* amplification during progression in a patient with adenocarcinoma of the ovary. *Cancer Res.* **45**, 4468-72.

47. Fukumoto, M., Estensen, R.D., Sha, L. *et al.* (1989). Association of Ki-*ras* with amplified DNA sequences detected in human ovarian carcinomas by a modified in-gel renaturation assay. *Cancer Res.* **49**, 1693-7.

48. Haas, M., Isakov, J. and Howell, S.B. (1987). Evidence against *ras* activation in human ovarian carcinomas. *Mol. Biol. Med.* **4**, 265-75.

49. Liehr, T., Tulusan, H.T. and Gebhart, E. (1993). Amplification of proto-oncogenes in human ovarian carcinomas. *Int. J. Oncol.* **2**, 155-60.

50. Masuda, H., Battifora, H., Yokota, J. *et al.* (1987). Specificity of proto-oncogene amplification in human malignant diseases. *Mol. Biol. Med.* **4**, 213-27.

51. Scambia, G., Catozzi, L., Panici, P.B. *et al.* (1993). Expression of ras oncogene p21 protein in normal and neoplastic ovarian tissues, correlation with histopathological features and receptors for estrogen, progesterone and epidermal growth factor. *Am. J. Obstet. Gynecol.* **168**, 71-8.

52. van't Veer, L.J., Hermens, R., van den Berg-Bakker, L.A.M. *et al.* (1988). *Ras* oncogene activation in human ovarian

carcinoma. *Oncogene* **2**, 157-65.

53. Yokota, J., Tsunetsugu-Yokota, Y., Battifora, H. *et al.* (1986). Alterations of *myc*, *myb* and *Ha-ras* proto-oncogenes in cancers are frequent and show clinical correlation. *Science* **231**, 261-5.

54. Zhou, D.J., Gonzales-Cadavid, N., Ahuja, H. *et al.* (1988). A unique pattern of proto-oncogene abnormalities in ovarian carcinomas. *Cancer* **62**, 1573-6.

55. Baker, V.V., Borst, M.P., Dixon, D. *et al.* (1990). *c-myc* amplification in ovarian cancer. *Gynecol. Oncol.* **38**, 340-2.

56. Kohler, M., Janz, I., Wintzer, H.-O. *et al.* (1989). The expression of EGF receptors, EGF-like factors and *c-myc* in ovarian and cervical carcinomas and their clinical significance. *Anticancer Res.* **9**, 1537-48.

57. Schreiber, G. and Dubeau, L. (1990). *c-myc* proto-oncogene amplification detected by polymerase chain reaction in archival human ovarian carcinomas. *Am. J. Path.* **137**, 653-8.

58. Serova, O.M., Nikiforova, I.F., Yurkova, L.E. *et al.* (1990). Alterations of the *c-myc* and *c-Ha-ras* oncogenes in ovarian carcinomas. *Eksper. Onkologiya.* **12**, 47-9.

59. Tashiro, H., Miyazaki, K, Okamura, H. *et al.* (1992). *c-myc* overexpression in human primary ovarian tumours, its relevance to tumour progression. *Int. J. Cancer* **50**, 828-33.

60. Katsaros, D., Zola, P., Theillet, C. *et al.* (1991). Amplification and/or overexpression of *c-myc* and *c-erbB-2* oncogenes is associated with aggressive biological behaviour in human ovarian carcinomas. *Proc. Am. Assoc. Cancer Res.* **32**, 291.

61. Sasano, H., Comerford, J., Silverberg, S.G. and Garrett, C.T. (1990). An analysis of abnormalities of the retinoblastoma gene in human ovarian and endometrial carcinoma. *Cancer* **66**, 2150-4.

62. Sasano, H., Garrett, C., Wilkinson, D.S. *et al.* (1990). Proto-oncogene amplification and tumour ploidy in human ovarian neoplasms. *Hum. Pathol.* **21**, 382-391.

63. Serova, O.M. (1993) Amplification of *c-myc* proto-oncogene in primary tumours, metastases and blood leukocytes of patients with ovarian cancer. *Eksper. Onkologiya.* **9**, 27.

64. Berchuck, A., Kamel, A., Whitaker, R. *et al.* (1990). Overexpression of HER-2/neu is associated with poor survival in advanced epithelial ovarian cancer. *Cancer Res.* **50**, 4087-91.

65. Tyson, F.L., Soper, J.T., Daly, L. *et al.* (1988). Overexpression and amplification of the *c-erbB-2* protooncogene in epithelial ovarian tumours and cell lines. *Proc. Am. Assoc. Cancer Res.* **29**, 471.

66. Lichenstein, A., Berenson, J., Gera, J.F. *et al.* (1990). Resistance of human ovarian cell lines to tumor necrosis factor and lymphokine-activated killer cells, correlation with expression of HER2/*neu* oncogenes. *Cancer Res.* **50**, 7364-70.

67. Slamon, D.J., Godolphin, W., Jones, L.A. *et al.* (1989). Studies of the HER2/*neu* proto-oncogene in human breast and ovarian cancer. *Science* **244**, 707-12.

68. Zhang, X., Silva, E., Gershenson, D. and Hung, M.-C. (1989). Amplification and rearrangement of *c-erbB* proto-oncogenes in cancer of human female genital tract. *Oncogene* **4**, 985-9.

69. Haldane, J.S., Hird, V., Hughes, C.M. and Gullick, W.J. (1990). *c-erbB-2* oncogene expression in ovarian carcinoma. *J. Pathol.* **162**, 231-7.

70. Rubin, S.C., Finstad, C.L., Wong, G.Y. *et al.* (1993). Prognostic significance of HER2/*neu* expression in advanced epithelial ovarian cancer, a multivariate analysis. *Am. J. Obstet. Gynecol.* **168**, 162-9.

71. Simpson, B.J.B., Weatherill, J., Miller, E.P.

et al. (1995). *c-erbB3* protein expression in ovarian tumours. *Br. J. Cancer* **71**, 758-62.

72. Kacinski, B.M., Carter, D., Mittal, K. *et al.* (1990). Ovarian adenocarcinomas express *fms*-complementary transcripts and *fms* antigen, often with co-expression of CSF-1. *Am. J. Pathol.* **137**, 135-47.

73. Lammie, G.A. and Peters, G.(1991). Chromosome 11q13 abnormalities in human cancer. *Cancer Cells* **3**, 414-20.

74. Ragoussis, J., Senger, G., Trowsdale, J. and Campbell, I.(1992). Genomic organisation of the human folate receptor genes on chromosome 11q13. *Genomics* **14**, 423-30.

75. Rosen, A., Sevelda, P., Klein, M. *et al.* (1993). First experience with FGF-3 (INT-2) amplification in women with epithelial ovarian cancer. *Br. J. Cancer* **67**, 1122-5.

76. Barletta, C., Lazzaro, D., Prosperi-Porta, R. *et al.* (1992). *c-myb* activation and the pathogenesis of ovarian cancer. *Eur. J. Gynaecol. Oncol.* **13**, 53-8.

77. Berek, J.S. and Martinez-Maza, O. (1995). Molecular and biological factors in the pathogenesis of ovarian cancer. In *Ovarian Cancer 3*. (eds. F. Sharp, P. Mason, T. Blackett and J. Berek). Chapman & Hall, London. pp 77-87.

78. Lee, J.H., Park, S.Y., Saya, H. *et al.*(1991). Chromosome 17 deletions and p53 gene mutations at codon 72 in human ovarian carcinomas. *Proc. Am. Assoc. Cancer Res.* **32**, 304.

79. Marks, J.R., Davidoff, A.M., Kerns, B.J. *et al.* (1991). Overexpression and mutation of p53 in epithelial ovarian cancer. *Cancer Res.* **51**, 2979-84.

80. Okamoto, A, Sameshima, Y., Yokoyama, S. *et al.* (1991). Frequent allelic losses and mutations of the p53 gene in human ovarian cancer. *Cancer Res.* **51**, 5171-6.

81. Eccles, D.M., Brett, L., Lessels, A.M. *et al.* (1992). Over-expression of the p53 protein and allele loss at 17p13 in ovarian carcinoma. *Br. J. Cancer.* **65**, 40-44.

82. Vila, V., Cheng, J. and Haas, M. (1989). Deleted retinoblastoma tumor suppressor gene in metastatic nodes but not in the primary tumor of an ovarian carcinoma. *Proc. Am. Assoc. Cancer Res.* **30**, 443.

83. Li, S.-B., Schwartz, P.E., Lee, W.H. and Yang-Feng, T.L. (1991). Allele loss at the retinoblastoma locus in human ovarian cancer. *J. Nat. Cancer Inst.* **83**, 637-40.

84. Wooster, R., Neuhausen, S.L., Mangion ,J. *et al.* (1994). Localisation of a breast cancer susceptibility gene, BRCA2, to chromosome 13q12-13. *Science* **265**, 2088-90.

85. Smith, S.A., Easton, D.F., Evans, D.G.R. and Ponder, B.A.J. (1992). Allele losses in the region 17q12-21 in familial breast and ovarian cancer involve the wild type chromosome. *Nat. Genet.* **2**, 128-31.

86. Merajver, S.D., Phan, T.M., Caduff, R.F. *et al.* (1995). Somatic mutations in the BRCA1 gene in sporadic ovarian tumours. *Nat. Genet.* **9**, 439-43.

87. Narod, S.A., Ford, D., Devilee, P. *et al.* (1995). An evaluation of genetic heterogeneity in 145 breast-ovarian cancer families. *Am. J. Hum. Genet.* **56**, 254-64

88. Prosser, J., Porter, D., Coles, C. *et al.* .(1992). Constitutional p53 mutation in a non-Li-Fraumeni family. *Br. J. Cancer* **65**, 527-8.

89. Sidransky, D., Tokino, T., Helzlsouer, K. *et al.* (1992) Inherited p53 mutations in breast cancer. *Cancer Res.* **52**, 2984-6.

90. Peltomaki, P., Aaltonen, L.A., Sistonen, P. *et al.* (1993). Genetic mapping of a locus predisposing to human colorectal cancer. *Cell* **75**, 1215-25.

91. Wooster, R., Cleton-Jansen, A.-M., Collins, N. *et al.* (1994). Instability of short tandem repeats (microsatellites) in human cancers. *Nat. Genet.* **6**, 152-6.

92. Swift, M., Morrell, D., Massey, R.B. and Chase, C.L. (1991). Incidence of cancer in

161 families affected by ataxia telangiectasia. *N. Engl. J. Med.* **325**, 1831-6.

93. Cramer, D.W., Hutchison, G.B., Welch, W.R. *et al.* (1983). Determinants of ovarian cancer risk. I. Reproductive experiences and family history. *J. Nat. Cancer Inst.* **71**, 711-6.

94. Harding, M., McIntosh, J., Paul, J. *et al.* (1990). Oestrogen and progesterone receptors in ovarian tumours. *Cancer* **65**, 486-92.

95. Krontiris, T.G., Devlin, B., Karp, D.D. *et al.* (1993). An association between the risk of cancer and mutations in the ras minisatellite locus. *N. Engl. J. Med.* **329**, 517-23.

96. Runnebaum, I., Tong, X.W., Konig, R. *et al.* (1995). p53-based blood test for p53PIN3 and risk of sporadic ovarian cancer. *Lancet* **345**, 994.

97. Lazar, V., Hazard, F., Bertin, F. *et al.* (1993). Simple sequence repeat polymorphism within the p53 gene. *Oncogene* **8**, 1703-5.

98. McKenna, N.J., Kieback, D.G., Carney, D.N. *et al.* (1995). A germline *Taq1* restriction fragment length polymorphism in the progesterone receptor gene in ovarian carcinoma. *Br. J. Cancer* **71**, 451-5.

99. Aldhous, P. (1994). Fast tracks to disease genes. *Science* **265**, 2008-10.

100. Kallioniemi, O.-P., Kallioniemi, A., Piper, J. *et al.* (1994). Optimising Comparative Genomic Hybridisation for analysis of DNA sequence copy number changes in solid tumours. *Genes Chrom. Cancer* **10**, 231-43.

101. Mok, S., Wong, K., Chan, R. *et al.* (1994). Molecular cloning of differentially expressed genes in human epithelial ovarian cancer. *Gynecol. Oncol.* **52**, 247-52.

Chapter 7

The inherited contribution to ovarian cancer

Bruce PONDER

7.1 INTRODUCTION

The inherited contributions to ovarian cancer are now being carefully elucidated. The UK Familial Ovarian Cancer Register has been an important means by which management of high-risk families can be studied and a realistic strategy for intervention developed.

7.2 PREDISPOSING GENES

Some families demonstrate a very high risk of developing ovarian cancer, such as the one shown in Figure 7.1. Through linkage analysis, the defect in this pedigree was localized to chromosome 17 [1] then to the BRCA1 gene locus [2]. BRCA1 predisposes to both breast and ovarian cancer. In addition, there are undoubtedly several other loci that account for these high-risk pedigrees. There may also be other loci that produce some of what we now call sporadic ovarian cancer. Although this is speculative, the proportion of ovarian cancer associated with some of these supposed defects may be higher than that associated with mutations in high-risk genes such as BRCA1.

Another gene which predisposes to breast cancer is BRCA2, which has been located to chromosome 13. BRCA2 has not been cloned. Initially, it appeared that BRCA2 is intriguingly different from BRCA1, because in BRCA2 families both female and male breast cancer were apparently observed. Male breast cancer had not initially been reported in BRCA1 families, while on the other hand, ovarian cancer was though to be uncommon or perhaps absent in BRCA2 families. However it is now becoming clear that, while this is broadly true, there are some BRCA1 families with male breast cancers and there is a predisposition to ovarian cancer in BRCA2 families, although the likelihood of these occurrences is unclear. Goldgar and Easton (personal communication) have studied two large BRCA2 families and the risk of ovarian cancer in those families is about 17-fold increased which gives a 15-20% life-time risk. BRCA2 is thought to be a suppressor gene.

Analysis of allele losses in tumours may give some indication of the involvement of BRCA2 in sporadic ovarian cancers, as well as further information to localize the gene. Because BRCA2 is close to RB on chromosome 13, there is some difficulty distinguishing losses driven by events at the BRCA2 locus from losses attributable to the RB locus. In a study of 50 ovarian cancers, Jacobs (personal communication) has indicated that, of three tumours with allele losses on chromosome 13, two of them are located near the RB gene but do not include RB, and one of them had a loss confined to the BRCA2 region. These findings suggest,

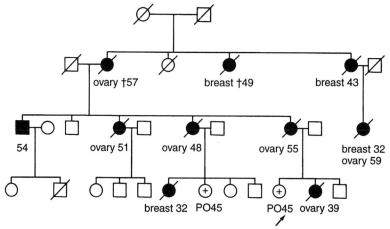

Figure 7.1 Family with breast/ovarian cancer syndrome, due to mutation in BRCA1. (PO = prophylactic oophorectomy; 55 = age at diagnosis; †57 = age at death).

but do not prove, that BRCA2 is involved in the genesis of sporadic ovarian cancers.

Another pattern involving familial ovarian cancer is seen in a family with the nonpolyposis colon cancer (Lynch II) syndrome with cancers of the ovary, colon, ureter and stomach (Figure 7.2). In many of these families, a mutation in one of the DNA repair genes, *e.g.* MSH2, hasbeen found. It is unclear what the mutation is in the family in Figure 7.2, and there are families like this in which ovarian cancer is not part of the family pattern. Furthermore, it is not clear to what extent these genes contribute to either sporadic or familial ovarian cancer. In sporadic ovarian cancers, the characteristic microsatellite instability that occurs with mutations in these genes is uncommon, so it is unlikely that these genes are very important in sporadic ovarian cancer.

Further indications of the familial patterns of ovarian cancer come from a preliminary review of data from the UK Familial Ovarian Cancer Registry. The pattern of other cancers in families defined by having sister-sister or mother-daughter ovarian cancer was studied. Of 221 such families in the registry,

there were 146 where there was only a pair of ovarian cancers and no other cancers. There were 63 pedigrees in which there were breast cancers, but only five with colorectal cancer diagnosed below the age of 60 and four with endometrial cancer below the age of 60 in first degree relatives. There are some uncommon families that have site-specific ovarian cancer, and analysis of nine such families suggests that most are associated with mutations in BRCA1 [3].

In summary, the currently known strong predisposing genes for ovarian cancer are as follows:
1. The predisposing alleles of BRCA1 are responsible for the great majority of breast and ovarian cancer families, including site-specific ovarian cancer families with two or more ovarian cancers in the pedigree.
2. The BRCA2 and the HMS2 genes are involved to some extent (but to what extent is currently unresolved) with a predisposition to ovarian cancer. However, at this time it appears that they account for only a minor component of predisposition.

In addition, it is likely that there are several much commoner genes which confer

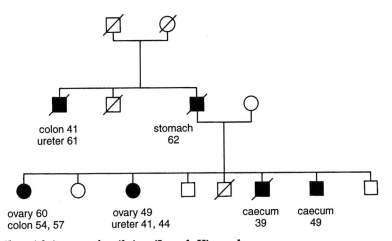

Figure 7.2 Family with 'cancer family' or 'Lynch II' syndrome.

a low level of predisposition. Because the predisposition is weak, multiple-case families are likely to be uncommon. One cannot therefore look for these genes easily by linkage analysis, so one has to search for them by taking candidate genes and testing the frequency of variants in these genes. We have been pursing the possibility that common polymorphisms in the BRCA1 gene are responsible for a low level of predisposition to ovarian cancer. By looking at the frequency of these polymorphisms in a consecutive series of women with breast cancer or ovarian cancer and comparing the frequency in matched controls (250 ovarian cancer patients and 420 controls), we will determine whether any of the polymorphisms are associated with significantly increased risk of these cancers. So far, the results are negative; but the analysis is incomplete.

7.3   UKCCCR FAMILIAL OVARIAN CANCER REGISTER

In the UKCCCR (United Kingdom Coordinating Committee for Cancer Research) Familial Ovarian Cancer Register, there are 275 families with at least two individuals confirmed by pathology report or death certificate to have epithelial ovarian cancer who are first-degree relatives of one another. There are another 285 families in progress of being entered into the register. There are 437 unaffected individuals between the ages of 25 and 65 who are first degree relatives of an affected individual who have signed consents to be followed up, and 212 women who are second-degree relatives of an affected individual. The purpose of the register is to accumulate data and material for study design. Anyone can suggest a study that can be applied to this database. Pedigrees can be printed out and sent out for study. The pedigrees show the family structure, the evidence for the diagnosis, the date of diagnosis, whether the individual is alive or dead, the date, what materials exist from the individual in terms of blood samples and tumour samples, information about other cancers, prophylactic oophorectomies and the presence of benign ovarian disease. Thus one can determine whether a study can potentially be done.

7.4 MOLECULAR GENETICS

Using the information and samples from the register, we are now studying families in which there are two individuals with ovarian cancer. We take a sample of blood from those individuals and test to see whether they have BRCA1 mutations or MHS2 mutations so we can determine what proportion of the families have which mutations in each gene. Once one determines what gene is present in a family, then there are a number of other questions that can be asked, provided that there are a sufficient numbers of individuals available in the pedigree. Unaffected individuals in the family can be typed to see whether they have the mutation, and from the proportion that have it, and the ages of these individuals, one can derive an estimate of the penetrance of the mutation. If one has data about oral contraceptive use in gene carriers, for example, whether they are affected or unaffected, one can derive some evidence of the interaction between oral contraceptive use and the mutation of the gene. If one has individuals in the family who have other cancers or who have benign disease, such as ovarian cysts for example, one can determine whether or not these conditions are also due to the mutation. Thus, on average, it is expected that 50% of first degree relatives of an individual with the mutant gene will themselves have inherited the gene. Individuals with other conditions – such as ovarian cysts – can be tested to determine the frequency with which they have inherited the predisposing mutation. If the frequency is significantly greater than the 50% expected rate, ovarian cysts are likely to be causally associated with the predisposing gene.

Examining the preliminary figures from the follow up conducted of the women in the register, there are 573 women-years of risk for ovarian cancer in individuals between the ages of 41 and 65. These are unaffected women who have not had an oophorectomy and who are 50% genetic risk. In those 573 women-years of risk there have been three ovarian cancers. This corresponds to 0.5 cancers per 100 women-years. This roughly represents a cumulative risk for ovarian cancer of one in eight between the ages of 41 and 65. However, this analysis includes all the families in the register, which are a heterogeneous collection, and so the risk may differ between families with differing types of family history.

For breast cancer, the age range of risk is greater so that one can use wider age limits than with ovarian cancer. There are fewer women who have had mastectomies than have had oophorectomies. There have been eight cancers in 1350 women-years of risk, which is roughly six cancers per 100 women-years, a cumulative risk of roughly one in four. The family set on which this figure is based contains many families in which there have already been cases of breast cancer, in addition to ovarian cancer. At present, it is not known what the risk of breast cancer is in a woman in a family in which the history is only of ovarian cancer. Ideally, the register population might form the basis for a study to evaluate screening strategies, such as blood markers or ultrasound. However, because there are expected to be only about five ovarian cancers per 1000 women-years in the set, 1000 women must theoretically be followed up for five years before 25 events can be observed. Therefore, at present the available sample size is still below that which would have sufficient power to accomplish these studies over a reasonably short time interval.

The policy of the register is that, when a family history is confirmed and the unaffected women in the family are therefore known to be at risk, they get a letter explaining their family history and its implications in general terms. They are also given some general recommendations for their follow up. Their doctor gets a letter with more detailed recommendations, and the local doctor must determine what is appropriate for the individual, such as screening with vaginal ultrasound on an annual basis. Of 240 such women between the ages of 30 and 65 to whom information was sent out, 170 actually went to their general practitioner and 70 did not go for various reasons. Of the 170 who saw their doctors, 121 actually ended up being screened, and 49 were not screened. Of the 121 who were screened, only 61 had a vaginal ultrasound (the recommended screening procedure) and others had various combinations of abdominal ultrasound, CA125 and physical examination while 40 individuals had physical examination only. Of the 49 who were not screened, the doctor was reluctant to perform any tests in 28. While it is unclear what sort of screening should be done in these patients, this study shows that it is difficult to predict what is going to happen when patients are managed *ad hoc* by their general practitioner. An important approach now is to organize the screening strategy prospectively and arrange a small number of centres where screening can be done. Ironically, since it is focussed on 'evidence-based medicine', the current reorganisation of the UK Health Service has placed several difficulties in the way of evaluating screening and deciding what should be done in the future.

7.5 MANAGEMENT OF FAMILIES

What should one do with women who have a family history of ovarian cancer? Since it is still of unproven benefit, screening should wherever possible be done as part of a research study.

1. If there is only one affected relative, and the family history has been carefully taken in order to determine that that is the case, the risk of ovarian cancer is only slightly increased. In this group, it is inappropriate for women to have screening or genetic testing, unless they are part of a research study. The cumulative risk by age 70 of ovarian cancer in the general population is about 1%. The cumulative risk by age 70 for all women who have a first-degree relative with ovarian cancer, is only about 3%, that is 1 in 30.

2. A woman who has two or more relatives, first-degree to each other and one of them first-degree to herself, with epithelial ovarian cancer may be at 15–30% risk of ovarian cancer by age 70. In this group, screening (and consideration of prophylactic oophorectomy after the late 30s, when her family is complete) is appropriate - although ideally it should be part of a research study. Gene-based prediction of risk may become available within the next two-to-five years for some families; it is not available as a service at the time of writing.

3. For a woman who has two affected close relatives with breast cancer diagnosed under the age of 50, it is difficult to give a firm recommendation. While we have a reasonable ability to predict the likelihood of breast cancer, particularly in those whose family members were diagnosed at an early age, the risk of ovarian cancer is less clearly known. Using an epidemiologically-derived estimate of the proportion of sister pairs with breast cancer under the age of 40 that might be due to the BRCA1 gene for example, there may be a 30% chance that a third, so far unaffected, sister might carry a BRCA1 mutation, and so have an approximately 10-15% lifetime chance of ovarian cancer. If the family history is of early onset breast cancer plus one case of epithelial ovarian cancer, the probability of BRCA1 mutation, and so of ovarian cancer, is likely to be considerably higher. There is therefore a case that ovarian

cancer screening should be offered to women who have at least two close relatives with breast cancer under the age of 40, or one relative with ovarian cancer at any age, plus at least one with breast cancer under 50 years.

4. In women who have only a single first degree relative with breast cancer, the risk of ovarian cancer is low. Screening for ovarian cancer should not at present be recommended in those families.

The timing and frequency of screening is still controversial. Because fewer than 10% of ovarian cancers in multiple case ovarian/breast cancer families occur before the age of 40, it may be best to initiate the screening in families of this type at 30–35 years. Prophylactic oophorectomy in women at risk should not normally be considered until 35–40 years.

7.6 CONCLUSION

What is the likely future role of gene testing in the management of familial ovarian cancer? One can only make such a prediction if one knows what the predisposing gene is in the family and can test for the specific mutation in unaffected individuals. The first step, therefore, is to obtain blood from an affected family member to search for a mutation (or failing a blood sample, stored pathology material from paraffin blocks – though this may present considerable technical difficulties in the analysis). If no mutation can be found, genetic prediction is impossible. Since there are probably many different predisposing genes, and moreover some families will be due to chance, it is quite likely that the attempt to offer

prediction will be frustrated at this stage, and family members should be aware of this at the outset so that they are not disappointed. If a mutation can be found which is clearly responsible for the familial predisposition, predictive testing is in principle possible. The important question to face then is what use will the individual make of the information, whether it is positive or negative, and is the testing likely, on balance, to be of benefit? The clearest situation in which benefit can be envisaged is when a clinical decision – for example, whether or not to proceed to oophorectomy – is to be made. It is less clear that, for example, a 20 year old will benefit from knowing that she has inherited the predisposition; and indeed the knowledge may cause psychological and social difficulty. Each individual must be considered separately; and no decision about genetic testing should be taken without the involvement of a clinical geneticist with experience of familial cancer.

REFERENCES

1. Hall, J.M., Lee, M.K., Newman, B. *et al.* (1990) Linkage of early onset familial breast cancer to chromosome 17q. *Science* **250**, 1684-9.
2. Miki, Y., Swensen, J., Shattuck-Eidens, D. *et al.* (1994) A strong candidate for the breast and ovarian cancer susceptibility gene BRCA1. *Science* **266**, 66-71.
3. Steichen-Gersdorf, E., Gallion, H.H., Ford, D. *et al.* (1994) Familial site specific ovarian cancer is linked to BRCA1 on 17q12-21, *Am. J. Hum. Genet.* **55**, 870-5.

Chapter 8

Clinical and ethical dilemmas in familial ovarian cancer

James MACKAY, Aileen E.C. CROSBIE, C. Michael STEEL, George E. SMART and John F. SMYTH

8.1 INTRODUCTION

The concept that a proportion of cases of the common cancers of the breast, ovary and colon have a genetic component has been accepted by the medical community over the last few years [1,2]. The recent identification of one of the genes responsible for some cases of inherited breast and ovarian cancer (BRCA1) has focused attention on a vital area of public health medicine [3]. The media, sometimes encouraged by publicity hungry researchers, has portrayed many of the recent advances in the understanding of the inherited components of breast and ovarian cancer in a very optimistic light. The general public are now very aware that these findings enable the medical profession to pick out certain groups of individuals who are at a higher risk than the general population of developing breast and/or ovarian cancer. The public is now starting to demand that provision be made, as part of the public health service, to inform individuals of their risk as accurately as up-to-date information allows, and those individuals who are found to be at increased risk are expecting access to the most effective clinical screening methods available, as it is now apparent that earlier treatment of

ovarian cancer improves survival [4].

This movement has now effectively started, and one of the greatest challenges facing our health care system over the next two decades will be how to handle the massive explosion of knowledge about the molecular genetics of the common cancers. These issues will have to be faced by society as a whole and many ethical dilemmas will remain outside the remit of cancer geneticists. Several possible pitfalls are already apparent and in this chapter we would like to build on the knowledge and experience gained in running a clinic for the screening and counselling of women with a family history of ovarian cancer in the South East of Scotland, in an effort to highlight some of these pitfalls. We hope that open discussion in a public forum will eventually bring us to a consensus on how the medical profession is going to meet this challenge.

8.2 THE EDINBURGH FAMILIAL OVARIAN CANCER CLINIC

We describe the staffing and running of the Edinburgh clinic as a basis for discussion and criticism rather than to hold it up as the perfect paradigm on which to model a familial cancer clinic. This clinic, initially

Table 8.1 Criteria for referal to a familial ovarian cancer clinic

Any woman who has:
1. One or more first degree relatives with epithelial ovarian cancer under 55 years of age.
2. One or more first degree relatives with both breast and epithelial ovarian cancer at any age.
3. One first degree relative with epithelial ovarian cancer at any age and one or more additional first or second degree relative with breast or ovarian cancer.
4. An actual or perceived family history of cancer causing undue anxiety.

NB: In this context a first degree relative is mother or sister and a second degree relative is grandmother, aunt or first cousin.

piloted for two years in the Royal Infirmary of Edinburgh is now held in an 'out of hospital' setting in a family planning centre and is staffed by cancer geneticists, community gynaecologists, gynaecological oncologists and clinical psychologists.

The referral criteria are illustrated in Table 8.1. Referrals come from general practitioners, other hospital clinics, hospital based gynaecologists and the 'well woman' gynaecology clinics. All women referred are seen by a genetic nurse specialist, often at a home visit, and a detailed family history taken, prior to the first clinic appointment with a geneticist and a gynaecologist. The distinction between genetic and sporadic ovarian cancer is explained, an estimate of the individual's risk given to her, the advantages and disadvantages of different screening strategies discussed, and a pelvic examination performed. The criteria used for risk assessment and the screening strategies employed are shown in Table 8.2.

All those who are screened are sent written confirmation of their results within three weeks, given the telephone number of the Clinical Genetics department, and are encouraged to make contact if they wish. Those who have a family history which satisfies the UKCCCR National Study of Familial Ovarian Cancer criteria are asked to consent to registration. The possibility of performing BRCA1 mutation testing is introduced to those with three or more relatives with breast and/or ovarian cancer. Prophylactic oophorectomy is discussed with those who have finished their families, and who have a strong family history. The fact that oophorectomy does not prevent the rare possibility of a primary abdominal carcinomatosis indistinguishable from ovarian cancer is also mentioned [5-7], but at the present moment we usually suggest waiting until direct gene testing is available if appropriate.

8.3 STAFFING FAMILIAL CANCER CLINICS

There is no doubt that a variety of different skills are required in running a familial cancer clinic. The difference between providing a first class service and running a clinic on a 'shoe-string' is clear, and financial constraints might encourage providers to opt for the cheapest-looking solution. We find that many of the women coming to our clinic want in-depth information on the diagnosis and treatment of breast and ovarian cancer. Many have been traumatized by their previous contacts with medical personnel who looked after their seriously ill and dying relatives [8]. They often wish to discuss various aspects of their relatives' care. Although these individuals often approach the discussion with a rather negative outlook initially, a well informed and sympathetic analysis of the problems of treating advanced cancer may have a cathartic effect.

Table 8.2 Risk assessment and screening strategy

Risk	Assessment Criteria	Pelvic Ultrasound	CA125
High	Those with a family history suggesting an autosomal dominant susceptibility gene.	Every 6 months	Annually
Intermediate	Those with one relative with ovarian cancer below 55 or more than one affected relative, who do not otherwise fit the criteria.	Annually	Annually
Low	Those who do not fit either of the above criteria.	Discharged	Discharged

There are other individuals, often very well informed, who come to the clinic seeking up to date information on the latest treatment advances and screening modalities. Both these groups undoubtedly benefit from meeting health professionals with modern oncological knowledge.

8.4 TRAINING CANCER GENETICISTS AND CANCER GENETICS NURSES

In the United Kingdom at present there is no structure for a formal training in cancer genetics, and it is not recognised as a subspecialty. In the 'post-Calman' era when training will be formalized [9,10] we suggest that this problem must be urgently addressed. Once an appropriate training has been agreed by the relevant bodies, it is imperative that we attract doctors either from clinical genetics, with its paediatric bias, or clinical oncology and supply the other half of the training to become cancer geneticists in a relatively short time. These changes are likely to be slower than the public will accept. In addition we should attract oncology nurses to do a truncated genetics training or genetics nurses or associates to do a truncated oncology training. This would result in the provision of adequately trained cancer genetics nurses, with appropriate counselling skills. This training can only be provided in cancer centres, where both the oncology department and the clinical

genetics department are willing to make the commitment in both teaching time and resources.

8.5 REFERRAL CRITERIA

Clear and straightforward referral criteria are essential for familial cancer clinics, to allow general practitioners to sift out those with a significant family history. These criteria must not be so complicated or written in so much jargon that a reasonably intelligent person cannot understand them nor must they be so wide as to swamp a limited resource, thus compromising the care of those truly at risk. Part of the raison d'être of these clinics is to reduce anxiety and we therefore feel it is desirable to accept those who are very anxious even if their cancer family history is not considered significant.

Studies are continuing into the different referral criteria used by clinics in various parts of the country, but as the number of clinics is relatively small, it should be possible to agree a set of common referral criteria. An incentive is required to reach such a consensus and the international forum provided by the Helene Harris Memorial Trust may well be the most appropriate way to generate the necessary momentum.

8.6 SCREENING CRITERIA

The importance of trying to develop standardized referral criteria across the country has been emphasized above, but the advantages of agreeing to a national policy on screening criteria will be an even greater step forward. We stratify each individual into a high, medium or low risk category according to the criteria in Table 8.2.

Low risk patients we discharge. Those who have a family history suggestive of an autosomal dominant trait conferring susceptibility to ovarian cancer are considered high risk and are offered transabdominal and/or vaginal ultrasound every six months and annual CA125 estimation. Ultrasonography, particularly if performed transvaginally and combined with Doppler colour flow imaging is relatively sensitive at identifying early disease [11-13] but is not particularly good at differentiating benign from malignant lesions. It is highly likely that adding in CA125 estimation will improve specificity, as demonstrated in two population based studies using CA125 as first line screen with ultrasonography as second line [14,15].

Those considered to be at intermediate risk are offered annual ultrasonography and CA125 estimation. All those who are at high or intermediate risk are reviewed annually in the clinic. The responsibility of identifying abnormal results, ensuring that regular investigations are performed when planned, and informing all individuals of their results rests with the cancer geneticist. The most controversial point in the above protocol is the screening of those who have only one relative with ovarian cancer [16].

The overall relative risk of breast or ovarian cancer in first degree relatives of individuals affected at the same site is two-to three-fold [17-20], but is higher in those with breast cancer at a young age [21]. An age at onset effect has not yet been clearly established in ovarian cancer [22]. The risk of developing ovarian cancer in the United Kingdom up to the age of 70 is 1:90, and we

are therefore offering screening to those at a risk of 1:30 or greater. In the familial breast cancer clinic in Edinburgh we offer early mammographic screening to those at more than twice the age specific population risk [23].

Those with a family history containing two or more affected individuals are generally agreed to be at high enough risk to justify the offer of some sort of screening. Many purists argue that the efficacy of screening those with a family history of ovarian cancer will only be proved by a randomized controlled trial. While accepting that those without a strong family history would accept such a trial with a no screen option, there have been continued worries amongst those who run family clinics about telling individuals that they are at high risk of developing ovarian cancer, and then trying to recruit them into such a trial. As the definitive evidence that screening high risk individuals remains equivocal, such a randomized trial is probably ethically justifiable, and most worries centre on the complete impracticality of attempting to set up such a trial. It is likely that the vast majority of high risk women would refuse to be randomized, and indeed might see such a trial as either unethical or reprehensible, thus damaging the rather fragile credibility of these clinics.

8.7 PSYCHOSOCIAL ASSESSMENT

The possibility of raising anxiety in some as well as allaying it in others is a well recognized danger of these clinics [24], and is one of the disadvantages that detractors of cancer genetics clinics have highlighted. While accepting that the exact instruments used in the psychosocial assessment remain contentious, we believe it is mandatory to have some form of assessment either originated by a professional psychologist or, at least, checked by a psychologist. Our early data originating from the Edinburgh familial breast cancer clinic, in agreement with published data [25,26], has suggested that it is possible to inform people accurately about their breast cancer risk, and increase their understanding of that risk, without significantly increasing their anxiety levels. Attendance at the familial breast cancer clinic was associated with a significant decrease in anxiety levels, but this was relatively short lived [27].

Any study which attempts to measure anxiety levels in a group of well people is likely to identify at least a few individuals who are in significant psychological distress, which may not be directly related to the focus of the study. Those mental health professionals who institute such studies are morally bound to provide a clear channel for offering help to significantly distressed individuals. Funding bodies who support such studies should be obliged to ensure that such a channel is clearly and unequivocally outlined in the overall program. We question whether merely referring the problem back to the general practitioner is sufficient.

We propose that the funding bodies should not release funds to projects which do not make this commitment, and would be interested to hear whether others support this proposal.

8.8 THE CLINIC POPULATION

The recent cloning of BRCA1 [3,28,29] opens up the possibility of offering a direct gene test to unaffected individuals in families with a known BRCA1 mutation. There are several large kindreds in the United Kingdom with a high frequency of breast and ovarian cancer. Members of these kindreds have often grown up knowing about the family history, and are often aware through relatively frequent contact with various health professionals that an abnormal gene may well be identified in

their particular family. It is clear that these individuals have a level of knowledge about cancer genetics far above that of the general public and are therefore atypical. The conclusions of studies which have looked at the psychosocial reactions of members of these families must be viewed with caution [30,31]. They certainly cannot be extrapolated to the general public. The only way to ascertain the true effect of such clinics whether for good or ill, is to study a relatively non-selected population.

The technical complexity of identifying mutations in the BRCA1 gene has forced clinics into offering such tests, in the first instance, to those with four or more affected individuals in the family. As we have argued above this is a self selecting situation, and the early studies will not be representative. To get a true understanding of the feelings and expectations of those with a family history of the common cancers, clinics along the lines of the Edinburgh clinic must be set up and financed, at least for an experimental period. The source of such funding remains controversial, but must be addressed.

8.9 CLINIC FUNDING

Informal discussion with several fund holding general practitioners have suggested that many would welcome the establishment of such clinics to take-over the management, counselling and screening of those with significant cancer family histories. Such clinics have not yet entered the service arena, but it now seems to have been accepted that several of the public health questions raised by the explosion in knowledge of the molecular biology of the common cancers must be answered. Several calls have been issued for proposals to look at the psychosocial consequences of these clinics as part of the NHS Research and Development initiative but there is a danger that the basic funding of these clinics will fall between two stools – 'pure research' or 'pure service' – when in fact they serve both purposes to some extent. A task force of the Advisory Council on Science and Technology has highlighted this problem and has stated that the organisation and funding of screening research has been a problematical area that requires a special solution [32].

A degree of permanence in the funding of these clinics would certainly give the staff and the public more confidence that their local service would continue. After all one of the main points of reassurance to those individuals who are at high risk is the knowledge that they will be offered a place on a screening program. Should that program be forced to close after two years these individuals will rightly feel aggrieved. This may well be a significant factor in persuading Health Boards to fund clinics through individual Trusts. The major cancer research charities may wish to make the case that these clinics have moved out of their research field and that public demand now obligates the National Health Service to respond by providing at least pilot funding.

Table 8.3 Pre-symptomatic testing for the BRCA1 gene. A protocol

First step after referral	Interview with Cancer Geneticist to explain:	The accuracy of the test
		How the test is done
		The implications of a positive result
		The implications of a negative result
		The test procedure
		Written information given with contact name and number.
Approximately one month later.	Interview with Cancer Genetic Nurse/Associate to assess:	Understanding of the implications of the test
		Reasoning behind decision-making
		Knowledge of the disease
		Understanding of preventative surgery
		Offer of session with surgeon.
Approximately two weeks later.	First clinic appointment	Blood sample taken
		Appointment given for result in two weeks time.
Two weeks later.	Second clinic visit	Result given at clinic appointment
		Follow-up plan with appropriate professional made.
Follow-up plan	If mutation NOT present	Discussion about further screening
		Letter stating result and offer of appointment if any further discussion wanted
Follow-up plan	If mutation IS present	If mutation present - discussion about further action
		Letter sent with test result and explanations about discussion.

8.10 DIRECT GENE TESTING

The technical and scientific ability to perform direct gene testing on certain individuals is now available in a number of centres in the United Kingdom. No clear guidelines on the protocols to be followed have yet been agreed. We have suggested, along with others, a modification of the Huntington's disease direct gene testing protocol [33,34], which is set out in Table 8.3.

While different centres in the United Kingdom may well adopt slightly varying protocols, there are unlikely to be any major differences. We would draw attention to the importance of the following points:
1. Each individual being seen alone.
2. Two 'thinking' periods before blood is taken for testing.
3. A genetic nurse or genetic associate seeing the individual alone for one consultation prior to the test.
4. The offer of an interview with a surgeon.
5. A precise date and time being specified for a face to face discussion about the test result.
6. No results being given over the telephone.
Many of these points need no clarification for those professionals with experience of direct gene testing in other diseases.

One novel aspect of BRCA1 testing which differentiates it from many of the single gene disorders already identified is the range of options available to those proven to be gene carriers. The existence of these options may make the counselling process easier, and may eventually result in the uptake of testing being higher than previously expected. It should not be allowed to encourage the clear danger of the professionals involved being more directive.

Prophylactic surgery ranks high on the list of possible options, and certainly in large breast/ovarian families our anecdotal impression is that quite a number of individuals would opt for prophylactic oophorectomy and/or prophylactic mastectomy. In this setting it is imperative that the appropriate surgeons have agreed a course of action prior to a test being performed. This is particularly important in the context of prophylactic mastectomy. A specialist breast surgeon skilled in the techniques of breast reconstruction must have given an undertaking to perform the surgery if asked, and to set aside the theatre time to do so. If an individual has already indicated her wishes in this direction, any unnecessary delay may well provoke anxiety or distress [30]. We believe that the onus is on the cancer genetics team involved in offering the test to ensure this does not happen, and we therefore favour offering an early appointment with a specialist breast surgeon prior to direct gene testing. It has been said that the surgical workload is too high to allow this in some areas. If so, serious consideration should be given to restricting the performance of direct gene tests to centres where the surgical input is sufficient to provide a more efficient service.

It is important to remember that no matter how intellectually satisfying a laboratory test is, or how long the scientific struggle to make that test available has been, it may not be the right test to offer a particular individual at a particular time.

8.11 CONCLUSIONS

The general public and the medical profession are now aware that there is a genetic component involved in ovarian cancer, and many individuals are demanding the right to be informed accurately about their risk. Individuals deemed to be at high risk are understandably eager to enter any screening program which may diminish the mortality from ovarian cancer. There is now clear public pressure to establish familial ovarian cancer clinics. While the final endpoint of the screening program is reduced mortality, we believe that a secondary endpoint of reduced anxiety in those with a family history is a reasonable public health goal. We have outlined several of the foreseeable problems involved in the running of these clinics and in direct gene testing. This chapter is written in an attempt to provoke discussion and to stimulate the movement towards consensus in the hope that the combined voices of an international forum will be more effective than a few lone zealots crying in the wilderness.

We have not attempted to cover all the dilemmas but have highlighted a few areas of concern. We believe that the recent explosion in the knowledge of the molecular biology of several common cancers has transformed the face of cancer genetics and represents one of the greatest challenges to face public health medicine over the next decade. The scientists have thrown down the gauntlet and it is up to us all, to cancer geneticists, to the medical profession, to the charities and public health service funding bodies, to the public and to society at large to respond.

ACKNOWLEDGEMENTS

The authors wish to thank: Dr B.B. Muir and Dr S.E. Chambers for performing the ultrasound scans, Dr J.R.B. Livingstone, Dr Farquharson, D. G.J. Beattie, the staff of the Well Woman and Family Planning Centre and the staff of the Clinical Genetics Department, particularly Ms Gillian Clement.

REFERENCES

1. Hall, J.M., Lee, M.K. and Morrow, J. (1990) Linkage of early-onset familial breast cancer to chromosome 17q21. *Science* **250**, 1684-9.
2. Vasen, H., Mecklin, J.P., Meera-Khan, P. and Lynch, H.T. (1991) Hereditary non-polyposis colorectal cancer. *Lancet* **338**, 887.
3. Miki, Y., Swensen, J., Shattuck-Eidens, P. et al. (1994) A strong candidate for the breast and ovarian cancer suceptability gene BRCA1. *Science* **266**, 66-71.
4. Young, R.C., Walton, C.A., Ellenberg, S,S. et al. (1990) Adjuvant therapy in stage I and stage II epithelial ovarian cancer. Results of two prospective randomised trials. *N. Eng. J. Med.* **322**, 1021-7.
5. Tobacman, J.K., Tucker, M.A., Kase, R. et al. (1992) Intra-abdominal carcinomatosis after prophylactic oopherectomy in ovarian cancer-prone families. *Lancet* **ii**, 795-7.
6. Kemp, G.M., Hsiu, J.G. and Andrews, M.C. (1993) Papillary peritoneal carcinomatosis after prophylactic oopherectomy. *Gynecol. Oncol.* **47**, 395-7.
7. Piver, M.S., Jishi, M.F., Tsukada, Y. and Nava, G. (1993) Primary peritoneal carcinoma after prophylactic oopherectomy in women with a family history of ovarian cancer. A report of The Gilda Radna Familial Ovarian Cancer Registry. *Cancer* **71**, 2751-5.
8. Wellisch, D.K., Gritz, E.R., Schain, W. et al. (1991) Psychological functioning of daughters of breast cancer patients. Part 1: daughters and comparison subjects. *Psychosomatics* **32**, 324-36.
9. NHS Executive. (1994) *Report of the working party on unified training grade.* Department of Health, London.
10. Calman, K., (1993) Hospital doctors: training for the future, in Working group in specialist medical training, Department of Health, London.
11. Campbell, S., Roysten, P., Bhan, V. et al. (1990) Novel screening strategies for early ovarian cancer by transabdominal ultrasonography. *Br. J. Obstet. Gynaecol.* **97**, 304.
12. Bourne, T.H., Campbell, S., Reynolds, K.M. et al. (1993) Screening for early familial ovarian cancer with transvaginal ultrasonography and colour blood flow imaging. *BMJ* **306**, 1025.

13. Van Nagell, J., DePriest, P.D., Gallion, H.H. and Pavlik, E.J. (1993) Ovarian cancer screening. *Cancer* **71**, 1523-8.

14. Jacobs, I., Davies, A.P., Bridges, J. *et al.* (1993) Prevalence screening for ovarian cancer in post-meopausal women by CA125 measurement and ultrasonography. *BMJ* **306**, 1030-4.

15. Einhorn, N., Sjovall, K., Knapp, R.C. *et al.* (1992) Prospective evaluation of serum CA125 levels for early detection of ovarian cancer. *Obstet. Gynecol.* **80**, 14-8.

16. Austoker, J. (1994) Screening for ovarian, prostatic and testicular cancers. *BMJ* **309**, 315-20.

17. Schildkraut, J.M. and Thompson, W.D. (1988) Familial ovarian cancer: a population-based case-control study. *Am. J. Epidemiol.* **128**, 456-66.

18. Hildreth, N.G., Kelsey, J.L., Li, V.A. *et al.* (1991) An epidemiologic study of epithelial carcinoma of the ovary. *Am. J. Epidemiol.* **114**, 398-405.

19. Easton, D.F. and Peto, J. (1990) The contribution of inherited predisposition to cancer incidence. *Cancer Surv.* **9**, 395-416.

20. Houlston, R.S. and Peto, J. (1995) Genetics and the common cancers. In *Genetic predisposition to cancer* (eds. R. Eeles, B. Ponder, D. Easton, A. Horwich) Chapman & Hall, London.

21. Claus, E.B., Risch, N. and Thompson, W.D. (1990) Age of onset as an indicator of familial risk of breast cancer. *Am. J. Epidemiol.* **131**, 961-72.

22. Ford, D. and Easton, D.F. (1995) The genetics of ovarian and breast cancer. *Br. J. Cancer.* in press.

23. Wardle, J. and Pope, R. (1992) The psychological costs of screening for cancer. *J. Psychosom. Res.* **36**, 609-24.

24. Anderson, E.D.C., Smyth, J., Mackay, J. *et al.* (1994) Clinic for genetic counselling and screening women with a family history of breast cancer - the Edinburgh experience. *Cancer Family Study Group*, oral presentation.

25. Ellman, R., Angeli, N., Christians, A. *et al.* (1989) Psychiatric morbidity association with screening for breast cancer. *Br. J. Cancer* **60**, 781-4.

26. Gram, I.T., Lund, E. and Slenker, S.E. (1990) Quality of life following a false positive mammogram. *Br. J. Cancer* **62**, 1018-22.

27. Cull, A., Anderson, A., Mackay, J. *et al.* (1994) The effect of attending a breast cancer family clinic on women's estimates of risk and levels of psychological distress. *Cancer Family Study Group*, oral presentation.

28. Simard, J., Tonin, P., Durocher, F. *et al.* (1994) Common origins of BRCA1 mutations in Canadian breast and ovarian cancer families. *Nat. Genet.* **8**, 392-8.

29. Friedman, L.S., Ostermeyer, E.A., Szabo, C.I. *et al.* (1994) Confirmation of BRCA1 by analysis of germline mutations linked to breast and ovarian cancer in ten families. *Nat. Genet.* **8**, 399-404.

30. Pernet, A.L., Wardle, J., Bourne, T.H. *et al.* (1992) A qualitative evaluation of the experience of surgery after false positive results in screening of familial ovarian cancer. *Psycho-Oncology* **1**, 217-33.

31. Wardle, F.J., Cillins, W., Pernet, A.L. and Whitehead, M.I. (1993) psychological impact of screening for familial ovarian cancer. *J. Nat. Cancer Inst.* **85**, 653-7.

32. Advisory Council on Science and Technology (1993) *A report on medical research and health.* Cabinet Office, HMSO, London.

33. Kessler, S., Field, T., Worth, C. *et al.* (1987) Attitudes of persons at risk from Huntington's Disease towards predictive counselling. *Am. J. Med. Genet.* **26**, 259-70.

34. Baraitser, M. (1990) Huntington's Chorea. In *The genetics of neurological disorders.* Oxford Univ. Press, Oxford. pp 308-23.

Chapter 9

Epidemiological and biological interactions

Peter BOYLE and Robin E. LEAKE

9.1 EPIDEMIOLOGY OF OVARIAN CANCER

Ovarian cancer is the most frequent cause of death from gynaecological malignancy world-wide. Overall, ovarian cancer is the sixth most frequent form of cancer world-wide with an estimated 162 000 incident cases in 1985 [1]. Epithelial cystadeno-carcinomas constitute the large majority of ovarian malignancies although reliable population-based incidence rates for different histological sub-types of disease are absent. The less frequent germ cell tumours have a younger age distribution. The range of geographical variation for this disease is rather small. For example, in Northern Europe, the estimated incidence rate for 1985 is 12.2/100 000/annum (based on 8300 cases); in Western Europe it is 11.0 per 100 000 (14 000 cases); in Central and Eastern Europe it is 10.7/100 000 (83 000 cases) and in Southern Europe it is 7.8/100 000 (7800 cases).

From knowledge of risk factors for ovarian cancer at the present time, it is difficult to envisage good prospects for prevention. It is, however, very clear that there is a genetic component to ovarian cancer risk which is particularly important at younger ages. It has been estimated that women who carry mutations to the BRCA1 gene (on chromosome 17q) have a 60% lifetime risk of ovarian cancer. A recent series of 30 Canadian families with either breast or ovarian cancer, identified 12 (40%) with BRCA1 mutations [2]. The topic of genetics and ovarian cancer is discussed in much more detail elsewhere in this volume (see chapters 5–8). Knowledge of such a large genetic component to ovarian cancer risk is problematic when it comes to the interpretation of epidemiological studies, which have been based on cases not homogenous for ovarian cancer risk. Thus, identification of susceptibles in epidemiological studies and proper investigation of the interaction of lifestyle factors with susceptibility will be an important area for future research strategies in understanding ovarian cancer causation.

9.1.1 DESCRIPTIVE EPIDEMIOLOGY

The highest incidence rate of cancer of the ovary is 17.3 per 100 000 in Ardeche, France, followed by St. Gall in Switzerland (17.0 per 100 000). High rates are also recorded from four Scandinavian countries: Iceland (16.6 per 100 000), Denmark (14.9), Sweden (14.6) and Norway (14.6) (the other country is Finland with the 82nd highest rate of 9.9). Again, this shows that there is little

Table 9.1 Relative incidence of ovarian cancer by geographical site

Registry	Cases	Rate
Switzerland, St Gall	307	17.0
Iceland	118	16.6
Israel: Born Eur. Amer.	742	15.2
Denmark	3058	14.9
Canada, N W T & Yukon	15	14.7
UK, N.E. Scotland	300	14.6
Sweden	507	14.6
Norway	2300	14.6
UK, S.E. Scotland	680	14.0
Czech., Boh. & Morav.	5195	13.6
Italy, Latina	38	4.3
US, Los Angeles: Korean	10	4.1
India, Ahmedabad	190	4.0
Kuwait: Kuwaitis	28	3.7
France, Martinique	30	3.2
Israel: Non-Jews	27	2.4
Algeria, Setif	22	1.6
China, Qidong	45	1.5
The Gambia	7	1.4
Mali, Bamako	7	1.0

geographical pattern to the regions with the highest or lowest rates (see Table 9.1).

Hawaiians and Pacific Polynesian Islanders have higher rates than Maoris in whom the incidence is similar to that of non-Maoris in New Zealand. Rates around 15 are reported in Israel for women born in Europe or America. Most rates in Europe and North America range between 8 and 12. Rates for United States Afro-Americans are about two thirds of those for Caucasian women in the same community. While women in Asia have a relatively low incidence of ovarian tumours, in the range of 5 to 7 per 100 000, Chinese and Japanese who reside in the United States tend to have slightly higher rates, although less than in the white population.

A recent study of migrants from Cyprus, Egypt, Iran, Iraq, Israel, Lebanon, Syria and Turkey to Australia demonstrated lower rates of ovarian cancer in this group than in those born in Australia [3].

9.1.2 TEMPORAL TRENDS IN INCIDENCE

There are few long time series of ovarian cancer incidence statistics available. In the Nordic countries [4], there here have been small increases in incidence rates since the late 1940s. In Denmark, the incidence rate increased from 11.5 per 100 000 in 1946-1950 to 14.9 per 100 000 in 1983-1987. In Finland, the rates have always been lower than in Denmark but they increased from 6.4 per 100 000 in 1953-1955 to 9.9 per100 000 in 1983-1987. In Norway the increase was from 10.6 per 100 000 in1953-1955 to 14.6 per 100 000 in 1983-1987, while in Sweden the increase was from 12.5 per 100 000 in 1958-1960 to 14.6 in 1983-1987. The incidence rates in Norway, Sweden and Denmark for the latter period are very similar and higher than the incidence rate recorded in Finland. The increases in incidence in all countries are small.

9.1.3 TEMPORAL TRENDS IN MORTALITY

More data are available to investigate temporal trends in mortality. While these data are very useful and give good information about the failure in many instances they cannot reflect the underlying incidence rate of the disease. They are open to influences of variation in the quality of diagnosis and recording on the death certificate as well as the influences of differences and changes in the outcome of treatment. Nine countries were chosen to give a representative selection of international trends:

In Canada, ovarian cancer mortality rates remained stable between 1955 and 1973; however, they declined thereafter, especially the truncated rates. Birth cohort examination suggests quite similar rates in successive birth cohorts born before 1925. For cohorts born after that, rates decreased in successive birth cohorts.

In Japan, both the truncated and overall age-adjusted mortality rates have been increasing rapidly since 1955. Birth cohort examination shows a rapid increase in rates in successive birth cohorts for all age groups examined, particularly those aged over 50.

In Czechoslovakia, a consistent increasing trend was observed for both truncated and overall age-adjusted mortality rates since 1955. Birth cohort examination suggests a slow but steady increase in rates in successive birth cohorts for age groups over 40.

In Poland, both the truncated and overall age-adjusted mortality rates increased rapidly after 1955 and peaked in 1977. There then followed a decline between 1978 and 1981. Since that time an increase in rates has again occurred. Birth cohort examination shows an increase in rates in successive birth cohorts. However, the rates in different age groups have shown inconsistent changes in the last time period.

In Germany, although the overall age-adjusted mortality rates remained relatively stable between 1968 and 1988, the truncated rates have been decreasing since the early 1970s. Birth cohort examination indicates a slight increase in rates in successive birth cohorts until 1920 and a decreasing trend for cohorts born thereafter.

In Denmark, there has been a small increase in the overall age-adjusted mortality rates of ovary cancer between 1955 and 1972, and thereafter a small decrease. Although subject to greater variation, this pattern is also evident in the truncated rates.

Examination of rates by median year of birth shows no systematic change by birth cohort.

In Italy, both the truncated and overall age-adjusted mortality rates have been increasing rapidly since 1955. Examination by birth cohorts shows an increase in rates in successive birth cohorts for almost all the age groups examined.

In the United Kingdom, the truncated rates of ovary cancer remained relatively stable until 1978. Since then, a small decrease in rates has occurred. The overall age-adjusted mortality rates, however, showed a slight increase before 1970 and remained relatively stable thereafter. Consequently, examination of rates by birth cohorts suggests an increase in rates in successive birth cohorts until the 1920 birth cohort, and a decrease for cohorts born thereafter.

In Australia, neither the truncated nor the overall age-adjusted mortality rates showed clear time trends before 1965 but they started to decline thereafter. Birth cohort examination shows a relatively stable rate in successive birth cohorts for those born before 1930, and a rapid decrease thereafter.

9.1.4 TEMPORAL TRENDS IN SURVIVAL

Interpretation of mortality trends should also include discussion of temporal trends in survival. Most data available on this topic are from special hospital series or clinical trials. In Denmark and Scotland there are population-based ovarian cancer survival data available for over twenty years. In Denmark [5], the five-year survival rate increased from 24.5% for women diagnosed in 1953-1957 through 25.7% for women diagnosed in 1968-1972 to 29.4% in 1983-1987. In Scotland, where the national cancer registration and follow-up are of similar quality to that of Denmark, survival rose from 26.5% in women diagnosed between 1968-1972 to 29.4% among women diagnosed between 1983 and 1987. These improvements in 5-year survival are thought to be the result of introduction of platinum-based drugs.

9.1.5 ANALYTICAL EPIDEMIOLOGY

Epithelial ovarian cancer is the commonest type of ovarian neoplasia [6] and the leading cause of death from gynaecological neoplasms in most western countries. This term contains a very wide and diverse range of pathological entities, although by grouping these under a limited number of headings (serous, mucinous endometrioid, clear cell and undifferentiated) no one group stands out as being different from the rest in epidemiological terms. As for other female-hormone related neoplasms, its age curve tends to flatten off around menopause.

The risk of ovarian cancer is increased approximately two fold in nulliparous women compared to parous women. An increased risk has been suggested for late age at first birth, early menarche and late menopause, but the evidence is inconsistent. Typical findings are those of Franceschi *et al.* [7] from a large study conducted in Northern Italy. With the referent group consisting of those women with a parity of three or higher, the risk rose to 2.1 (95%CI(1.2, 3.5)) among nulliparous. Those women who had a first birth after age 25 had a relative risk of 2.0 (1.2, 3.1) compared to the referent category of women who had a first birth before 25. Girls who had a menarche at 11 years or younger had an increased risk of 1.5, which was not statistically significant, compared to those who had menarche after 15 (referent category). Age at menopause was a very important factor in this study. Using women who had a menopause before age 45 as referent, the risk rose among women aged 45-49 at menopause (OR=2.9 (1.1, 7.9)) to a peak among women who had menopause after the age of 50 years (OR=4.7 (1.8, 11.5)).

There have been at least fifteen case-control studies which have uniformly indicated that oral contraceptive use is protective against ovarian carcinogenesis [8]. The incidence of epithelial invasive cancer being reduced by approximately 30% in ever users of oral contraceptives, and to a greater extent in long-term users: five or more years of use is associated with a 50% reduction in risk, while the relative risk for users of 97 months duration, or more, was only 0.3 (95%CI(0.1-0,7))[9]. The protective effect of oral contraceptives persists for ten or more years after its use is discontinued and becomes apparent several years after beginning use. Reduced risks of ovarian cancer have been observed for all major histological types of ovarian cancer and among users in developing and developed countries. The little information available suggests that the effects of oral contraceptives appear to be similar for malignant and borderline malignant epithelial tumours. Thus, on a population scale, combined oral contraceptives have probably been the major determinant of the (favourable) decrease in ovarian cancer rates observed in several western countries. The open question is whether this effect, only seen so far at pre-menopausal ages, will continue to protect against ovarian cancer at post-menopausal ages.

Among gravid women, a reported history of infertility has been associated with an odds ratio of 0.86 (95%CI(0.61, 1.2)) from a meta-analysis [10,11]. When analysis was made according to drug use for infertility (or, more correctly, sub-fertility), there were differences between those who reported drug treatment (OR=1.4(0.52,3.6)) and those who did not (OR=0.84 (0.58, 1.2)): these odds ratios were based on 8 cases and 10 controls. Among nulligravid women, the overall odds ratio associated with a history of infertility was 2.1 (1.0,4.2). When this nulligravid population was limited to women who reported drug treatment but continued infertility, the odds ratio rose to 27.0 (2.3, 315.6), though it is important to note that this was based on only 12 cases and one control. Among those who reported no drug treatment, the odds ratio was 1.6 (0.74, 3.3) based on 22 cases and 22 controls. These results are of considerable interest but deserve to be interpreted cautiously.

The twelve studies entered into this meta-analysis were considered after they had been analysed and published and there was no opportunity for coordination in either study design or exposure assessment. Infertility was based on a report from the women that they had been told by a physician that they were infertile: the definition of infertile encompasses both a reduced ability to conceive and to maintain a pregnancy and they may have different aetiologies. The findings are based on relatively small numbers of cases and controls in some strata in whom the basis of the diagnosis is unknown. Subsequently, the potential association with ovarian cancer risk and a history of infertility was investigated in a study in Italy. Based on 195 epithelial ovarian cancers and 1339 controls, fewer ovarian cancer cases reported use of fertility drugs than controls (OR=0,7, 95%CI(0.2-3.3)). Among nulligravid women, five (out of 177) control women compared with zero (out of 36) cancer cases reported having ever used fertility drugs [7]. These null findings were also essentially similar to those reported in a similar study from Toronto [12].

These findings constitute a good basis for the development of a study hypothesis but require confirmation before being accepted as causal. A prospective study designed to explore the hypothesis is being launched in the UK, along with corresponding studies in France and Australia.

As for breast and endometrial cancer, nutrition and diet are the major open questions in ovarian cancer epidemiology. The American Cancer Society One Million Study showed an elevated risk of ovarian cancer among obese women [13], but the evidence from case-control studies is largely negative, possibly on account of loss of weight secondary to the neoplastic process. Ecological studies found positive correlations with fats, proteins and calories, although these are less strong than for endo-metrial cancer. Case-control studies showed a possible association with total fat intake and some protection by green vegetables, but further research is required in the area, particularly because diet may be more amenable to intervention than reproductive or menstrual history. The protective effects of fruits and vegetables seen widely for many forms of cancer seem weaker or absent for ovarian cancer [14]. *In vitro* work on the inhibitory effects of various retinoic acid derivatives has been reported by Bast *et al.* [15].

Lactose has been proposed on biological grounds to be potentially associated with the risk of ovarian cancer. A recent large case-control study from Canada has found that neither lactose intolerance nor average daily intake of lactose or free galactose was found to be associated with the risk of ovarian cancer. Lactose intake or intolerance did not appear to modify the protective effects of parity and oral contraceptive use [16].

There is no evidence that cigarette smoking affects the risk of ovarian cancer in women of any age [17]. Four studies have investigated the association between ovarian cancer risk and alcohol consumption. No study has demonstrated an increased risk of ovarian cancer among alcohol drinkers, with two studies suggesting a protective effect of heavy alcohol consumption against ovarian cancer in young women [18].

In all seven case-control studies which examined the issue, coffee users had an increased risk of ovarian cancer although the elevation in risk was statistically significant in only two studies [19]. Comparing users to non-users, the odds ratio was between 1.1 and 1.3 in five studies, 1.4 in a further study and 1.9 in the remaining study. A Mantel-Haenszel analysis produced a (conservative) estimate of the pooled odds ratio of 1.3 (95%CI(1.1, 1.5)). Although the overall analysis reveals a marginal, significant increase in risk of ovarian cancer, bias from unidentified sources or chance cannot yet be ruled out [19].

Occupational factors have been investigated in a cross-sectional study of 159 000 women in Torino who have been followed [20]. Metal, wood and clothing manufacturers showed a significantly increased risk of ovarian cancer.

Risk factors for benign ovarian teratomas, histologically confirmed in women aged below 65 years, have been investigated in a case-control study conducted in Milan [21]. Four of 77 cases and two of 231 controls reported a history of infertility, the corresponding odds ratio being 8.3 (95%CI(1.3, 54)). This gives some support to the association found with infertility and malignant tumours of the ovary. There was no clear association between parity and the risk of benign ovarian teratoma: in comparison with nulliparae, the estimated relative risks were 1.1 and 0.7 respectively for women reporting one or two-or-more births. No relation emerged between marital status, age at menarche, menstrual cycle pattern, menopausal status, abortion history, age at first pregnancy, oral contraceptive use and risk of benign ovarian teratomas [21]. These findings differ markedly from those found with malignant disease.

9.2 BIOLOGICAL AND EPIDEMIOLOGICAL INTERACTIONS

The normal ovary is a complex structure which is designed primarily to make available a mature follicle such that fertilization of the egg cell can take place. In addition to ovulation, the main role of the ovary is to synthesize and secrete the female sex steroids oestradiol and progesterone. The principal reproductive function of the sex steroids is to prepare the endometrium for implantation of the fertilized egg and then maintain the pregnancy, once established. In evolutionary terms, the healthy women was designed to be pregnant. Given that ovulation does not occur in women who are breast feeding, one can argue that ovulation was designed to occur as rarely as once every two years - giving a lifetime value of about twenty ovulations (*i.e.* 10 per ovary) and, therefore, only this number of subsequent repairs of the surface ovarian epithelium. In contrast, a woman who goes through life with normal menstrual cycles, but does not become pregnant, is likely to undergo 480 ovulations and repairs (240 per ovary).

Because the vast majority of ovarian cancers are epithelial cancers, the working hypothesis is is that ovarian cancer arises because of promotion of transformed epithelial cells during the course of the repair of surface epithelium damaged by ovulation. Work on point mutations in p53 has provided strong evidence that ovarian cancer is monoclonal, rather than arising from many different transformations of surface epithelial cells (or inclusions).

To explore the possibilities of prevention of ovarian cancer through endocrine manipulations, it is first necessary to review the endocrine control of the functional ovary. Follicular maturation is under the control of the gonadotrophins, follicle stimulating hormone (FSH) and luteinizing hormone (LH). These glycoproteins act through the plasma membrane receptors on their target cells. Simplistically, in the follicular phase of the ovarian cycle, FSH can be said to prime the maturing follicle (an event begun prior to the previous menstruation). Concurrently, LH acts on the theca cells to induce androgen synthesis. The androgens are secreted across to the neighbouring granulosa cells, where these are converted to oestrogens by the enzyme aromatase. Aromatase action is stimulated by FSH in a process which is activated by the active androgen-receptor complex [22,23]. The LH surge that promotes ovulation involves local release of prostaglandins, together with FSH and LH induced release of plasminogen activator [24]. The plasmin, released by the action of plasminogen activator (uPA), is thought to mediate the release of the oocyte from the follicle wall [24]. This whole process appears to be under the control of transforming growth factor-beta (TGF-β) and a critical part of the malignant transformation may relate to changed response of uPA secreting cells to TGF-β [25]. The role of uPA, as an important controlling element in the process of invasion, is now well established not only in ovarian cancer, but also in breast and many other cancers [26,27].

A further action of FSH on the granulosa cells is to induce synthesis of LH receptors. Thus, once ovulation is successfully completed, the granulosa cells can give rise to the corpus luteum which, under the continued action of LH, synthesizes and secretes the progesterone. Although the principal role of progesterone is to induce differentiation of, and invagination into, the endometrial epithelial cells, there is a secondary role of progesterone in the ovary itself. This action is, of course, mediated by the progesterone receptor.

Progesterone receptor (PR) activity in the ovary is unusual. In most reproductive tissues, oestrogens act through their receptor (ER) to induce synthesis of PR. However, PR is found in the ovary often in the absence of

ER [28]. Indeed, it is thought that activated PR actually primes the differentiation of the epithelial cells. Breakdown of this control may be another step in the malignant process since ovarian cancer is associated with a decrease in PR and an increase in ER [29].

The role of paracrine agents, such as TGF-β, has already been alluded to. Normal ovarian thecal cells synthesize and secrete TGF-α (an analogue of epidermal growth factor - EGF - which binds to and activates the EGF receptor with similar affinity to EGF). Since both thecal and granulosa cells have adequate EGF receptors [30], it is assumed that TGF-α causes growth responses in both cell types. Normal ovarian surface epithelium also stains strongly for both EGF and its receptor [30]. This supports the hypothesis that the post-ovulation repair mechanism is, at least in part, EGF-driven. Interestingly, TGF-α levels are detectable in almost all ovarian epithelial cell cancers (over 90%) and very much elevated in some [31] suggesting loss of normal growth control. However, EGF receptor is only detected in about 45% of ovarian epithelial cell cancers [32] so that EGF/TGF-α induced growth promotion is not the only mechanism in ovarian cancer. TGF-β is also synthesized and secreted by the thecal cells. However, thecal cells do not appear to have TGF-β receptors and the main target is thought to be the granulosa cells, though ovarian cancer cells in culture show marked growth inhibition by TGF, leading to the concept of a balance of control by TGF α and β in at least some ovarian cancers [15,33]. A dose dependent effect of LH on ovarian cancer cells *in vitro* has shown that the inhibitory process is blocked if anti-TGF antibody is added prior to LH.

Ovarian cancer is complex because of the large number of cell types. Even if attention is confined to epithelial cancers, classification is difficult. Malkasian and colleagues [34]

have concluded (from a study of 1938 women) that the behaviour of different cell types was similar when compared stage-for-stage and grade-for-grade. For example, mucinous cystadeno-carcinomas tended to be low grade and low stage, whereas serous cystadenocarcinomas tended to be high grade and high stage. Nevertheless, Stage 1/Grade 1 survival at 20 years was very similar for serous and mucinous tumours. Our own studies have failed to demonstrate any dramatic differences between the different histological sub-groups of ovarian cancers in terms of contents of either growth factors or their receptors [31,32].

There are differences in the incidence of ER and PR according to histological type [29,35]. If the tumour contains both functional ER and PR, then the survival chance is better irrespective of cell type [29,36]. Unfortunately, ER and PR are only found together in about 20% of ovarian cancers and so ER-mediated approaches to therapy have, at best, limited application. Almost all ovarian cancers contain androgen receptor (AR). This may be a consequence for the requirement of AR to mediate the FSH-induced aromatase conversion of androgens to oestrogens in the granulosa cells. Aromatase activity is retained in only about one third of ovarian epithelial cell cancers [37,38]. Thus, if local oestrogen synthesis and/or functional oestrogen receptor is required for the early promotion of ovarian cancer, this requirement is lost by most tumours before they are clinically detectable.

About 90% of ovarian cancers also contain glucocorticoid receptors (GR)[39]. Ovarian cancer cells grown in culture respond to the synthetic glucocorticoid dexamethasone [40]. The responses include 95% inhibition of uPA secretion, 50% inhibition of growth and pronounced morphological changes. The clinical significance of these *in vitro*

observations is not clear since, *in vivo*, there is presumably a physiologically-effective supply of glucocorticoid.

9.3 PREVENTION

Our baseline information is that:
1. Most ovarian cancers are cancers of the surface epithelium or inclusions thereof.
2. Procedures which reduce the numbers of ovulations are associated with reduced risk of ovarian cancer.

Putting these two together, it follows that the repair mechanisms which are activated after ovulation, may also be the mechanisms involved in the promotion of transformed cells into tumour. These mechanisms are thought, at least in part, to involve EGF receptor activation by either EGF or, more likely, TGF-α. Regulation of these growth factors by steroid hormones has been shown *in vitro* and the most effective known agent for reducing incidence of ovarian cancer is the contraceptive pill. However, it is not clear whether the effect of the pill is direct action of the steroids or is due to feedback onto the hypothalamic-pituitary axis, resulting in reduced levels of gonadotrophins. Further, another anterior pituitary hormone, prolactin may also have a role. Ovarian cancer is higher in sub-fertile patients and a proportion of these have hyperprolactinaemia.

There may be as much as a four-fold increased risk of ovarian cancer for women who enter menopause after the age of 50, compared with women who become menopausal at 45 years. This suggests that the older the ovary, the more likely it is that the ovarian epithelial cells will contain transformations which, when promoted by post-ovulation growth repairs, will lead to ovarian cancer. Thus, prevention measures - application of agents to reduce cell division in surface epithelium - should be applied before the age of 45.

Possible additive endocrine/paracrine strategies include:

1. Blocking gonadotrophin secretion.
2. Blocking EGF receptor function.
3. Promoting apoptosis.
4. Promoting selective TGF-β down-regulation of surface epithelium.

The contraceptive pill is the most obvious agent to use. However, some people may have clinical or ethical reasons for not wishing to go on the pill. An additional complication is that taking the pill in this late stage of reproductive life may raise the incidence of breast cancer. Because of the relative incidence rates, a small rise in incidence of breast cancer could give a net balance of an excess of total cancers, even if the reduction of ovarian cancer is large. Another approach might be use of LHRH agonists, though there would be objections to giving such agents to 'well women' of 45 years of age. As our understanding of the cell biology of the ovary improves, so it may become more possible to select a specific intervention which does not have undesirable side-effects. This would tend to exclude strategies aimed at cell signalling intermediates (*e.g.* EGFR-related tyrosine kinase has been shown to be elevated in platinum resistant ovarian cancer cells [41]). Steroid and gonadotrophin regulation of apoptosis in normal ovarian cells requires investigation.

However, the priority for prevention strategies should continue to revolve around the potential for oral contraceptive use to halve the risk of ovarian cancer. There is a need to confirm that this protection continues in the long-term, *i.e.* after use ends. It is also important to establish whether the protective effect is maintained after the menopause. Identification of the biological mechanisms underlying this association could serve to greatly increase the prospects for ovarian cancer prevention.

REFERENCES

1. Parkin, D.M., Ferlay, J. and Pisani, P. (1993). Estimates of the worldwide incidence of eighteen major cancers in 1985. *Int. J. Cancer* **54**, 594-606.
2. Simard, J., Tonin, P., Durocher, F. *et al.* (1994) Common origins of BRCA1 mutations in Canadian breast and ovarian cancer families. *Nat. Genet.* **8**, 392-8.
3. MacCredie, M., Coates, M. and Grulich, A. (1994) Cancer incidence in migrants to New South Wales from the Middle East. *Cancer Causes Control* **5**, 414-21.
4. Hakulinen, T., Andersen, A.A., Malker, B. *et al.* (1986) Trends in cancer incidence in the Nordic countries. *Acta Pathol. Microbiol. Immunol. Scand.* **94**, Suppl.228.
5. Kruger, K.S. and Storm, H.H. (1993) Female genital organs. *APMIS* **101**, 107-21.
6. Scully, R.E. (1985) Ovary. In: *Pathology of incipient neoplasia*. Eds. D.E.Hempson and J. Albores-Saavedra. W.B.Saunders, Philadelphia, pp 279-93.
7. Franceschi, S., La Vecchia, C., Negri, E. *et al.* (1994) Fertrility drugs and risk of epithelial ovarian cancer in Italy. *Hum. Reprod.* **9**, 1673-5
8. Stanford, J.L. (1991) Oral contraception and neoplasia of the ovary. *Contraception* **43**, 543-56.
9. Vessey, M.P. and Painter, R. (1995) Endometrial and ovarian cancer and oral contraceptoves - findings in a large cohort study. *Br.J.Cancer* **71**,1340-2.
10. Whittemore, A.S., Harris, R. and Itnyre, J. (1992) Collaborative Ovarian Cancer Group. Characteristics relating to ovarian cancer risk: collaborative analysis of 12 US case-control studies. II invasive ovarian cancers in white women. *Am. J. Epidemiol.* **136**, 1184-1203.
11. Harris, R., Whittemore, A.S. and Itnyre, J. (1992) Collaborative Ovarian Cancer Group. Characteristics relating to ovarian

cancer risk: collaborative analysis of 12 US case-control studies. III Epithelial tumours of low malignant potential in white women. *Am. J. Epidemiol.* **136**, 1204-11

12. Risch, H., Marret, L.D. and Howe, G.R. (1994) Parity, contraception, infertility and the risk of epithelial ovarian cancer. *Am. J. Epidemiol.* **140**, 585-97.

13. Lew, E.A. and Garfinkel, L. (1979). Variations in mortality by weight among 750,000 men and women. *J. Chron. Dis.* **32**, 563-76.

14. Steinmetz, K.A. and Potter, J.D. (1991). Vegetable, fruit, and cancer: I.Epidemiology, *Cancer Caus. Control* **2**, 325-58.

15. Bast, R.C., Boyer, C.M., Xu, F.J. *et al.* (1995) Cell growth regulation in human epithelialovarian cancer, In, 'The Biology of Gynaecological Cancer' (eds. R.Leake, M.Gore, R.H. Ward), RCOG Press, London. pp 109-13.

16. Risch, H., Jain, M., Marret, L.D. and Howe, G.R. (1994) Dietary lactose intake, lactose intolerance and the risk of epithelial ovarian cancer in southern Ontario. *Cancer Caus. Control* **5**, 540-8.

17. IARC (International Agency for Research on Cancer) (1986). Monographs on the Evaluation of the Carconogenic Risk of Chemicals to Man. Vol. 38. Tobacco Smoking, IARC, Lyon.

18. IARC (International Agency for Research on Cancer) (1988). Monographs on the Evaluation of Carcinogenic Risk to Humans. Vol. 44. Alcohol Drinking, IARC, Lyon.

19. IARC (International Agency for Research on Cancer) (1991). Monographs on the Evaluation of Carcinogenic Risk to Humans. Vol. 51. Coffee, tea, mate, methylxanthines (caffeine, theophylline, theobromine) and methylglyoxal. IARC, Lyon.

20. Costantini, A.S., Piratsu, R., Lagorio, S. *et al.* (1994) Studies in cancer among female workers, methods and prelimary results from a record-linkage system in Italy. *J. Occup. Med.* **36**, 1180-6.

21. Parazzini, F., La Vecchia, C., Negri, E. *et al.* (1995) Risk factors for benign ovarian teratomas. *Br. J. Cancer* **71**, 644-6.

22. Daniel, S.A.J. and Armstrong, D.T. (1980) Enhancement of FSH induced aromatase activity by androgens in cultured rat granulosa cells. *Endocrinology* **107**, 1027-33.

23. Hillier, S.G. and De Zwart, F.A. (1985) Evidence that granulosa cell aromatase induction/activation by follicle-stimulating hormones is an androgen receptor regulated process *in vitro. Endocrinology* **109**,1303-5.

24. Beers, W.H., Strickland, S. and Reich, E. (1985) Ovarian plasminogen activator, relationship to ovulation and hormonal regulation. *Cell* **6**, 387-94.

25. Laiko, M. and Keski-Oja, J. (1989) Growth factors in the regulation of pericellular proteolysis, A review. *Cancer Res.* **49**, 2533-53.

26. Janicke, F., Scmitt, M., Hafter, R. *et al.* (1990) Urokinase-type plasminogen activator (uPA) antigen is a predictor of early relapse in breast cancer. *Fibrinolysis* **4**, 69-78.

27. Pedersen, H., Brunner, N., Francis, D. *et al.* (1994) Prognostic impact of urokinase receptor and type 1 plasminogen activator in squamous and large cell lung cancer tissues. *Cancer Res.* **54**, 120-3.

28. Soutter, W.P. and Leake, R.E. (1987) Steroid hormone receptors in gynaecological cancers. *Rec. Adv. Obstet. Gynecol.* **15**, 175-94.

29. Harding, M., Cowan, S., Hole, D. *et al.* (1990) Oestrogen and progesterone receptors in ovarian cancer. *Cancer* **65**, 486-91.

30. Scurry, J.P., Hammand, K.A., Astley, S.B. *et al.* (1994) Immunoreactivity of antibodies to epidermal growth factor, transforming growth factors alpha and beta and epidermal growth factor receptor in the premenopausal ovary. *Pathology* **26**, 130-3.

31. Owens, O.J., Stewart, C. and Leake, R.E. (1991a) Growth factor concentration and distribution in ovarian cancer. *Br. J. Cancer* **64**, 1177-81.

32. Owens, O.J., Stewart, C., Brown, I. and Leake, R.E. (1991b) Epidermal growth factor receptors in human ovarian cancer. *Br. J. Cancer* **64**, 907-10.

33. Hurteau, J., Rodriguez, G.C., Berchuck, A. and Bast, R.C. (1994) Transforming growth factor beta inhibits proliferation of human ovarian cancer cells obtained from ascites. *Cancer* **74**, 93-9.

34. Malkasian, G.D., Melton, L.J., O'Brian, P.C. and Greene, M.H. (1984) Prognostic significance of histologic classification and grading of epithelial malignancies of theovary. *Am. J. Obstet. Gynecol.* **149**, 274 84.

35. Topila, M., Tyler, J.P.P., Fay, R. *et al.* (1986) Steroid receptors in human ovarian malignancy. A review of 4 years tissue collection. *Br. J. Obstet. Gynaecol.* **93**, 986-92.

36. Iversen, O.E., Skaarland, E. and Utaaker, E. (1980) Steroid receptor content in human ovarian tumours, survival of patients relative to steroid receptor content. *Gynecol. Oncol.* **23**, 65-76.

37. Kuknel, R., Dellemarre, J.F.M., Rao, B.R. and Stolk, J.G. (1986) Correlation of aromatase activity and steroid receptors in human ovarian carcinoma. *Anticancer Res.* **6**, 889-92.

38. Rao, B. and Slotman, B.J. (1994) Endocrine factors in common epithelial ovarian cancer. *End. Rev.* **12**, 175-87.

39. Galli, M.C., De Giovanni, C., Nicoletti, G. *et al.* (1981) The occurrence of multiple steroid hormone receptors in disease-free and neoplastic human ovary. *Cancer* **47**, 1297-302.

40. Amin, W., Karlan, B.Y. and Littlefield, B.A. (1987) Glucocorticoid sensitivity of OVCA433 human ovarian carcinoma cells, Inhibition of plasminogen activators, cell growth and orphological alterations. *Cancer Res.* **47**, 6040-5.

41. Leake, R., Barber, A., Owens, S. *et al.* (1995) Growth factors andreceptors in ovarian cancer. In, *'Ovarian Cancer 3'* (eds F. Sharp, P. Mason, T. Blackett and J. Berek) Chapman & Hall, London, pp 99-108.

Part Three

Optimizing Treatment

I - Surgery

Chapter 10

Primary and interval debulking surgery for advanced disease

Sergio PECORELLI, Franco ODICINO and Antonella TESSADRELLI

10.1 INTRODUCTION

In the majority of publications on therapy of epithelial ovarian cancer primary cytoreductive surgery is regarded as the milestone of the therapeutic approach. However, only retrospective studies have shown that advanced ovarian cancer patients do benefit from primary debulking (or cytoreductive) surgery.

10.2 RATIONALE FOR DEBULKING

Primary cytoreductive surgery can be defined as the removal of as much tumour as possible at the time of the first operation in a patient with advanced ovarian cancer. The theoretical basis and therefore the rationale for performing tumour debulking is mainly based on the kinetics of tumour growth and on the observation that epithelial ovarian cancer is fairly chemosensitive, even if not as sensitive as ovarian germ cell tumours or gestational trophoblastic disease. Ovarian cancers are more chemosensitive than other solid tumours such as gastric or pancreatic. A summary of the rationale for debulking surgery has been presented [1]:
1. Presence of pharmacological sanctuaries, that could be eliminated by the removal of poorly perfused bulky tumour masses.
2. Higher growth fraction in the better perfused small residual tumour masses,

which favours an increased cell kill by chemotherapy or radiation therapy.
3. Small tumour masses require fewer cycles of chemotherapy, so there is less opportunity for induced drug resistance.
4. Host immunocompetence is enhanced by the removal of large tumour masses.
5. Clones of phenotypically resistant cells may possibly be removed, particularly if all gross macroscopic disease can be eliminated. Moreover, the removal of large intra-abdominal masses sometimes results in the relief of bowel obstruction and, therefore, in the improvement of the patient's gastrointestinal function and nutrition, with obvious advantages toward chemotherapy tolerance.

10.3 MUTATIONS AND RESISTANCE TO CHEMOTHERAPY

It is well known that the development of tumour resistant clones to chemotherapy in untreated patients is mainly due to spontaneous mutation; and this occurs as an intrinsic property of genetically unstable tumour cells. This is a random event that depends on the growth curve of the tumour and on the mutation rate. Therefore the probability of resistant clones increases as the size of the tumour mass increases. The size of the disease at the opening of the abdominal cavity and not only the size of the

105

residual disease after surgery may thus play an important role. The removal of large tumour masses not only reduces the likelihood that drug resistant clones will appear as a result of spontaneous mutations, but smaller tumours will require fewer cycles of chemotherapy, thus decreasing the probability of drug-induced resistance [2].

10.4 CRITICISMS OF CYTOREDUCTIVE SURGERY

Historically, the concept of *maximal surgical effort* and better survival goes back to the 1960s [3], and in 1975 Griffiths reported that the survival of 102 patients with advanced ovarian cancer correlated with the tumour residuum at the end of primary surgery and before the medical treatment [4]. Since that study, multiple reports have shown that the diameter of the largest residual disease is directly related to response rate, progression-free interval, likelihood of being negative at second-look operation and survival.

Today there are two main criticisms of the concept of cytoreductive surgery in advanced ovarian cancer: The first is the lack of randomized prospective studies and the second is whether the improved prognosis in patients with small residual tumour masses is related to the surgical resection of the bulky disease or to the surgical resectability of the disease. The Gynecologic Oncology Group tried to answer the first question with a randomized study (GOG #80) comparing primary debulking surgery to six courses of chemotherapy in stage III patients. The study was closed due to the low accrual of patients. This was due both to ethical and medico-political reasons and it is reasonable to believe that even today such a study cannot have a good chance of successful accrual. The only prospective randomized study addressing a surgical question and successfully terminated is the EORTC (European Organisation for Research and

Treatment of Cancer) study on interval debulking, which showed a survival benefit with a reduced risk of progression and death for patients in the surgical arm of the study. These were patients with tumours that could not be optimally cytoreduced (to less than 1 cm) at first surgery and were later debulked after only three courses of platinum-based chemotherapy, if having no clinical evidence of progressive disease. In this study interval debulking surgery was not associated with death, severe morbidity and major intraoperative complications. In addition, surgery did not have a negative effect on subsequent chemotherapy. Even if the study was not designed to address the quality of life issue, the above mentioned remarks would not suggest a negative impact of repeated operations upon the quality of life of patients. Moreover the six months median increase in survival represents an important result that deserves immediate confirmation [5]. In fact the GOG has just started a similar study addressing also the issue of quality of life.

10.5 RESECTION AND RESECTABILITY

Concerning the issue of resection *versus* resectability, the earliest publications were in accordance with the thoughts of Griffitths, claiming that patients whose tumours could be surgically reduced to *optimal* status had the same prognosis as those with *optimal* metastatic disease *de novo* [6]. It was Hacker and colleagues who first reported in 1983 that patients with large metastatic disease (more than 10 cm in diameter) had a worse prognosis than patients with a small initial tumour burden regardless of the extent of cytoreduction [7].

Similar conclusions were reached also by Hoskins in a retrospective analysis of some GOG data, in which patients found to have small volume disease survived longer than patients cytoreduced to small volume disease

[8]. All these observations, although they do not negate the effectiveness of cytoreductive surgery, do indicate that intrinsic factors within the tumour itself are of prognostic significance, the so-called 'biology of the tumour'.

10.6 PERITONEAL METASTASES

Another factor related to tumour biology is the presence of peritoneal carcinomatosis, shown by Heintz *et al.* in 1988 [9] and later by Farias-Eisner *et al.* [10] to be an adverse prognostic factor. A high number of tumour nodules was related to a poorer prognosis [10], and this was also demonstrated by neural network analysis to predict treatment outcome [11]. In a case-control study of patients with minimal residual disease Eisenkop *et al.* suggested that the removal of all small metastatic nodules by whatever means (CO_2 laser, CUSA, electrocautery, Argon beam coagulator or sharp dissection) can significantly improve survival over those patients in whom such small lesions were not resected [12].

10.7 SURGERY AND CHEMORESISTANT TUMOURS

In 1992 a meta-analysis of surgery in advanced ovarian carcinoma suggested that surgery had only a small effect on survival, the type of chemotherapy being the most important variable [13]. Although the meta-analysis included almost 7000 patients entered in 58 studies, it suffers from grave methodological problems, the most serious one being that it compared the survival of patients with 'optimal' (less than 3 cm!) and sub-optimal cytoreduction, which is hampered by unavoidable and serious bias when patients with different prognostic factors are compared. In 23 cohorts 'optimal' cytoreduction was achieved in 20% or less of the cases, thus making it impossible to weigh the value of tumour debulking. Moreover, only half of the patients received effective platinum-based chemotherapy.

We think it is reasonable to say that approximately 25% of patients with ovarian cancer present with chemoresistant tumours. In such patients cytoreductive surgery does not play the same therapeutic role as in chemosensitive tumours, but unfortunately this group of patients cannot be identified pre-operatively. It is clear that as long as we include these patients in any analysis or even meta-analysis of primary cytoreductive surgery, it will be difficult to draw objective conclusions, while we cannot deny a significant survival advantage to the group with chemosensitive tumours In the future we should concentrate on studies of the biology of the tumour in order to identify the chemoresistant tumours pre-operatively and possibly plan a different therapeutic strategy. Until that time, all patients should be offered the possibility of aggressive cytoreductive primary surgery. Data suggest that a serious attempt to debulk all possible tumour masses prior to the start of chemotherapy should always be made [12,14,15]. At the Royal Hospital for Women in Sydney, Hacker reported a very high percentage of survival (greater than 50% at 4 years) in patients with no macroscopic residual after primary surgery [14] and Schwartz had similar results in a study of 100 patients, in which the group with no residual disease had a significantly better survival; patients with residual tumour nodules < 2 cm in diameter did not show any survival advantage over those with larger lesions, unless the former group included the patients with no macroscopic residual masses [15].

In good gynaecological oncology centres optimal cytoreduction (to < 1 cm diameter) should be achievable in at least 70% cases. All other patients and those that were referred to these centres after 'suboptimal' surgery could be offered a second surgical attempt in an 'interval cytoreductive' set, that is during chemotherapy as demonstrated by the EORTC study [5].

10.8 LYMPHADENOPATHY

Finally, the value of pelvic and para-aortic lymphadenectomy in otherwise optimally debulked tumours is yet to be assessed. Systematic lymphadenectomy is strongly advocated by Burghardt *et al.* [16], who reported approximately 70% positivity in stage III and IV disease, with actuarial 5-year survival rates of 69%, 58% and 28%, depending on the number of positive lymph nodes (0, 1, >1 respectively). In order to establish whether or not we should perform pelvic and para-aortic lymphadenectomy, a randomized prospective study is ongoing as a result of a cooperation between European, North American and Australian centres. Patients with stage III disease will be randomized to receive either systematic lymphadenectomy or just resection of bulky pelvic nodes prior to six courses of cisplatin-based chemotherapy. One hundred and seventy patients are required in each arm of the study.

10.9 CONCLUSIONS

In conclusion, there seems to be no doubt that the ultimate fate of the patient is linked to the biology of her tumour, but she should be offered a serious attempt at primary cytoreductive surgery and the best available chemotherapy treatment. Moreover, the removal of large tumour masses from the abdominal cavity very often results in an improved quality of life of the patient.

REFERENCES

1. Hacker, N.F. (1989). Controversial aspects of cytoreductive surgery in epithelial ovarian cancer. In *Operative treatment of ovarian cancer.* (eds. E.Burghart and J.M.Monaghan) *Baillere's Clin. Obstet. Gynecol.* 3, 49-57.
2. Goldie, J.H. and Coldman, A.J. (1979) A mathematic model for relating the drug sensitivity of tumors to their spontaneous mutation rate. *Cancer Treat. Rep.* 63, 1727-33.
3. Munnell, E.W. (1968) The changing prognosis and treatment of in cancer of the ovary, A report of 235 patients with primary ovarian cancer 1952-1961. *Am. J. Obstet. Gynecol.* 100, 790-805.
4. Griffiths, C.T. (1975) Surgical resection of tumor bulk in the primary treatment ovarian cancer. *Monogr. Natl. Cancer Inst.* 42, 101-4.
5. van der Burg, M.E.L., van Lent, M., Buyse, M. *et al.* (1995) The effect of debulking surgery after induction chemotherapy on the prognosis in advanced epithelial ovarian cancer. *N. Engl. J. Med.* 332, 629-34.
6. Griffiths, C.T., Park, L.M., Fuller, A.F. (1979) Role of cytoreductive surgical therapy in the management of advanced ovarian cancer. *Cancer Treat. Rep.* 63, 235-40.
7. Hacker, N.F., Berek, J.S., Lagasse, L.D. *et al.* (1983) Primary cytoreductive surgery for epithelial ovarian cancer. *Obstet. Gynecol.* 61, 413-20.
8. Hoskins, W.J., Bundy, B.N., Thigpen, J.T. *et al.* (1992) The incidence of cytoreductive surgery on recurrence free interval and survival in small-volume stage III epithelial ovarian cancer, a Gynecologic Oncology Group study. *Gynecol. Oncol.* 47, 159-66.
9. Heintz, A.P.M., van Oosterom, A.T., Trimbos, J.B.M.C. *et al.* (1988) The treatment of advanced ovarian carcinoma (1) Clinical variables associated with prognosis. *Gynecol. Oncol.* 30, 347-58.
10. Farias-Eisner, R., Oliviera, M., Teng, F. *et al.* (1992) The influence of tumor

distribution number and size after optimal primary cytoreductive surgery for epithelial ovarian cancer. Abstract, *Gynecol. Oncol.* **46**, 267.

11. Serbouti, S., Neijt, J., ten Bokkel Huinink, W. *et al.* (1994) Neural network analysis to predict treatment outcome in patients with gynecologic cancer. *Found. Neur. Net.* Report **10**.

12. Eisenkop, S., Nalick, R. and Teng, N. (1992) Peritoneal implant excision or ablation during cytoreductive surgery. The impact on survival. Abstract, *Gynecol. Oncol.* **45**, 97.

13. Hunter, R.W., Alexander, N.D.E. and Soutter, W.P. (1992) Meta-analysis of surgery in advanced ovarian carcinoma: Is maximum cytoreductive surgery an independent determinant on prognosis? *Am. J. Obstet. Gynecol.* **166**, 504-11.

14. Hacker, N.F., Wain, G.V. and Trimbos, J.P. (1992) *Management and outcome of stage III epithelial ovarian cancer.* Chapman & Hall Medical, London, pp 351-6.

15. Schwartz, P.E., Chambers, J.T., Kohorn, E.I. *et al.* (1989) Tamoxifen in combination with cytotoxic chemotherapy in advanced epithelial ovarian cancer. A prospective randomized study. *Cancer* **63**, 1074-9.

16. Burghardt, E., Girardi, F., Lahousen, M. *et al.* (1991) Patterns of pelvic and para-aortic lymph node involvement in ovarian cancer. *Obstet. Gynecol.* **40**, 103-106.

Chapter 11

Interventional surgery

John M. MONAGHAN

11.1 INTRODUCTION

Interventional surgery in patients with advanced ovarian cancer includes not only the immediate re-exploration in patients whose initial operation was incomplete, but also the secondary operations, interval debulking operations, secondary debulking and palliative intervention for progressive disease, especially operations for the correction of intestinal obstruction. The impact of these operations on patient outcome and survival is less well understood than that of primary operations. While it is generally accepted that a maximal primary debulking operation is associated with an improved survival [1], the role of these secondary surgeries remains controversial. Their purpose is to intervene when the effects of chemotherapy have been incomplete or unsuccessful. However, if primary and metastatic tumours were not removed at the first surgery, either because of the sheer extent of disease or because of the inexperience or inability of the surgeon, then a subsequent attempt might be appropriate and theoretically beneficial in some patients.

Retrospective analyses have shown the limited value of intervention debulking surgery (i.e. secondary cytoreductive surgery) when performed at the end of a full chemotherapy course [2]. However, in a pilot study that analysed interval debulking surgery performed after an initial several cycles of chemotherapy, a high proportion (89%) of tumours became optimally resectable although they were unresected or thought to be unresectable at the first surgery [3]. Whilst this experience sought to demonstrate the technical feasibility of these operations and not an improvement in survival, other studies have shown mixed results from interval and secondary debulking surgery [4]. Attempts at tumour resection have not always been aggressive.

In an analysis of patient care in the United States between 1983 and 1988, it was found that patients presenting with ovarian cancer had the ovaries removed in 80% of cases. A total abdominal hysterectomy was performed in only 50%, omentectomy in 60%, node sampling in 23% and optimal debulking (i.e. removal of tumour to less than 2 cm maximum diameter of residual disease) in only 52% of patients. Interestingly 18% of these patients had had previous total abdominal hysterectomy. Only 25% of patients had had adequate surgical staging. Clearly, there are major difficulties in achieving initial optimal debulking, the inevitable consequence being that many patients will present for chemotherapy with significant amounts of residual disease. Thus, a strategy for subsequent intervention must be developed, and these interventional surgeries need to be carefully scrutinized and their indications properly categorized.

111

11.2 TYPES OF INTERVENTIONAL SURGERY

Interventional surgery for patients with advanced stage epithelial ovarian cancer falls into four general categories [5]:

1. Re-exploration immediately after incomplete or failed primary surgery.
2. Interval debulking performed in patients who undergo several cycles of chemotherapy after an incomplete primary surgery.
3. Secondary debulking performed at the completion of a complete course of chemotherapy.
4. Palliative operations for progressive disease associated with symptoms, typically intestinal obstruction.

11.3 RE-OPERATION FOLLOWING INADEQUATE PRIMARY SURGERY

Approximately 25% of patients with ovarian cancer are operated on by general surgeons who tend to have a sceptical view of the value of debulking surgery in patients who appear to have widespread peritoneal cancer. This scepticism exists principally because the pattern of growth of intestinal cancer is such that it is not amenable to debulking surgery. Uniquely, ovarian cancer spreads along the surfaces of the intestinal serosa rather than invading the lumina of the intestines as do primary carcinomas of intestinal origin. This growth pattern permits debulking of tumours that have metastasized throughout the peritoneal cavity. Because most general gynaecologists are not trained to effectively perform debulking operations, routine resection of the pelvic tumour and upper abdominal disease may not be done even though it is indicated. In those patients when there has not been an adequate attempt to debulk the cancer, a gynaecological oncologist must decide whether a second operation should be done immediately or after a period of induction chemotherapy.

One of the potentially most valuable roles of early re-operation is the assessment and performance of lymphadenectomy which has been perported to produce a survival advantage in patients with advanced ovarian cancer [6–8]. However, there have been considerable reservations expressed about the role of lymphadenectomy, the most critical being that patients who are amenable to the performance of a full radical lymphadenectomy, by the very nature of their cancer pattern may have a survival advantage [4]. Furthermore, the patients in whom it is impossible to perform satisfactory lymphadenectomy are those who, because of the nature of their disease, have extensive disease throughout the peritoneal cavity. There is currently a multinational randomized trial underway to determine if radical lymphadenectomy actually improves survival.

11.4 INTERVAL DEBULKING SURGERY

The theoretic rationale for interval debulking is the same as that for primary debulking, *i.e.* to reduce the residual tumour to minimal residual disease in order to facilitate a response to chemotherapy and a prolongation in survival. While tumours that have incompletely responded may be inherently insensitive to chemotherapy, and it is logical to change chemotherapy to a different regimen, interval bulk reduction may theoretically facilitate the response to the subsequent treatment. It is often a difficult decision to immediately re-explore some patients who have had an incomplete initial operation as an alternative to giving 'induction' chemotherapy followed by an interval debulking.

Interventional debulking surgery should be done by a gynaecological oncologist skilled in the performance of retroperitoneal dissections and in the performance of bowel resection and by-pass procedures [4]. It is essential that, prior to any surgical procedure, where there is the possibility of bowel resection or formation of a colostomy, the risks associated with such surgery have to be outlined clearly to the patient who understands these risks and is prepared to accept them.

One of the few randomized studies to determine whether interventional debulking surgery improves survival in patients with advanced ovarian cancer who have greater that 2cm residual disease after primary surgery was done by Redman *et al.* in 1994 [9]. Although this study showed a slight survival advantage in the group that had initial chemotherapy followed by interval debulking, the differences in the two groups were not statistically significant. However, a recent EORTC study suggested that interval debulking may actually improve survival [10]. In this study, progression-free and overall survival were both significantly lower in the group that underwent interval debulking surgery. The results of this randomized prospective trial convincingly demonstrate that debulking surgery can reduce the risk of death from advanced cancer. Furthermore, while these data are encouraging, it is likely that a primary debulking would produce an even greater decrement in the risk of death [5].

11.5 SECONDARY DEBULKING SURGERY

Patients with advanced ovarian cancer have tended to undergo at least two operations during the course of their disease treatment. In addition to the primary surgery performed to stage, resect and debulk the disease, secondary operations may be necessary. As new chemotherapeutic agents were being introduced over the past two decades, it was felt necessary to perform a surgical assessment of response. 'Second-look' surgery was used extensively and demonstrated its value in identifying the responses to chemotherapy.

Frequently, patients who were undergoing second-look surgery had further interventional surgery when it was thought to be technically feasible; these were initially called 'second-chance' procedures but later became known as 'secondary debulking' surgery. However, the

role and value of secondary debulking interventional operations remains controversial [5]. For the patient who has a persistent visible or palpable mass after chemotherapy, the removal of the mass might be beneficial. The use of debulking surgery in patients at the time of correction of intestinal obstruction can be of value in carefully selected patients when the obstruction is caused by focal lesions and not by diffuse carcinomatosis.

An important indication for secondary surgical intervention is in patients with persistent mucinous tumours associated with pseudo myxoma peritonei. These tumours tend to grow slowly and are often associated with normal serum CA125 levels. Patients often present with extensive recurrent disease and intervention debulking surgery can extend survival even though patients will ultimately succumb to their disease. The management of pseudomyxoma peritonei was reviewed by Carter *et al.* [11] who concluded that, although this condition is generally accepted to be a benign disease, its frequent association in the majority of cases with a malignant primary tumour requires intermittent surgical intervention to maintain the quality of life. The five year survival is 68% with a ten year survival of 52%. The mainstay of treatment remains complete surgical debulking at the initial presentation followed by palliative interventional debulking for symptomatic relief as needed.

11.6 MANAGEMENT OF RISING CA125

There are many patients in whom a tumour marker (*e.g.* CA125) may be slightly elevated without clear evidence of tumour recurrence as demonstrated by radiological or clinical examination, which are relatively insensitive. The clinician may be presented with a tumour marker which was initially normal and is now rising. It is not certain what the best strategy should be in these situations. In general, if a measurable tumour is detected on pelvic examination or CT scan, the persistent or recurrent tumour appears to be resectable and diffuse carcinomatosis is not detected, then the patient should be considered a candidate for a secondary resection of her disease. With a rising CA125 level, it is not appropriate to routinely perform a laparotomy to determine what is happening to the patient.

An alternative surgical approach for the evaluation of these patients is to use laparoscopy. This approach can be facilitated by the use of techniques such as the Hassan open laparoscopy technique or with Visaport® (US Surgical). In some patients, these techniques allow the evaluation of the contents of the abdominal cavity and clearer decisions can then be made as to the role and application of intervention debulking. Using the laparoscope, peritoneal cytology can be obtained, tissue can be sampled and a determination of the patient's tumour status can be made. While there is a theoretical risk of tumour implantation in port sites, it is uncertain if this phenomenon, when it does occur, worsens prognosis.

11.7 PALLIATIVE SURGICAL INTERVENTION

Palliative intervention surgery clearly has a role in patients where there is evidence of obstruction. By-pass procedures can both improve the quality of life and perhaps prolong survival in carefully selected patients . In some patients who have isolated recurrences, such as in the pelvis, resection of tumour is often feasible and can improve outcome [4].

Often the patients who are most amenable to palliative bowel surgery are those where the tumour is slow growing, and is causing obstruction by local pressure rather than invasion. Thus, these patients tend to live longer and are suitable for intestinal resection and by-pass procedures. Some patients live for many years following palliative interventional surgery with a very much better quality of life.

11.8 THE PATIENT AND HER FAMILY

Although the patient may not be a good candidate for surgery there is often pressure from the family to undertake surgical intervention. Indeed, the decision to operate or not is difficult. The clinician has to balance the value of interventional surgery against the prospect of hastening her demise. If the surgeon determines that the likelihood of benefit is low, then he must clearly present this to the patient and her family. If surgery is performed, care must be taken to minimize the morbidity and the procedure should be discontinued if it becomes obvious that the operative objectives cannot be met.

11.9 CONCLUSIONS

One of the great challenges with ovarian cancer is a product of the wide range of surgeons who operate on these women, as well as the variable chemotherapeutic regimens that are used. Probably the most important factor is the enormous variability of individual patients. A meta-analyses suggested that our initial premise that maximal debulking is the cornerstone of survival in ovarian cancer is questionable [12]. Because of the positive result from the interval debulking trial, which is a randomized prospective study, we can now conclude that debulking surgery is essential for the proper treatment of women with advanced ovarian cancer. Until we have more uniform and aggressive primary surgical procedures being done and until our primary chemotherapies are more successful and 'curative', we must better define a strategy and guidelines for the use of all interventional surgeries. The key to success will now be the more widespread application of appropriate surgical techniques to maximize patient outcome.

REFERENCES

1. Griffiths, C.T. (1975) Surgical resection of tumor bulk in the primary treatment of

ovarian carcinoma. *Monogr. Nat. Cancer Inst..* **42**, 101-4

2. Luesley, D.M., Lawton, F.G., Blackledge, G. *et al.* (1988) Failure of second look laparotomy to influence survival in epithelial ovarian cancer *Lancet* **ii**, 599-603.

3. Lawton, F.G., Redman, C.W.E., Luesley, D.M. *et al.* (1989) Neoadjuvant (cytoreductive) chemotherapy combined with intervention debulking surgery in advanced unresected epithelial ovarian cancer. *Obstet. Gynecol.* **73**, 61-5.

4. Monaghan, J.M. (1989) Surgical Techniques used in achieving optimal resection of stage III cancer of the ovaries. In *Operative Treatment of Ovarian Cancer, Clinic in Obstetrics and Gynaecology* (eds. E. Burghardt and J.M.Monaghan), Bailliere Tindall, London.

5. Berek, J.S. (1995) Interval debulking of ovarian cancer - an interim measure. *N. Engl. J. Med.* **332**, 675-7.

6. Burghardt, E., Pickel, O., Lahousen, M. and Stettner, H. (1986) Pelvic lymphadenectomy in operative treatment of ovarian cancer. *Am. J. Obstet. Gynecol.* **155**, 315.

7. di Re, F., Fontanelli, F., Raspagliesi, F. and di Re, E. (1989) Pelvic and paraaortic lymphadenectomy in cancer of the ovary.In *Operative Treatment of Ovarian Cancer, Clinics in Obstetrics and Gynaecology* (eds E. Burghardt and J.M. Monaghan), Bailliere Tindall, London.

8. Wu, P.C., Qu, J.Y., Lang, J.H. *et al.* (1986) Lymph node metastasis of ovarain cancer. A preliminary survery of **74** cases of lymphadenectomy. *Am. J. Obstet Gynecol.* **155**, 1103.

9. Redman, C.W.E., Warwick, J., Leusley, D.M. *et al.* (1994) Intervention debulking surgery in advanced epithelial ovarian cancer. *Br. J. Obstet. Gynaecol.* **101**, 142-6.

10. van der Burg, M.E.L., van Lent, M., Buyse, M. *et al.* (1995) The effect of debulking surgery after induction chemotherapy on the prognosis in advanced epithelial ovarian cancer *N. Engl. J. Med.* **332**, 629-34.

11. Carter, J., Carson, L.F., Moradi, M.M. *et al.* (1991) Pseudomixoma peritonei, a review. *Int. J. Gynecol. Cancer* **1**, 243-7.

12. Hunter, R.W., Alexander, N.D.E. and Soutter, W.P. (1992) Meta-analysis of surgery in advanced ovarian carcinoma, is maximum cytoreductive surgery an independent determinant on prognosis? *Am. J. Obstet. Gynecol.* **166**, 504-11.

Chapter 12

Immediate post-surgical tumour growth

Sean KEHOE, Peter VAN GEENE, Kim WARD, David LUESLEY

and K.K. CHAN

12.1 INTRODUCTION

The concept that surgical trauma influences residual tumour proliferation has corroborative evidence from animal and now human studies. It is accepted as fact that normal tissues respond to trauma by the initiation of repair mechanisms which include tissue growth. As malignant cells have abnormal growth patterns intuition would suggest that similar, or indeed excessive, proliferative responses would result from trauma. This concept has received little attention even with the knowledge, for some time, from animal studies linking trauma and enhanced tumour growth [1]. In a clinical trial by Fielding and Wells [2] examining two- *versus* one-stage operations for excision of colonic carcinomas, a poorer survival was recorded in those undergoing two-stage procedures. This lead the authors to hypothesize enhanced growth and metastatic potential of residual tumour subsequent to the primary operation as a potential cause of reduced survival patterns.

In ovarian carcinoma, primary intervention consists of surgery. This permits histological confirmation and staging of disease, along with tumour resection. The removal of all macroscopic tumour affords cure for many patients with early stage disease. Most patients though, present with widespread disease rendering complete excision of all visible tumour impossible. If residual tumour is affected by surgery, then investigating this area further could lead to a greater understanding of tumour biology, possibly influence our present concepts in respect of surgery, and direct the introduction of new therapeutic modalities. The bulk of evidence indicating that increased tumour proliferation follows surgery is from animal studies, though recent work in our laboratory on patients with ovarian carcinoma would corroborate the findings from such models.

12.2 EVIDENCE FROM ANIMAL STUDIES

A variety of animal experiments are reported in the literature employing different tumour cells and methods of determining cellular proliferation. It is pertinent to review some of this work. Excision of the primary tumour in C57BL/6 mice injected subcutaneously (s.c.) with Lewis lung carcinoma cells resulted in larger spontaneous lung tumours (as measured by callipers), when compared to controls [3]. In the same study, evaluation of cell kinetics by thymidine indices (TI) revealed that in control mice TI levels of lung nodules fell from 0.37 on day 17 following implantation to 0.26 on day 31. In those mice exposed to surgical removal of the primary tumours on day 14, TI levels in lung nodules rose on day 16 and only reduced to 0.48 by day 30. Even surgical insult, without tumour excision, influenced TI levels, with the indices in both primary tumours and lung metastases elevated. TI levels of lung nodules in this latter study rose to 0.55 on the fourth post-operative day, the highest index achievable in such studies, indicating the important impact of trauma.

More relevant to ovarian cancer are studies addressing intraperitoneal tumour growth. Tumour deposits developed in 89% of Fischer rats following intraperitoneal inoculation with colonic cancer cells at laparotomy. This compares with only 47% developing deposits with injection and no surgery, indicating again that factors related to trauma assist in malignant cell growth [4]. It was also noted by the authors, that anaesthesia played a role in enhancing tumour proliferation, though exposing the rats to repeated surgery resulted in a proportional increase in tumour growth. Others reported similar findings using C57BL/6 mice, and MCA-105 sarcoma and B16 melanoma cell lines placed intraperitoneally [5]. Numerical evaluation of peritoneal deposits was undertaken following a laparotomy, splenectomy, sham surgery and skin incisions. The conclusion from this work was that any incision of the peritoneal cavity increased the number of peritoneal deposits, irrespective of the surgery undertaken. Skin trauma alone did not affect tumour deposition. The authors also noted that the response persisted for some days. When mice were inoculated four days after surgery, enhanced growth occurred, though the effect ceased if inoculation was 14 days after surgery. The timing coincides with the duration of tissue repair, and it was found that scar tissue was particularly receptive to malignant cell deposition.

If factors involved in repair mechanisms

are important in inducing tumour growth, then scar tissue would seem an ideal site for metastatic deposition. Skipper et al. . [6] have investigated this by injecting syngeneic MC 28 sarcoma cells and OES5 breast carcinoma cells into the hearts of hooded Lister rats. When incision and repair of a section of colon was undertaken, preferential tumour growth occurred at these sites. The maximum effect was during the second to eighth post-operative days, peaking between days five and seven. Subsequent work from the same group [7], found greater growth at damaged sites following both intraperitoneal and intraluminal colonic injections. The probability of intracardiac injected cells depositing and developing tumour nodules in damaged tissue was estimated to be 1000 times more likely as compared to such an occurrence in normal tissue. One can only surmise as to whether these influences partly explain tumour growth reported to occur at trocar sites when a laparoscope is used in patients with intraperitoneal malignancies [8].

A multiplicity of factors are probably involved. The suppression of fibrinogen-related proteins present in wound sites with plasminogen activators decreases malignant cell deposition at areas of hepatic damage in mice [9]. Angiogenic factors also seem to have a role in regulating metastatic tumour proliferation. Recent work by Holmgren et al. [10] on C57BL6/J mice inoculated with Lewis lung carcinoma, found that metastases grew after excision of the primary tumour. The interesting finding in this report is that bromodeoxyuridine (BrdU) labelling and proliferating cell nuclear antigen (PCNA) revealed similar levels in growing metastases and those from controls, but that the apoptotic indices were 75% lower in the growing metastases. Treating the metastases with angiogenic inhibitors maintained metastases in a dormant phase. The group postulated that excision of the primary tumour interfered with angiogenesis, altering the balance between apoptosis and proliferation in metastases.

Yet another variable in the complex picture of malignant proliferative response to surgery is the inherent biology of the tumour itself. When Wag/Rij rats were subcutaneously inoculated with different tumours – MCR 83 (a slow growing mammary tumour), EMR86 (a fast growing mammary tumour) and MCR 86 (a rapidly but autonomously growing carcinoma) – the responses were notably different [11]. Removal of the bulk of primary tumour in MCR83 cases caused increased proliferation of residual and distant metastases (estimated by BrdU). Sham surgery had no effect. The increase in BrdU labelling in metastases commenced 33 hours following primary tumour resection and persisted until the seventh post-operative day. EMR 86 tumours responded earlier with increased proliferation detected 33 hours post-operatively, and also maintained for the seven days. Again no significant response to sham surgery was noted. The response in the MCR 86 model was enhanced metastatic proliferation achieved with both primary tumour removal and sham surgery. This proliferation lasted for four days, followed by a fall in BrdU levels.

All these animal studies have employed the spectrum of acceptable tumour growth measurements and concur that surgical insult enhances residual tumour proliferation. The consistent finding that the response approximates with the period of maximum tissue healing, with injured sites particularly susceptible to deposition, strongly suggests the involvement of factors responsible for healing. The impact of injury on the host must also be considered, in particular the immunosuppressive response to injury [12]. A reduction in metastases has been recorded in mice when the cell-mediated immune system is stimulated after surgery [13], and

indeed in patients with colonic cancer such therapy has been introduced to ameliorate surgery-induced immunosuppression [14].

12.3 OVARIAN CARCINOMA

The evidence from animal studies indicating that surgery enhances residual tumour growth is convincing. In an ideal world, assessing residual tumour kinetics in humans as performed in animal models, would give more conclusive answers as to whether or not surgical trauma affected tumour growth. The tendency for ovarian cancer to remain confined to the intra-peritoneal environment, a region easily accessible, makes collection of peritoneal fluid, and at least limited evaluation of residual tumour cell dynamics, possible. We undertook studies to examine any changes within malignant peritoneal cells, following primary surgical intervention. A further study addressed the influence of peritoneal fluids on tumour growth.

12.4 EVALUATION OF INTRA-PERITONEAL ANEUPLOID POPULATIONS FOLLOWING PRIMARY SURGERY

The initial studies undertaken in our centre, involved flow cytometric DNA analysis of aneuploid cells in malignant peritoneal fluids [15]. Work from others has shown that increasing S-Phase fractions of ascitic aneuploid cells in patients with relapsed disease correlates with poorer survival [16], supporting the application of this methodology. Aneuploid cells were specifically targeted as they are a well recognized subgroup of malignant cells. Diploid malignant cells do occur but attempting to incorporate this population would result in the inclusion of normal cells with the possibility of error therefore being increased. Ethical approval and informed consent was obtained for the study; 43 patients with histologically proven ovarian

Table 12.1 Patient Characteristics

Malignant		Number	Control		Number
Total number		43	**Total number**		20
Age	Mean 59 years (range 41-81)		**Age**	Mean 50 yrs (range 36-87)	
Stage			**Indication**		
	I	5		Ovarian cyst	
	II	2		(ascites = 2, both < 1l)	12
	III	32		Fibroids	4
	IV	4		Dysfunctional uterine	
Histology				bleeding	4
	Serous	16	**Histology**		
	Mucinous	4		Serous cystadenoma	6
	Carcinosarcoma	2		Mucinous cystadenoma	5
	Endometrioid	4		Fibroma	1
	Clear cell	1		Fibroids	4
	Mixed Müllerian	1		Normal findings (occasional	
	Adenocarcinoma (unspec.)	15		patches ademomyosis)	4
Differentiation			**Procedure**		
	Borderline	3		TAH, BSO, omentectomy	11
	Well	7		BSO, omentectomy	1
	Moderate	12		TAH, BSO	8
	Poor	13			
	Unknown	8			
Procedure					
	TAH, BSO, omentectomy	21			
	Oophoectomy, biopsy	22			
Residual Tumour					
	No residual tumour	11			
	< 2 cms (max. diameter)	9			
	> 2 cms (max. diameter)	23			
Ascites					
	None	14	**NB:**		
	< 5 lit.	14	TAH = total abdominal hysterectomy		
	> 5 lit.	15	BSO = bilateral salpingo-oophorectomy		

carcinoma and a control group of twenty patients were enrolled. The patient characteristics are shown in Table 12.1. The first specimen was collected at incision of the peritoneal cavity. On completion of the appropriate surgical procedure, a wide bore drain was left in the abdomen, with the tip placed on the pelvic floor. Samples were obtained each morning prior to 09:00h, by flushing the cavity with normal saline and collecting as clear a sample as possible. As circadian proliferation is reported to occur in ovarian cancer [17], the time of sampling was kept constant. Specimens were freshly analysed using propidium iodide staining on a flow cytometer (Coulter EPICS Profile II). All samples were coded to permit blinded analysis. The coefficient of variation (CV) was ≤ 5% in all the specimens. CV values greater than this were considered inaccurate and excluded. The operative sample (day 0) acted as the control for each patient and subsequent samples compared with this using the Wilcoxson signed rank test and corrected t-test.

Three patients with malignancy had only diploid cells detected and were excluded from the analyses. As is evident in Figure 12.1, an increase in aneuploid populations occurred following surgery, reaching a significant level (p<0.008) on the fourth day. S-phase fraction was assessable in 37/40 patients with ovarian cancer. Three patients were excluded as accurate estimate of S-phase was not possible, due to the proximity of aneuploid and diploid peaks. S-phase fraction levels fell significantly on the first post-operative day (p<0.02), followed by a continuing non-significant rise in the values (Figure 12.2). Seven patients in the control population had aneuploid cells detected on day 0 and in three of these, aneuploid cell patterns were similar to those of patients with ovarian cancer. Interestingly two of these patients had ovarian cysts with benign ascitic fluid.

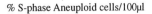

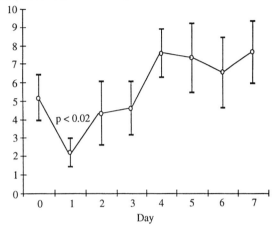

Figure 12.2 Mean S-phase of aneuploid cells (n=32; day 0=control day, subsequent results compared with this).

To determine the presence of malignant cells in specimens examined, cytological evaluation was undertaken and in the malignant group 79% had tumour cells present at levels of 30% or more. Cytological investigations of the control samples were all negative. When the patients were grouped depending on residual tumour load, the greatest increase in aneuploid cells was found in those with no macroscopic tumour (Figure 12.3). Whether this reflects tumours with differing inherent biology remains to be confirmed or refuted as the presently insufficient numbers prevent statistical analysis.

12.5 SERIAL CELL FREE PERITONEAL FLUIDS AND GROWTH OF PRIMARY TUMOUR EXTRACTS

Assuming that intraperitoneal fluids could contain stimulatory factors a second study, examining the influence of serial post-operative cell free peritoneal fluids on

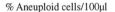

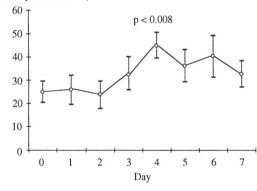

Figure 12.1 Mean aneuploid population (n=40; day 0=control day, subsequent results compared with this).

% Aneuploid cells/100µl

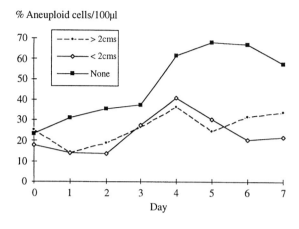

Figure 12.3 Mean aneuploid count and residual disease.

Table 12.2 Patient Characteristics

Malignant population (n=10)
Mean age = 58 (28-81) yrs
Stage III = 10
Histology:
Serous = 7
Mucinous = 3

Control population (n=7)
Mean Age = 50 (37-69) yrs
Histology:
Leiomyoma = 2
CIN III = 1
DUB = 4

DUB = dysfunctional uterine bleeding

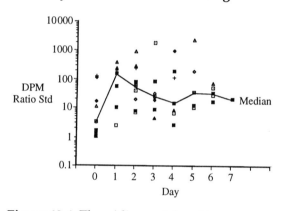

Figure 12.4 Thymidine uptake of tumours.

tumour explants, was embarked upon to investigate any variations in stimulatory effect with time.

The collection of peritoneal fluid specimens in this study was performed as described above. Explants of the primary tumour were exposed to these peritoneal fluids. Cell kinetics were evaluated by tritiated thymidine incorporation [18].

Results are available on seventeen patients, ten with ovarian cancer and seven control patients (Table 12.2). Explants from primary tumour tissue obtained at surgery were prepared and grown for nine days until 80% confluent and then quiesced for three days. Serial peritoneal fluid specimens were collected each morning until the seventh post-operative day in ovarian cancer patients and the fifth day in controls. Fluid samples were spun down and passed through Ficoll hypaque and through step-wise procedures the tumour cells and lymphocytes were removed resulting in a cell free suspension. These samples were then standardized for protein content. The prepared specimens

were kept on ice until the tumour explants were ready.

Tumour explants prepared from at least 10 000 cells were exposed to 100µl of the cell free suspension. After 16 hours, tritiated thymidine incorporation was undertaken followed by cell harvesting for 24 hours. A scintillation counter measured the radioactive content in the tumour cells. Statistical methods employed were the Wilcoxson sign rank test, with the sample at operation acting as control for each patient.

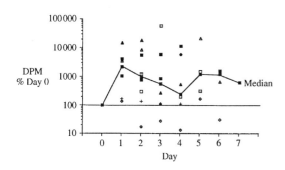

Figure 12.5 Thymidine uptake of tumours as percentage of day 0 values.

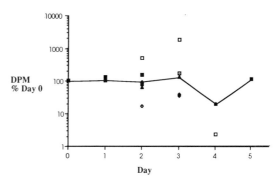

Figure 12.7 Thymidine uptake of controls as percentage of day 0 values.

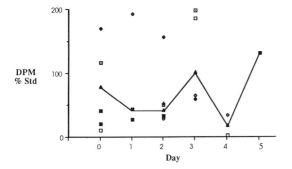

Figure 12.6 Thymidine uptake of controls.

These early investigations suggest that factors present in the peritoneal fluids are responsible for inducing growth of primary tumour cell explants. As the effect was seen only in fluids from patients with ovarian cancer the source of these factor(s) would seem to be malignant cells. Continued work in this area is attempting to target possible causative factors.

12.6 CONCLUSIONS

The conclusion from these original experiments, which attempted to evaluate the response of residual intraperitoneal malignant cells to surgery, suggest that the proliferative activity of these cells is enhanced by factors within the peritoneal fluids. Their source would seem to be malignant cells, though exactly what they are needs to be identified. Further research and advances in methodology should expand the information available from *in vivo* models. Even accepting the present inherent faults, the studies support those found in animals. Other variables which are probably involved include blood transfusion [19] or the host immune suppression following surgery [20]. Indeed we have investigated cellular immunity in ovarian cancer and noted a reduction intra-peritoneal cellular immune

The median uptake of tumour cells exposed to peritoneal fluids from patients with ovarian cancer is shown in Figure 12.4, and described as a percentage of the control value in Figure 12.5. Post-operative values rose compared with the day 0 (operation) value, with a significant peak on day 1 (p=0.014).

The single patient with values persistently below the control level had undergone insertion of a Tenkhoff catheter. Explanations for the finding could be the lack of interference with any tumour or the fact that the patient had relapsed disease. Exposure of tumour explants to fluids from control patients did not impact on proliferative response (Figures 12.6 and 12.7).

components coinciding with the duration of increased aneuploid populations [21]. Although many questions require addressing prior to a complete understanding of the findings presented, this does not detract from the potential clinical application of the results. A time of high proliferative activity renders malignant cells more susceptible to cytotoxic agents, and cell kinetic-based therapy could be considered. Similarly, host immune stimulation may diminish the probability on residual malignant cells escaping surveillance. These are but two theoretical outcomes to the present findings, and hopefully ongoing research will reveal novel aspects of tumour biology and advance therapeutic strategies.

ACKNOWLEDGEMENTS

Permission for reproduction of some of the information in this chapter, along with Table 12.1 and Figures 12.1–12.3 was given by the Editor-in-Chief of the International Journal of Gynecological Cancer.

S. Kehoe was supported by the Cancer Research Campaign, and P. van Geene by Birthright.

REFERENCES

1. Deelman, H.T. (1927) The part played by injury and repair in the development of cancer. *BMJ* **1**, 827.
2. Fielding, L.P. and Wells, B.W. (1974) Survival after primary and after staged resection for larger bowel obstruction caused by cancer. *Br. J. Surg.* **61**, 16-8.
3. Simpson-Herren, L., Sanford, H.S. and Holmquist J.P. (1976) Effects of surgery on cell kinetics of residual tumour. *Cancer Treat. Rep.* **60**, 1749-60.
4. Weese, J.L., Ottery, F.D.and Emoto, S.E. (1986) Do operations facilitate tumour growth? An experimental model in rats. *Surgery* **100**, 273-6.
5. Eggermont, A. M., Steller, E. P. and Sugarbaker, P.H. (1987) Laparotomy enhances intraperitoneal tumour growth and abrogates the antitumour effects of interleukin-2 and lymphokine-activated killer cells. *Surgery* **102**, 71-8.
6. Skipper, D., Jeffrey, M.J., Cooper, A.J. and Alexander, P. (1988) Preferential growth of blood-borne cancer cells in colonic anastomoses. *Br. J. Cancer* **57**, 564-68.
7. Skipper, D., Jeffery, M.J., Cooper, A.J. *et al.* (1989) Enhanced growth of tumour cells in healing colonic anastomoses and laparotomy wounds. *Int. J. Colorectal Dis.* **4**, 172-7.
8. Nduka, C.C., Monson, J.R.T., Menzies-Gow, N. and Darzi, A.(1994) Abdominal wall metastases following laparoscopy. *Br. J .Surg.* **81**, 648-52.
9. Murthy, M.S., Summaria, L.J., Miller R.J. *et al.* (1991) Inhibition of tumour implantation at sites of trauma by plasminogen activators. *Cancer* **68**, 1724-30.
10. Holmgren, L., O'Reilly, M.S. and Folkman, J. (1995) Dormancy of micrometastases, Balanced proliferation and apoptosis in the presence of angiogenesis suppression *Nat. Med.* **1**, 149-53.
11. Van Dierendonck, J.H., Keijzer, R., Cornelisse, C.J. and Van De Velde, C.J.H. (1991) Surgically induced cytokinetic responses in experimental rat mammary tumour models. *Cancer* **68**, 759-67.
12. Lundy, J., Lovett, E.J., Hamilton, S. and Conran, P. (1978) Halothane, surgery, immunosuppression and artificial pulmonary metastases. *Cancer* **41**, 827-30.
13. Lundy, J., Lovett, E.J., Hamilton, S. and Conran, P. (1979) Immune impairment and metastatic tumour growth. *Cancer* **43**, 945-51.
14. Deehan, D.J., Heys, S.D., Simpson, W. *et al.* (1995) Modulation of the cytokine and acute-phase response to major surgery by

recombinant interleukin-2. *Br. J. Surg.* **82,** 86-90.

15. Kehoe, S., Ward, K., Luesley, D. and Chan, K.K. (1995) *In vivo* evidence of increased malignant cell proliferation following surgery in ovarian cancer. *Int. J. Gynecol. Cancer* **5,** 121-7.

16. Sahni, K., Tribukait, B and Einhorn, N. (1990) Development of ploidy and cell proliferation in serial samples of ascites from patients with ovarian carcinoma. *Acta. Oncol.* **29,** 193-7.

17. Klevecz, R.R. and Braly, P.S. (1991) Circadian and ultradian cytokinetic rhythms of spontaneous human cancer. *Ann. N.Y. Acad . Sci.* **618,** 257-76.

18. Van Geene, P., Kehoe, S. and Luesley, D.(1994) Proliferative response of tumour explants exposed to peritoneal fluids from ovarian cancer patients. *Proceedings of the Blair Bell Meeting, October 1994.*

19. McGehee, R.P., Dodson, M.K., Moore, *et al.* (1994) Effect of blood transfusion in patients with gynecologic malignancy. *Int. J. Gynecol. Obstet .* **46,** 45-52.

20. Lennard, T.W.J., Shenton, B.K., Borzotta, A. *et al.* (1985) The influence of surgical operations on components of the human immune system. *Br. J. Surg.* **72,** 771-6.

21. Kehoe, S. (1995) Cellular immunity and immunotherapy in ovarian cancer. *Int. J. Oncol.* **6,** 451-8.

Part Three

Optimizing Treatment
II - Chemotherapy

Chapter 13

Serum CA125 to define response

Gordon J.S. RUSTIN, Anne NELSTROP and Patrick McCLEAN

13.1 INTRODUCTION

Assessment of response to cancer therapy is an essential part of care and a major endpoint in clinical research. Precise definitions have been produced by the World Health Organisation (WHO) and the Eastern Co-operative Oncology Group (ECOG) [1,2] which are accepted by the regulatory authorities when evaluating a new anticancer agent. These definitions rely upon measurable tumours. Unfortunately most patients with advanced ovarian carcinoma have disease which cannot be adequately monitored by computer tomography (CT) or by ultrasound (U/S) scans. However over 90% of these women have an elevated level of serum CA125 [3]. Falling levels of this marker have been shown to be associated with response and rising levels with progression [4]. Serial CA125 measurements are used by many to monitor ovarian cancer patients and, therefore, precise definitions of response using serum CA125 are necessary. If accurate enough, CA125 could be accepted as another method to measure response. We describe how definitions for response using CA125 have been derived and how they compare to standard response criteria.

13.2 REQUIREMENTS OF CA125 BASED DEFINITION

Proposed definitions were produced with the following considerations:
1. The definition needs to have similarities to the standard criteria such as maintenance of response for one month.
2. There needs to be a minimal number of three CA125 measurements. If only two measurements are made, one could be falsely high or low due to factors such as laboratory error, inflammation, influence of surgery or tumour lysis
3. The definition needs to be easy enough to be used in the clinic but precise enough for clinical trials.
4. It needs to be sensitive enough to be applicable to at least 50% of patients, but specific enough so that it produces a false positive prediction of response in less than 10% of patients.

Several definitions were considered but discarded:
1. Complete tumour marker response was discarded for two reasons. Some patients with advanced ovarian carcinoma have substantial volumes of active tumour but normal CA125 levels. Also, it would be inappropriate to place into the same complete response group a patient whose CA125 levels had fallen from just above the upper limit of normal to within the normal range, with a patient whose levels had fallen from several thousand U/ml to the normal range.
2. The measurement of a serial decrease in CA125 without a specified percentage is not precise enough. Serial determinations of CA125 based on regression analysis are too complicated to be practical in the clinic.

129

3. A log fall in the CA125 levels was discarded because it automatically excluded all patients whose initial CA125 value was less than ten times the upper limit of normal. We also found that fewer than a third of all patients with a clear-cut, sustained fall of CA125 levels, actually had a fall to less than 10% of the initial level.

13.3 DEFINITIONS OF RESPONSE ACCORDING TO CA125

The definitions of CA125 response were initially produced after analysing serial CA125 levels from 277 patients in the North Thames Ovary Trial '3' which consisted of five courses of carboplatin followed by whole abdominal irradiation or five further courses of carboplatin (Trial A). It soon became apparent that (to include as many obviously responding patients as possible) more than one definition was required. Also, to prevent mistakes, the definitions had to be quite complicated. For example, a simple definition would not elucidate a method to describe patients with weekly CA125 levels that vary around a downwards trend because the amount of variation that was allowable was difficult to define. Therefore, it was decided to have two simple but correct definitions for use in the clinic and more precise definitions written in mathematical logic for use in clinical trials. Once the definitions were found to be acceptable, they were incorporated into a computer programme that analysed data from many patients using definitions based on mathematical logic. The programme was written in Microsoft Foxpro which could be run on an IBM-compatible personal computer. This programme could be use by assay laboratories to state whether the CA125 results indicated a 'response'.

To prevent the categorization of CA125 responses based on large percentage differences within the normal range (where assays are less reliable), all levels less than 15U/ml were re-

Table 13.1 Definitions giving earliest prediction of CA125 response

	Trial A	Trial B
Evaluable by CA125	118	186
50% alone	7 (10)	11 (11)
75% definition 1 alone	16 (22)	22 (22)
75% definition 2 alone	15 (21)	26 (26)
Combination simultaneously	35 (48)	43 (42)
Total CA125 response rate	73=62%	102=55%

Number in parentheses is percentage of responses predicted by each definition.

classified as 15U/ml..

To be evaluable for response according to CA125 the following criteria had to be met:
1. Patients had to have at least three CA125 levels.
2. At least one of these CA125 levels had to be > 40 U/ml.
3. At least one CA125 was obtained between nine days prior to and 35 days after the start of chemotherapy.
4. A response was only recognized if it occurred within six months from the start of chemotherapy.

Based on these criteria only 118 of 277 patients (43%) were evaluable and 57 patients were not evaluable because all levels were < 40 U/ml despite having three or more samples taken.

13.3.1 TWO PROPOSED DEFINITIONS FOR CA125 RESPONSE

50% response to a specific treatment has occurred if after two samples there has been a 50% fall of serum CA125 levels, confirmed by a fourth sample, or;

75% response has occurred if there is a serial fall of serum CA125 over three samples of more than 75%.

In each case the final sample has to be at

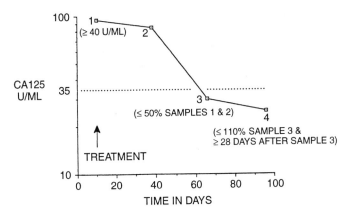

Figure 13.1 Example of 50% response definition.

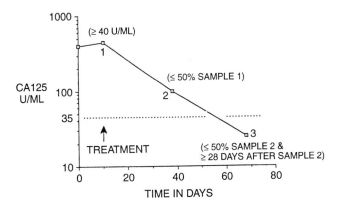

Figure 13.2 Example of 75% response definition 1.

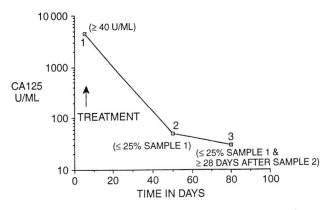

Figure 13.3 Example of 75% response definition 2.

least 28 days after the previous sample. These definitions are shown in Figures 13.1–13.3. The definitions in mathematical formulae are presented below. To detect as many responses as soon as possible, two 75% response definitions are required (Table 13.1).

13.4 CA125 RESPONSE DEFINITIONS

50% RESPONSE DEFINITION

Sample 1 = x and ≥ 40U/ml
Sample 2 = y
Sample 3 = ≤ 50% x and y
Sample 4 = ≤ 110% sample 3 and ≥ 28 days after sample 3. (If samples 3 and 4 are < upper limit of normal, intervening samples between 2 and 3, or 3 and 4 which are within the normal range, must be ≤ 150% sample 2 or 3 respectively. Intervening samples between 2 and 3, or between 3 and 4 which are outside the normal range, must be ≤ 110% sample 2 or 3 respectively and ≤ 110% preceding sample.)

75% RESPONSE DEFINITION, CRITERIA 1

Sample 1 = x and ≥ 40U/ml
Sample 2 = ≤ 50% x
Sample 3 = ≤ 50% sample 2 and ≥ 28 days after sample 2
(Intervening samples between 1 and 2 must be ≤ 110% sample 1, and between 2 and 3 must be ≤ 110% sample 2. All intervening samples must be ≤ 110% of the preceding sample. Intervening samples between 2 and 3 which are within the normal range must be ≤ 150% sample 2.)

75% RESPONSE DEFINITION, CRITERIA 2

Sample 1 = ≥ 40U/ml
Sample 2 = ≤ 25% sample 1
Sample 3 = ≤ 25% sample 1 and ≥ 28 days after sample 2
(Intervening samples between 1 and 2 must be < 110% sample 1, and between 2 and 3 must be < 110% sample 2. All intervening samples must

be < 110% of the preceding sample. If samples 2 and 3 are < upper limit of normal, sample 3 must be < 150% sample 2. Intervening samples between 2 and 3 which are within the normal range must be < 150% sample 2).

The upper limit of normal is 30U/ml and the lower limit of assay sensitivity is 15 U/ml for this analysis.

The start date for all response procedures must be in the range of < 10 days before or < 36 days after the start date of treatment.

13.5 TESTING THE CA125 RESPONSE DEFINITIONS

13.5.1 EVALUATION OF DIFFERENT DEFINITIONS

These CA125 response definitions were tested and refined by analysing data from the North Thames Ovary Trial '4' of five versus eight courses of cisplatin or carboplatin (Trial B). 254 patients entered this trial and 186 were evaluable by CA125. The definitions that gave the earliest prediction of response are shown in Table 13.1. The majority of responses were first detected by applying one of the definitions, however, in many cases more than one definition simultaneously predicted response. Approximately 10% of responses would be missed if the '50% response' definition was not used. The observation that the percentage of responses predicted by each definition is so similar in trials 'A' and 'B' suggests that they are highly reproducible.

13.5.2 CORRELATION BETWEEN CA125 AND STANDARD RESPONSE CRITERIA

Comparing CA125 with standard response is only possible in those patients who are evaluable by both modalities. While standard response assessment was not an endpoint of trials 'A' and 'B', the date of progression was accurately recorded. Only one patient clinically progressed prior to the date of CA125 response, a false positive rate of 0.3% (1/304 evaluable patients).

Data were made available from 451 patients entered into the dose intensity study GOG protocol 97. There were 343 patients evaluable according to CA125, but only 107 of these were also evaluable according to GOG criteria. None of these evaluable patients progressed clinically prior to CA125 response. However, 14 of the 34 patients recorded as 'stable disease' by GOG criteria were considered CA125 responders. It is obvious that some patients whose tumour measurements do not decrease enough to be classified as a responder by one criteria may be classified as a responder by another criteria, particularly as ovarian cancer tumour measurements are often subject to error. The fact that there were no cases of clinical progression seen in the days following CA125 response among these 34 patients suggests that these patients had durable stable disease.

The sensitivity of the CA125 response was 68% among those 71 patients responding according to GOG criteria. It could not be close to 100% for several reasons. Ten percent of the patients had all CA125 levels < 40 U/ml and were not evaluable. Another group had levels that were not high enough to permit a 50% or 75% fall. Another group may have had a response based on a CT scan and a fall in CA125 levels, but if the latter was not maintained for at least a month a CA125 response would not be recorded.

The response rate by CA125 was 62% in trial 'A', 55% in trial 'B' and 66% in the GOG trial; response rates which are similar to those recorded for most first-line chemotherapy regimens. The highest response rate of 66% was only seen in the trial using combination chemotherapy.

13.5.3 PHASE II TRIALS

The greatest value of these CA125 definitions will be if they can be used as a method for assessing response of patients in phase II trials.

This would allow far more patients to be evaluable for these trials and could lead to great cost savings. Clearly, five CA125 assays are much cheaper than three CT scans. To be accepted, the CA125 definitions must produce response rates of > 20% with drugs that are active and response rates of < 10% with drugs that are inactive. It is also necessary to demonstrate that the drugs do not interfere with the CA125 assay. Removal of ascites or administration of mouse antibodies may invalidate reliance on the CA125 response.

13.5.4 TAXOTERE AND HEXALEN

The CA125 response definitions are shown in Chapter 16. They correlate well with standard clinical response criteria in the phase II trial of Taxotere. An equally encouraging result was seen in the phase II trial of oral Hexalen in patients relapsing more than 6 months after initial chemotherapy [5]. Table 13.2 shows a matrix comparing clinical with CA125 response among those 41 patients who had both EORTC evaluable and CA125 evaluable disease.

There were no patients who responded by CA125 criteria yet were clinically progressing at the same time, but there were four patients who

Table 13.2 Comparison of standard response criteria with CA-125 defined response in Phase II trial of oral Hexalen in relapsed ovarian carcinoma

	Clinical Response		
	Yes	No	NM
CA125-defined response	11	4*	4
No CA125-defined response	4#	22	1
Not evaluable	2	1	

NM = Not Measurable
* = No change at time of CA125 response
# = Progressing according to CA125 at time of clinical response

had stable disease at the time of CA125 response. It is unclear which modality of response assessment is correct. However, the fact that the response rate according to CA125 was 41.3% (19/46, CI 26.5–56) and according to EORTC was 38.6% (17/44, CI 23.6–53.6) indicates that either modality gives a similar efficacy result.

We are currently analysing our CA125 response definitions in the following trials; EORTC and NCI Canada trial of Taxol, UK trial of Taxol, randomized trial of Taxol versus Topetecan, ECTG trial of gemcytabine, CRC trial of rhizoxin and Vancouver trial of etoposide. A high correlation is not likely because there will inevitably be patients who respond according to CA125 who have stable disease according to standard clinical criteria. The most important aspect as far as phase II trials are concerned is that the CA125 definition can distinguish between drugs that are active against ovarian carcinoma and drugs that are inactive. So far there has been close agreement between the modalities of assessing response. Providing there is a tight correlation between the CA125 response and standard clinical response rates with a variety of drugs, the CA125 definitions should be accepted by the regulatory authorities as a method of measuring tumour response.

ACKNOWLEDGEMENTS

The authors are grateful to all members of the North Thames Ovary Group, the Gynaecology Oncology Group and participants of the Hexalan phase II study, who contributed data to this study.

REFERENCES

1. Bast, R.C., Klug, T.L., John, E.S. *et al.* (1983) A radioimmunoassay using a monoclonal antibody to monitor the course of epithelial ovarian cancer. *N. Engl. J. Med.* **309**, 883-7.
2. van der Burg, M.E.L., Lammes, F.B. and Verweij, J. (1992) CA125 in ovarian cancer. *Neth. J. Med.* **40**, 36-51.
3. Miller, A.B., Hoogstraten, B., Staquet, M. *et al.* (1981) Reporting results of cancer treatment. *Cancer.* **47**, 207-14.
4. Oken, M.M., Creech, R.H., Tormey, D.C. *et al.* (1993) Toxicity and response criteria of the Eastern Cooperative Oncology Group. *Am. J. Clin. Oncol.* **5**, 649-55.
5. Rustin, G.J.S., Crawford, M., Lambert, J. *et al.* (1994) Phase II trial of oral Hexalen in patients with ovarian carcinoma relapsing 6 months after initial chemotherapy. *Ann. Oncol.* **5**, Suppl 8.

Chapter 14

Dose intensification

A. Hilary CALVERT, Nigel P. BAILEY, Neelam SIDDIQUE, Michael J. LIND,

D.R. Herbie NEWELL, Alan P. BODDY, Huw THOMAS and

Andrew HUGHES

14.1 INTRODUCTION

When alkylating agents were introduced in the 1950s they were administered to patients with a variety of malignant conditions. It was found that they would produce remissions in the tumours of a proportion of patients with ovarian cancer, although these remissions were usually of short duration. Many individual patients undoubtedly benefited from these remissions, but there was no good evidence that the overall survival of a population of patients with advanced ovarian cancer was enhanced [1]. It is generally agreed that the survival of patients with advanced ovarian cancer improved significantly following the introduction of cisplatin in the 1970s [2]. Recent overviews of the clinical trials data suggest that the use of cisplatin in combination with other agents (particularly cyclophosphamide) may be associated with a marginally improved long-term survival compared to the use of cisplatin as a single agent [3]. Carboplatin was introduced in 1986 as a less-toxic analogue of cisplatin. Most randomized studies have shown equivalence in efficacy between carboplatin and cisplatin although retrospective subset analyses of some studies have identified

groups of patients who appear to do better on cisplatin [4–9]. Recently a randomized trial comparing the combination of cisplatin plus paclitaxel with cisplatin plus cyclophosphamide has shown superior disease-free and overall survival for the paclitaxel-treated arm, suggesting a pivotal role for paclitaxel in the treatment of this disease [10].

In parallel with the development of better drugs and regimens has been the development of the concept of dose-intensity. Higher doses of an anticancer drug, although potentially more toxic, would be expected to have a better effect on the tumour. Similarly, the administration of more frequent courses of cytotoxic treatment, by reducing the recovery period for the tumour, should enhance the therapeutic effect. These ideas have been developed by Hryniuk and his colleagues and led to the concept of 'dose intensity' as an averaged dose per unit time, with scaling factors for the individual drugs. Retrospective studies have suggested a correlation between dose intensity and both tumour response and patient survival [11].

Increases in our understanding of the pharmacokinetics and pharmacodynamics of anticancer drugs have shown that the concept of 'dose' expressed in milligrams per square metre of body surface area is too simplistic. For many drugs the toxic and therapeutic effects are related to a measurable pharmacokinetic parameter, such as the area under the plasma concentration/time curve. Individual differences in the function of organs such as the kidneys and liver, which determine the pharmacokinetic disposition of the molecules, may lead to vast changes in the effective drug exposure experienced by the patient [12]. The use of dose (measured in mg/m^2) as an index of the intensity of treatment is at best a blunt instrument which, although it may produce correlations over a large group of patients, can be expected to have little relevance for the individual. In order to perform a trial to assess the role of dose-intensity it is therefore desirable to account for the confounding effect of pharmacokinetic variables. For many drugs the relevant pharmacological factors are not well understood or are hard to predict. However in the case of carboplatin and paclitaxel there are existing data linking pharmacokinetic parameters to myelotoxicity and in the case of carboplatin also to response [13-15].

14.2 RANDOMIZED TRIALS COMPARING DIFFERENT DOSES

14.2.1 CONVENTIONAL VERSUS LOW DOSES

A number of randomized trials have compared rather modest doses of anticancer drugs with more conventional doses. For example Wiltshaw *et al.* [16] compared cisplatin 100mg/m^2 every four weeks for five courses with cisplatin 20mg/m^2 in combination with chlorambucil 10mg per day for seven days every three weeks for 12 courses, followed by maintenance chlorambucil for up to two years. The high-dose cisplatin arm produced significantly better five-year survival than the less

intensive combination arm. A study that used identical drugs in each arm but compared the duration of treatment was performed by Murphy *et al.* [17]. They used a combination cyclophosphamide 600mg/m^2 and carboplatin 300mg/m^2 alternated every four weeks with doxorubicin 50mg/m^2 and ifosfamide 5g/m^2. The treatment was given either as 6 courses at these doses or as 12 courses at half dose. Although the total doses given were the same, the response rates were significantly improved and survival was better for the group who received the more intensive regimen.

14.2.2 LOW VERSUS HIGH DOSES

Both studies described above compared chemotherapy at what are now considered fairly conventional doses with a reduced-intensity regimen. Comparisons with more intensive regimens have not revealed such a clear-cut conclusion. Kaye and colleagues [18] compared a cisplatin dose of 50mg/m^2 or 100mg/m^2 every three weeks, both arms receiving cyclophosphamide at a dose of 750mg/m^2. Recruitment to this study was stopped early when an interim analysis showed a significant difference in survival. Median survival was 114 weeks in the high-dose arm and only 69 weeks in the low dose arm. However toxicity was considerably higher on the high-dose arm. A total of 165 patients were randomized and 25 were withdrawn for toxicity on the high dose arm compared with nine on the low dose arm. Longer follow up of these patients has also shown some convergence of the survival curves. A second study by McGuire and colleagues [19] randomized a total of 485 patients to receive either 'standard' therapy (cyclophosphamide 500mg/m^2 and cisplatin 50mg/m^2 intravenously every three weeks for eight courses) or intense therapy (cyclophosphamide 1000mg/m^2 and cisplatin 100mg/m^2 intravenously every three weeks for four courses). The doses administered were carefully monitored demonstrating that the high-dose patients did actually receive 1.97 times the dose intensity of the low dose group. However, the total doses received in each arm were the same. There was no significant difference in response or survival, although there was more toxicity in the high-dose group.

14.2.3 DISCUSSION OF PUBLISHED LITERATURE

The published data on old trials where 'low dose' regimens were extremely non-intensive, particularly with respect to the platinum (or carboplatin) exposure clearly show poorer survival, supporting the role of platinum drugs in this disease and suggesting that very protracted regimens (> 6 months) are inferior. In the two more recent trials the platinum doses were significantly higher. The study of Kaye *et al.* delivered the highest total dose of cisplatin (600mg/m^2) compared to 400mg/m^2 in the McGuire study and there is a suggestion that this may have led to an improvement in median, although not necessarily in long-term, survival. Both studies showed considerable cisplatin-related toxicity in the high-dose arm, particularly when prolonged to six courses, implying that it would not be feasible to evaluate regimens using even higher doses of cisplatin.

The use of carboplatin should allow a better evaluation of the role of dose and/or dose intensity. Carboplatin has reduced non-haematological toxicities allowing proportionately higher doses to be given with appropriate haematological support. Further, carboplatin doses can be calculated to give a relatively constant exposure in terms of the 'area under the curve' (AUC) [20], thus removing one confounding factor, that of pharmacokinetic variability, from the study.

14.3 RETROSPECTIVE STUDIES ON THE AUC-INTENSITY OF CARBOPLATIN

The most widely used dosing formula for carboplatin is,

$$Dose = AUC \times (GFR + 25)$$

where *Dose* is the total dose in mg, *AUC* is the desired area under the curve in mg/ml×min, *GFR* is the glomerular filtration rate (not normalized for surface area) and 25 is the average non-renal clearance for adults [20]. Providing that the pre-treatment GFR and the total dose given are known for a patient it is possible to calculate retrospectively the AUC to which the patient has been exposed by inverting the dosing formula,

$$AUC = (GFR + 25) / Dose$$

This technique has been used in a number of retrospective studies.

The most compelling data relating AUC to therapeutic efficacy have come from the study of male germ cell tumours. Childs *et al.* [21] studied 121 patients with testicular non-seminomatous germ cell tumours who had been treated with a combination of carboplatin, etoposide and bleomycin. The risk of treatment failure was significantly higher in 23 patients who had a calculated AUC of less than 4·5 (six relapses), than in the remaining 98 (three relapses, p < 0.05). There was no relationship between relapse and the dose measured in mg/m^2.

Studies in ovarian cancer have been performed by Jodrell and his colleagues [22], who obtained data on a large series of patients with advanced ovarian cancer included in a number of early Phase II studies. For previously treated patients, the response rate increased as the AUC increased to about four or five but increased little for AUCs above six. Similar results were obtained from trials of previously untreated patients, although the number of patients exposed to a high AUC was extremely low. The authors suggested that response in ovarian cancer is related to AUC up to an AUC of about five, but that above this there is no additional increase if the AUC goes higher. However the retrospective calculation of the AUC means in patients whose doses were calculated on the basis of mg/m^2 that only those patients with a low pre-treatment GFR would have a high AUC. This means that the population of patients with the higher AUCs will have a preponderance of patients with previous cisplatin treatment or bulky disease causing ureteric obstruction.

14.4 PROSPECTIVE STUDIES ON THE AUC INTENSITY OF CARBOPLATIN

Clearly a prospective randomized trial is needed to test the hypothesis of an effect of AUC on response and survival in ovarian cancer. It is worth noting that such a trial would have to compare two widely differing AUCs in order to be likely to show much difference between the two arms. Hills *et al.* [23] studied ten human ovarian tumour cell lines in cell culture and documented a 100-fold range of sensitivity. Other authors have also found a wide range of sensitivities [24]. It can be calculated that a difference in AUC of at least two-fold and preferably four-fold would be needed to demonstrate a significant (~50%) improvement in response or survival in the high AUC arm [25]. One current study has been reported in preliminary form [26]. Patients with stage III or IV ovarian cancer were randomized to receive either an AUC of six every four weeks for six courses or an AUC of 12 every four weeks for four courses. The AUC of 12 produced a 58% complete response rate compared with 36% for the AUC of six. However the high AUC was associated with almost universal grade III or IV myelo-toxicity necessitating extensive hospital

admission and supportive care.

If further prospective studies are to be designed which can compare two AUCs with a sufficiently large difference then some means of haematological support will be needed for the high dose arm. We have recently completed a study in which carboplatin was administered at escalating AUCs every two weeks, with haematological support provided by filgrastim and platelet transfusions [27]. It was possible to administer carboplatin in this regimen for four courses at an AUC of seven, roughly equivalent to 2–2.5 times the 'normal' AUC intensity. Although this was a small pilot study containing only 25 patients (19 were suboptimally debulked, six were optimally debulked) the response rate was high and survival was good. The median survival was in excess of three years for the whole group and was 34 months for the suboptimally debulked group. However the relatively modest increase in AUC obtained compared to that usually given without the haematological support suggests that further development of high dose intensity regimens is necessary. Possibilities would be the use of a platelet-sparing growth factor and the use of peripheral blood stem cell transplantation. In addition to these possibilities, recent data on the combination of carboplatin and paclitaxel raise the intriguing possibility that paclitaxel may alleviate the thrombo-cytopenia associated with carboplatin as well as being a useful therapeutic agent in its own right.

14.5 THE COMBINATION OF CARBOPLATIN AND PACLITAXEL

Reports of this combination have suggested, surprisingly, that the degree of thrombocytopenia seen was less than that expected from single agent carboplatin, suggesting a useful interaction between the two drugs [28]. However, several pharmacokinetic studies suggested that the AUC achieved was significantly less than expected, raising the possibility that the reduction in thrombocytopenia was merely an artefact of a pharmacokinetic interaction. However these studies used the Cockcroft or Jeliffe formulae based on the plasma creatinine level to calculate the GFR. Our data have suggested that these formulae significantly underestimate the GFR [29]. We have recently completed a study of carboplatin given at an AUC of seven every four weeks with escalating doses of paclitaxel [29]. The paclitaxel has been increased from 150mg/m² to 225mg/m² with only a limited amount of thrombocytopenia being observed. Pharmacokinetic studies showed that there was no evidence that the AUC of carboplatin was affected by the co-administration of paclitaxel, a mean AUC of seven being achieved. Further the pharmacokinetic parameters obtained for taxol were compatible with those seen in other studies and confirmed the marked non-linearity previously reported. Mean AUCs for taxol were 476µg/ml.min at 150mg/m², 690µg/ml.min at 175mg/m², 1461µg/ml.min at 200mg/m² and 1787µg/ml.min at 225mg/m². Thus modest dose increases for paclitaxel are associated with significant changes in exposure, at least as described by AUC, despite the fact that serious myelosuppression has not been seen. This study has confirmed the high response rates previously reported by others.

14.6 CONCLUSIONS

There is clear evidence in the published literature that the survival from advanced ovarian cancer is reduced when low doses, particularly of platinum, are used. Data from trials comparing doses of 50 with 100mg/m² of cisplatin are disparate, but suggest the possibility that the total dose administered may be important. However

the non-haematological toxicities of cisplatin limit the potential of trials designed to answer dose or dose intensity questions which are centred around this drug. In the case of carboplatin there is evidence of an AUC-response relationship although it is not clear how far this will extend as the AUCs are increased.

Consideration of the experimental data suggests that a large increase in carboplatin AUC will be necessary to impact significantly on outcome. Carboplatin is a more suitable drug for exploring dose-intensity/outcome relationships because its reduced non-haematological toxicities compared to cisplatin will allow a greater increase in the dose providing that suitable techniques for haematological support are used. Paclitaxel, already shown to be a useful addition to the first-line treatment of ovarian cancer, may also be useful in combination with carboplatin because of the apparent reduction in platelet toxicity seen.

REFERENCES

1. Smith, J.P. and Day, G.T. (1979) Review of Ovarian Cancer of the University of Texas Systems Cancer Center M.D. Anderson Hospital and Tumour Institute. *Am. J. Obstet. Gynecol.* **135**, 984-90.
2. Advanced Ovarian Trialists Group (1991) Chemotherapy in Advanced Ovarian Cancer, an overview of randomized clinical trials. *BMJ* 303, 884-93.
3. Allen, D.G., Baak, J., Belpomme, D. *et al.* (1994) Advanced Epithelial Ovarian Cancer - 1993 Consensus Statements. *Ann. Oncol.* **4** (suppl 4), 83-8.
4. Adams, M., Kerby, I.J., Rocker I. *et al.* (1989) A comparison of the toxicity and efficacy of cisplatin and carboplatin in advanced ovarian cancer. *Acta Oncol.* **28**, 57-60.
5. Alberts, D.S., Green, S., Hannigan, E.V. *et al.* (1992) Improved therapeutic index of

carboplatin plus cyclophosphamide versus cisplatin plus cyclophosphamide, Final report by the Southwest Oncology Group of a phase III randomized trial in stages III and IV ovarian cancer. *J. Clin. Oncol.* **10**, 706-7.

6 Swenerton, K., Jeffrey, J., Stuart, G. *et al.* (1992) Cisplatin-cyclophosphamide versus carboplatin-cyclophosphamide in advanced ovarian cancer, A randomized phase III study of the National Cancer Institute of Canada Clinical Trials Group. *J. Clin. Oncol.* **10**, 718-26.

7. ten Bokkel Huinink, W.W., van der Burg, M.E.L., van Oosterom, A.T. *et al.* (1988) Carboplatin in combination therapy for ovar-ian cancer. *Cancer Treat. Rev.* **15**, 9-15.

8. Mangioni, C., Bolis, G., Pecorelli, S. *et al.* (1989) Randomized trial in ovarian cancer comparing cisplatin and carboplatin. *J. Nat. Cancer Inst.* **81**, 1464-71.

9. Wiltshaw, E., Evans, B.D., Jones, A.C. and Baker, J.W. (1983) JM8, successor to cisplatin in advanced ovarian-carcinoma. *Lancet* **1**, 587.

10. Trimble, E.L., Arbuck, S.G. and McGuire, W.P. (1994) Options for primary chemotherapy of epithelial ovarian cancer, Taxanes. *Gynecol. Oncol.* **55**, S114-21.

11. Levin, L. and Hryniuk, W. (1987) The application of dose intensity to problems in chemotherapy of ovarian and endometrial cancer. *Sem. Oncol.* **14**, 12-9.

12. Reviewed in *Cancer Surveys*, (1993) Vol.17, Pharmacokinetics and Cancer Therapy.

13. Calvert, A.H. (1994) Dose optimisation of carboplatin in adults. *Anticancer Res.* **14**, 2273-8.

14. Gianni, L., Kearns, C.M., Gianni, A. *et al.* (1995) Nonlinear pharmacokinetics and metabolism of paclitaxel and its pharmacokinetic/pharmacodynamic relationships in humans. *J. Clin. Oncol.* **13**, 180-90.

15. Beijnen, J.H., Huizing, M.T., ten Bokkel Huinink, W.W. *et al.* (1994) Bioanalysis, pharmacokinetics, and pharmacodynamics of the novel anticancer drug paclitaxel (Taxol). *Sem. Oncol.* **21**, 53-62.

16. Wiltshaw, E., Evans, B., Rustin, G., *et al.* (1986) A prospective randomized trial comparing high-dose cisplatin with low-dose cisplatin and chlorambucil in advanced ovarian carcinoma. *J. Clin. Oncol.* **4**, 722-9.

17. Murphy, D., Crowther, D., Renninson, J. *et al.* (1993) A randomized dose intensity study in ovarian carcinoma comparing chemotherapy given at four week intervals for six cycles with half dose chemotherapy given for twelve cycles. *Ann. Oncol.* **4**, 377-83.

18. Kaye, S.B., Lewis, C.R., Paul, J. *et al.* (1992) Randomized study of two doses of cisplatin with cyclophosphamide in epithelial ovarian cancer. *Lancet*, **340**, 329-33.

19. McGuire, W.P., Hoskins, W.J., Brady, M.F. *et al.* (1995) Assessment of dose-intensive therapy in suboptimally debulked ovarian cancer, A Gynecologic Oncology Group study. *J. Clin. Oncol.* **13**, 1589-99.

20. Calvert, A.H., Newell, D.R., Gumbrell, L.A. *et al.* (1989) Carboplatin dosage, prospective evaluation of a simple formula based on renal function. *J. Clin. Oncol.* **7**, 1748-56.

21. Childs, W.J., Nicholls, J. and Horwich, A. (1992) The optimisation of carboplatin dose in carboplatin, etoposide and bleomycin combination chemotherapy for good prognosis metastatic nonseminomatous germ cell tumours of the testis. *Ann. Oncol.* **3**, 291-6.

22. Jodrell, D.I., Egorin, M.J., Canetta, R.M. *et al.* (1992) Relationships between carboplatin exposure and tumor response and toxicity in patients with ovarian

cancer. *J. Clin. Oncol.* **10**, 520-8.

23. Hills, C.A., Kelland, L.R., Abel, G. *et al.* (1989) Biological properties of ten human ovarian carcinoma cell lines, calibration *in vitro* against four platinum complexes. *Br. J. Cancer* **59**, 527-34.

24. Hill, B.T., Whelan, R.D.H., Gibby, E.M. *et al.* (1987) Establishment and characterisation of three new human ovarian carcinoma cell lines and initial evaluation of their potential in experimental chemotherapy studies. *Int. J. Cancer* **39**, 219-25.

25. Calvert, A.H., Newell, D.R. and Gore, M.E. (1992) Future directions with carboplatin, can therapeutic monitoring, high-dose administration, and hematological support with growth factors expand the spectrum compared with cisplatin? *Sem. Oncol.* **19**, 155-63.

26. Jones, A., Wiltshaw, E., Harper, P. *et al.* (1992) A randomized study of high versus conventional dose carboplatin forpreviously untreated ovarian cancer. *Br. J. Cancer* **65**, 15 (Abstract C8).

27. Calvert, A.H., Lind, M.J., Ghazal-Aswad, S. *et al.* (1994) Carboplatin and granulocyte colony-stimulating factor as first-line treatment for epithelial ovarian cancer, A Phase I dose-intensity escalation study. *Sem. Oncol.* **21**, suppl 12, 1-6.

28. Kearns, C.M., Belani, C.P., Erkmen, K. *et al.* (1995) Reduced platelet toxicity with combination carboplatin and paclitaxel; pharmaco-dynamic modulation of carboplatin associated thrombocytopenia. *Proc. 7th Int. Symp. on Platinum and other Metal Compounds in Cancer Chemotherapy,* Amsterdam, March 1-4 1995, Abstract. 70.

29. Calvert, A.H., Boddy, A., Bailey, N.P. *et al.* (1995) Carboplatin in combination with paclitaxel in advanced ovarian cancer, dose determination, pharmacokinetic and pharmacodynamic interactions. *Sem. Oncol.* - in press.

Chapter 15

The role of taxanes

Martin E. GORE

15.1 INTRODUCTION

In the 1960s as part of the National Cancer Institute's large scale screening programme, a crude extract from the Pacific yew, *Taxus brevifolia*, was found to have activity against several murine tumours [1]. In 1971 paclitaxel was isolated, found to be the active constituent of this crude extract and its structure described [1]. A compound for clinical use was not developed at that time because of problems obtaining the parent material and difficulties encountered in its extraction and formulation, partly due to its poor solubility in water. Phase I trials eventually got underway in 1983 but again development was relatively slow because patients experienced hypersensitivity reactions. However, early phase I data became available between 1985 and 1987 [2-7] and by 1990 a number of phase II studies had been completed and published [8-12].

Structurally, the taxanes are made up of a complex 8-membered ring linked to a 4-member oxetan ring and an ester chain. Paclitaxel and docetaxel, a semi-synthetic analogue, are the two compounds currently in clinical use, differing by virtue of their side chains. The needles of the European yew, *Taxus baccata*, provide the source of docetaxel and thus this analogue could potentially be a more convenient and readily available taxane. Taxanes act by promoting the polymerization of tubulin and inhibiting its depolymerization [reviewed in 13]. Tubulin is the natural structural component of microtubules which are responsible for spindle formation during mitosis. The microtubules become extremely stable and non-functional as a result of interaction with taxanes. Morphological changes in the microtubules correlating with cytotoxicity can be seen by electron microscopy and immunofluorescent light microscopy. These changes either consist of bundles of microtubules, often arranged in parallel with one another and seen in all phases of the cell cycle, or abnormal spindle asters which appeared during mitosis [13]. A number of interphase functions such as the maintenance of cell shape, mobility, attachment and intra-cellular transport, in addition to the transmission of transmembrane signals are also affected [13]. Several biological effects have been ascribed to taxanes including neutrophil function, TNF alpha secretion from macrophages, adrenal steroid production, hepatocyte protein secretion, mitogen- stimulated lymphocyte prolif-eration and the contractility of chorioretinal fibroblasts [13]. Cells become resistant to taxanes via a number of mechanisms. Chinese hamster ovarian cell lines with acquired paclitaxel resistance contain mutated alpha and beta tubulin which appears to require the presence of paclitaxel for normal function. Normal microtubules are absent during mitosis if these cells are

143

grown without paclitaxel in the medium [reviewed in 14]. A second mechanism involves a glycoprotein probably related to P-glycoprotein but with a molecular weight of 135kD [14]. This 135kD protein functions as a drug efflux pump in the same way as P-glycoprotein. Cells expressing the protein are up to 800 times more resistant to paclitaxel than their parents [14]. Another observation in resistant leukaemic cell lines suggests that paclitaxel resistance is related to the reversibility of microtubule bundle formation [14]. G0/G1 and S phases of the cell cycle were unaffected in these lines and the cells accumulated in G2/M with the formation of abnormal asters which contained polyploid DNA. These changes may provide a useful marker for both *in vivo* and *in vitro* studies of taxane resistance.

15.2 ADMINISTRATION OF TAXANES

Paclitaxel is formulated in 50% cremophor and 50% dehydrated alcohol because of its aqueous insolubility. Prior to administration it is diluted in 5% dextrose or 0.9% sodium chloride. Administration is slightly complicated by the fact that it can only be administered via non-PVC materials, glass or polyolefin containers and polyethylene-lined tubing must be used. Solutions of paclitaxel are slightly hazy and contain fibres, therefore in-line filters should always be included in the giving-set. These precautions are unnecessary with docetaxel but, the solution contain the drug requires vortexing when being made up and subsequently froths. It therefore needs to stand and settle before being finally diluted. In addition, it is advisable to keep the giving-set in the dark while the drug is being administered.

15.3 TOXICITY

The major problem encountered in the early phase I and II studies was that of hypersensitivity reactions, which included typical type I hypersensitivity manifestations such as hypotension, dyspnoea with bronchospasm, urticaria, angioedema and skin erythema. Less typical reactions such as abdominal pain were also reported [15]. Symptoms occurred very rapidly, within 10 minutes of administration in 13% of patients. The incidence of these hypersensitivity reactions was reduced by increasing the length of the infusion to 24h and by pre-medicating patients with corticosteroids, antihistamines and H2 blockers. Using a pre-medication regimen of dexamethasone 20mg orally, 12 and 6 hourly pre-treatment, diphenhydramine 50mg IV and cimetidine 300mg IV both 30 minutes prior to treatment, short infusions over 3h can be given safely with an incidence of severe hypersensitivity of 1% although about 40% of patients still get some reaction [16]. Whether these reactions are caused by paclitaxel or the cremaphor in the vehicle remains uncertain. Similar hypersensitivity occurs in dogs injected with cremaphor but hypersensitivity reactions have also been seen in 28% of patients given docetaxel when this drug is given without similar steroid-based cover.

The commonest dose-limiting toxicity in early phase I studies of paclitaxel was neutropenia with maximum tolerated doses in most studies being 200–250mg/m^2 [2–7]. Subsequent dose escalation studies in previously untreated patients suggest that doses up to 250mg/m^2 can be given safely but at higher doses haemopoetic growth factor support is required [17–20]. Neuropathy would appear to be the next dose-limiting toxicity as doses are further escalated and it is doubtful whether repeated courses of much more than 300mg/m^2 can be given safely [18,20]. An important side effect of the taxanes is alopecia, the significance of which should not be underestimated in the context of a woman's cancer which for many

Table 15.1 Non-haematological toxicity of paclitaxel in previously treated patients [16]

| | 135mg/m² | | 175mg/m² | |
	Total	≥G3	Total	≥G3
Alopecia	86%	0%	89%	0%
Arthralgia/myalgia	54%	4%	67%	7%
Neuropathy	36%	0%	52%	1%
Hypersensitivity	41%	1%	43%	1.6%
Stomatitis	26%	0.8%	27%	1%
Nausea/vomiting	-	9%	-	7%

G3 = Grade 3

Table 15.2 Toxicity of paclitaxel in previously treated patients [16]

	135mg/m²	175mg/m²
Granulocytopenia (> Grade 4)	43%	50%
Thrombocytopenia (> Grade 4)	1%	3%
Febrile neutropenia	6%	7%

is incurable and thus treatment is being given in the palliative context.

In previously treated patients who receive paclitaxel at 135mg/m² or 175mg/m², treatment is well tolerated and severe side effects are few. The results from a randomized study comparing these two doses in relapsed and refractory patients are shown in Tables 15.1 and 15.2. Cardiac events in this study of 391 patients were rare, asymptomatic brachycardia (1%) and transient hypotension (0.5%) were infrequently reported [16]. Paclitaxel was discontinued because of toxicity in 2% of patients, predominantly neurosensory symptoms or hypersensitivity reactions [16]. The objective toxicity profile of docetaxel [21] is very similar to that of paclitaxel except that fatigue is a feature of docetaxel therapy in most patients (82%) and nearly half the patients experience diarrhoea (≥grade 3, 10%). In addition there is a syndrome of peripheral oedema (≥grade 3, 8%) occasionally associated with pleural effusions (8%) whose aetiology is obscure [21]. Phlebitis at the infusion site is seen in almost a third of patients and conjunctivitis, albeit mild, occurs in almost 20% of patients [21]. In our own unit where both paclitaxel and docetaxel have been given to a large number of patients there is a subjective impression amongst nursing staff that docetaxel is a more toxic drug.

However, when the doses of docetaxel and paclitaxel that were given to the majority of patients on our unit are compared, namely 100mg/m² and 135–175mg/m² it is evident that docetaxel has been given at a dose much closer to its maximum tolerated dose than paclitaxel. This may be important when comparing the therapeutic ratios of these two drugs.

15.4 RELAPSED/RESISTANT DISEASE

It has been shown clearly that patients who relapse after platinum-based first line therapy may achieve a second response to a platinum drug particularly after a treatment-free interval of over one year [22,23]. This time-response relationship also exists for phase II drugs [24] and increasingly in phase II studies, patients are being stratified into three groups namely, patients who relapse within four months, patients who relapse between 4 and 12 months and those who relapse at an interval of greater than one year. Unfortunately, this trial design was not used during the early development of

Table 15.3 Duration of response following paclitaxel therapy (135mg/m^2) for relapsed/refractory epithelial ovarian cancer

	n	*Response duration*
Trimble *et al.* 1993 (25)	652	7.1 mos
Uziely *et al.* 1994 (27)	65	6.4 mos
Thigpen *et al.* 1994* (32)	3	4.5 mos
Athanassiou *et al.* 1994* (31)	19	≥5 mos
Eisenhauer *et al.* 1994[+] (16)	391	8.5 mos
Gore *et al.* 1995 (29)	140	9.8 mos

* 175 mg/m^2
[+] 175 and 135mg/m^2

Table 15.4 Response rate to paclitaxel therapy for relapsed/refractory epithelial ovarian cancer

Dose	Responders/Eval.	Resp. Rate	Ref.
135 mg/m^2	141/652		[25]
	0/13		[26]
	10/65	19%	[27]
	25/100	(232/1211)	[28]
	29/195		[16]
	22/140		[29]
	5/46		[30]
175 mg/m^2	6/19		[31]
	7/25		[26]
	6/43	24%	[32]
	37/187	(66/274)	[16]
250 mg/m^2	6/30	46%	[33]
	15/21	(42/95)	[34]
	21/44		[35]

paclitaxel and whether it is superior to other agents in patients with late relapse remains uncertain. In patients previously treated with platinum-based regimens the response rate to 135mg/m^2 of paclitaxel is 19% and there is a suggestion of a dose response relationship with 46% of patients treated at 250mg/m^2 responding (Table 15.4). However, the duration of response as measured from the start of treatment is between 4.5 and 9.8 months in recent studies (Table 15.3). Cumulative data from two studies show that for patients who relapse within 6 months of completing their previous therapy 29% of patients respond, whereas for those who relapse at an interval greater than six months the response rate is 42% [32,36]. The Early Clinical Trials Group of the EORTC, have been able to produce clear data on response rates to docetaxel in relation to the relapse-free interval.

The overall response rates were 22.6% and 27.5% for those patients with a progression-free interval of < 4 months and 4–12 months respectively [21]. The data on patients who relapse after one year is currently being analysed.

The median duration of response is very similar to that seen in paclitaxel studies, namely 6.7 months [21]. There have been suggestions that there may be a role for multiple courses of paclitaxel above the conventional 6–8 treatment cycles of chemotherapy. It has however been shown by Seewaldt and colleagues [28] that the response rate to paclitaxel falls with subsequent courses and these data do not suggest that more than six courses would be of benefit. Patients with relapsed and refractory disease were treated with 135mg/m^2 of paclitaxel and at course three and six the response rate was 25% and 24% respectively, but by courses nine and twelve the response rate had dropped to 17% and 9% respectively. We have examined the clinical evidence for platinum-paclitaxel non-cross-resistance by analysing the response rate to paclitaxel in patients who have objective evidence of progressive disease while on platinum therapy, as measured by computerized axial tomography scan. We found that only patients treated with 175mg/m^2 or above responded and that the overall response rate (non-cross-resistance rate) was 22% in 36 patients [37]. The duration of the remissions was however short, with median 7 months.

15.5 FIRST LINE CHEMOTHERAPY

There is very little data on the activity of single agent paclitaxel in previously untreated patients with epithelial ovarian cancer. Two studies, one from Sweden and the other from the London Gynaecological Oncology Group are ongoing. A preliminary analysis of the latter study suggests that the response rate to paclitaxel is perhaps slightly lower than might be expected 32% in the first 28 patients analysed [38]. This result is interesting because if paclitaxel platinum-based combinations are proven to be the most effective treatment for epithelial ovarian cancer then it is possible that there is synergy between the two drugs. Further randomized data on the use of single agent paclitaxel in epithelial ovarian cancer will be available from a recently closed Gynaecological Oncology Group study in sub-optimally debulked patients (Table 15.5).

There is only one study of paclitaxel-based chemotherapy as first line treatment in epithelial ovarian cancer that has been reported. The study was performed by the Gynaecology Oncology Group in sub-optimally debulked patients who were randomized to receive a combination of paclitaxel 135mg/m^2 over 24h plus cisplatin 75mg/m^2 or cyclophosphamide 750mg/m^2 plus cisplatin 75mg/m^2 (Protocol 111). A statistically significant survival advantage for the paclitaxel combination was reported, median survival 37.5 months against 24.4 months [39]. The Gynaecological Oncology Group have also recently closed a

Table 15.5 Completed trials of paclitaxel as first line therapy in epithelial ovarian cancer

Group	Regimen	Dose mg/m^2 (schedule)
GOG (Subopt.)	Taxol/Cisplatin	135(24h)/75
	Cyclophosphamide/Cisplatin	750/75
GOG (Subopt.)	Taxol/Cisplatin	135(24h)/75
	Taxol	200 (24h)
	Cisplatin	100
GOG (Opt.)	Taxol/Cisplatin	135(24h)/75
	(Cyclophosphamide/Cisplatin)	(750/75)
	Taxol/Carboplatin/IPCisplatin	135(24h)/AUC9/100
LGOG (IV)	Taxol	225(3h)

Subopt. = suboptimally debulked patients with advanced disease; Opt. = optimally debulked patients with advanced disease; IV = stage IV patients randomized study of paclitaxel/cisplatin, administered as in the previous study, against paclitaxel 135mg/m^2 plus carboplatin at AUC9 followed by intra-peritoneal cisplatin. This last study did have a third arm, cyclophosphamide/cisplatin but accrual was stopped following the preliminary analysis of their first trial. The EORTC, NCI-Canada and West of Scotland groups are repeating a very similar trial to the initial Gynaecology Oncology Group study, namely, paclitaxel given at 175mg/m^2 over 3h plus cisplatin given at 75mg/m^2 against cyclophosphamide plus cisplatin at 750mg/m^2 and 75mg/m^2 respectively. A collaborative group from Utrecht and Denmark is hoping to answer the question of equivalence between cisplatin and carboplatin in the context of combination

therapy with paclitaxel, by a trial of paclitaxel 175mg/m^2 over 3h and carboplatin AUC6 against paclitaxel 175mg/m^2 over 3h and cisplatin 75mg/m^2. The MRC has just launched a study of paclitaxel 175mg/m^2 over 3h plus carboplatin at AUC5 against either single agent carboplatin AUC5 every three weeks or cyclophosphamide plus adriamycin plus cisplatin given at 500mg/m^2, 50mg/m^2 and 50mg/m^2 respectively. These latter three studies involve the much more practical and cost-effective way of giving paclitaxel that is by 3h infusion as opposed to over 24h. The combination of paclitaxel and carboplatin is particularly important to investigate as this is potentially outpatient therapy. Much has been said of the initial Gynaecological Oncology Group study in sub-optimally debulked patients which has

Table 15.6 Current trials of paclitaxel given as first line therapy in epithelial ovarian cancer

Group	Regimen	Dose mg/m^2
GOG (Early stage)	Taxol/Carboplatin 3 *vs* 6 cycles	175(3h)/AUC7.5
GOG (Opt.)	Taxol/Cisplatin	135(24h)/AUC7.5
	Taxol/Cisplatin	120(96h)/AUC7.5
	Taxol/Carboplatin	175(3h)/AUC7.5
GOG (Subopt.)	Taxol/Cisplatin x6 *vs* x3 - surgery x3	135(24h)AUC7.5
EORTC/Scot/NCI-C	Taxol/Cisplatin	175(3h)/75
	Cyclophosphamide/Cisplatin	750/75
Utrecht/Denmark	Taxol/Carboplatin	175(3h)/AUC6
	Taxol/Cisplatin	175(3h)/75
MRC	Taxol/Carboplatin	175(3h)/AUC5
	Carboplatin or CAP	AUC5 or 500/50/50
Sweden	Taxol	175 - 225(3h)

produced a highly significant result in favour of the paclitaxel-cisplatin combination. In this author's view, it is not appropriate to conclude that, because of these data, paclitaxel must be included in any first line treatment schedule. The Gynaecological Oncology Group study is well performed but it is still only one result and must be confirmed. Clearly, the EORTC/NCI-Canada/Scottish study has taken on enormous importance in this context. Recently opened Gynaecological Oncology Group studies are shown in the Table 15.6.

15.6 FUTURE DIRECTIONS

The three major directions of clinical research into paclitaxel are dose escalations, scheduling and paclitaxel-based combinations. It seems that paclitaxel can be given at a dose of 225–250mg/m^2 without haemopoetic growth factor support but that beyond this figure, haemopoetic growth factors are necessary. At 300mg/m^2 15% of patients develop $\geq$ grade 3 peripheral neuropathy and 17% have significant myalgia/arthralgia [18]. The main combinations that have been investigated have included carboplatin, cisplatin, adriamycin, cyclophosphamide, etoposide and ifosfamide. Myelo-suppression is likely to be the dose-limiting toxicity for schedules involving carboplatin, adriamycin, cyclophosphamide, etoposide and ifosfamide, while neuropathy is likely to be dose-limiting for combinations including cisplatin, and there are concerns that cardiotoxicity may become evident with adriamycin-paclitaxel combinations. One study of paclitaxel given at 200mg/m^2 and cisplatin at 75mg/m^2 suggests that indeed neuropathy may well be a problem [40]. Several studies have investigated the combination of paclitaxel and carboplatin and it appears that G-CSF is not required for combinations of paclitaxel 135mg/m^2 and

carboplatin given at an AUC6 [41], but if carboplatin is given at an AUC9, then GCSF is required [42]. One study has been able to deliver paclitaxel 175mg/m^2 and carboplatin AUC6 with only 14% of patients developing > grade 3 myelosuppression [43] while another suggests that the maximum tolerated dose without GSCF is a combination of paclitaxel 135mg/m^2 and carboplatin AUC7.5 [44]. Many of these investigations are finding that far from paclitaxel having an additive myelosuppressive effect on carboplatin, it may afford a level of protection against carboplatin-induced thrombocytopenia. The maximum tolerated doses for paclitaxel-cyclophosphamide combinations appear to be 200mg/m^2 and 1250mg/m^2 respectively [45]. In another study, 44% of patients developed grade 4 myelosuppression when given paclitaxel 175mg/m^2 and cyclophosphamide 750mg/m^2 and it appears that if the dose of paclitaxel is lowered to 135mg/m^2 then this combination is very well tolerated [46].

One of the issues that is emerging is the scheduling of paclitaxel and the order in which drugs are given when combined with paclitaxel. A number of studies are investigating one hour schedules to increase the convenience of delivery of paclitaxel, while other groups are looking at prolonged infusions of paclitaxel up to 96 hours or bi-weekly administration. There is the theoretical consideration that for drugs such as the taxanes, whose main mechanism of action involves elements essential to mitosis, prolonged exposure may improve efficacy and there is some *in vitro* data to support this. Recently, there has been much interest in the observation that when paclitaxel is combined with other drugs, the sequencing of the combination is of importance, for instance, if cyclophosphamide or adriamycin are given after paclitaxel there appears to be an increase myelosuppression [45,47].

15.7 CONCLUSIONS

The taxanes are undoubtedly active in refractory and relapsed epithelial ovarian cancer. However, whether or not they are more active than other drugs in patients who have relapsed after an interval of greater than one year remains to be assessed. They cause alopecia and since treatment for patients with refractory and relapsed disease is palliative, the seriousness of this side effect should not be underestimated. No comparisons exist between paclitaxel and docetaxel and it remains to be seen which one proves the more useful.

Current attention has been focused on the use of paclitaxel as part of first line platinum-based combination therapy and although the results of the Gynaecological Oncology Group in sub-optimally debulked patients with advanced disease are extremely encouraging, they need to be confirmed. Meanwhile, many groups are focusing on developing paclitaxel combinations and investigating the possibility of dose escalations within these regimens with haemopoetic growth factor support. It should be remembered however, that currently it appears the dose of paclitaxel can only be escalated by a factor of approximately two and the benefit from such a small increase may well not outweigh the toxicity of such treatment.

REFERENCES

1. Wani, M.C., Taylor, H.L., Wall. M.E. *et al.* (1971) Plant antitumour agents VI. The isolation and structure of taxol, a novel antileukemic and antitumour agent from *Taxus brevifolia. J. Am. Chem. Soc.* **93**, 2325-9.
2. Donehower, R.C., Rowinsky, E.K., Grochow, L.B. *et al.* (1987) Phase I trial of taxol in patients with advanced cancer. *Cancer Treat. Rep.* **71**, 1171-7.
3. Wiernik, P.H., Schwartz, E.L., Strauman, J.J. *et al.* (1987) Phase I clinical and pharmacokinetic study of taxol. *Cancer Res.* **47**, 2486-93.
4. Wiernik, P.H., Schwartz, E.L., Einzig, A. *et al.* (1987) Phase I trial of taxol given as a 24-hour infusion every 21 days: Responses observed in metastatic melanoma. *J. Clin. Oncol.* **5**, 1232-9.
5. Kris, M.G., O'Connell, J.P., Gralla, R.J. *et al.* (1986) Phase I trial of taxol given as a 3-hour infusion every 21 days. *Cancer Treat. Rep.* **70**, 605-7.
6. Ohnuma, T., Zimet, A.S., Coffey, V.A. *et al.* (1985) Phase I study of taxol in a 24-hr infusion schedule. *Proc. Am. Assoc. Cancer Res.* **26**, 662.
7. Legha, S.S., Tenney, D.M. and Krakoff, I.R. (1986) Phase I study of taxol using a five-day intermittent schedule. *J. Clin. Oncol.* **4**, 762-6.
8. Einzig, A.L., Gorowski, E., Sasloff, J. *et al.* (1988) Phase II trial of taxol in patients with renal cell carcinoma. *Proc. Am. Assoc. Cancer Res.* **29**, 884.
9. Einzig, A.L., Trump, D.L., Sasloff, J. *et al.* (1988) Phase II pilot study of taxol in patients with malignant melanoma. *Proc. Am. Soc. Clin. Oncol.* **7**, 963.
10. McGuire, W.P., Rowinsky, E.K., Rosenshein, N.B. *et al.* (1989) Taxol: A unique antineoplastic agent with significant activity in advanced ovarian epithelial neoplasms. *Ann. Intern. Med.* **111**, 273-9.
11. Thigpen, T., Blessing, J., Ball, H. *et al.* (1990) Phase II trial of taxol as second-line therapy for ovarian carcinoma: A Gynaecologic Oncology Group study. *Proc. Am. Soc. Clin. Oncol.* **9**, 604.
12. Einzig, A.L., Wiernik, P.H., Sasloff, J. *et al.* (1989) Phase II study of Taxol in patients with advanced ovarian cancer. *Proc. Am. Soc. Clin. Oncol.* **8**, 158.
13. Slichenmyer, W.J. and Von Hoff, D.D.

(1991) Taxol: a new and effective anti-cancer drug. *Anti-Cancer Drugs* **2,** 519-30.

14. Rowinsky, E.K., Cazenave, L.A. and Donehower, R.C. (1990) Taxol: A novel investigational antimicrotubule agent. *J. Natl. Cancer Inst.* **82,** 1247-59.

15. Weiss, R., Donehower, R.C., Wiernik, P.H. *et al.* (1990) Hypersensitivity reactions from Taxol. *J. Clin. Oncol.* **8,** 1263-8.

16. Eisenhauer, E.A., ten Bokkel Huinink, W.W., Swenerton, K.D. *et al.* (1994) European-Canadian randomized trial of paclitaxel in relapsed ovarian cancer: high dose versus low-dose and long versus short infusion. *J. Clin. Oncol.* **12,** 2654-66.

17. Schrijvers, D., Wanders, J., Dirix, L. *et al.* (1993) Coping with toxicities of docetaxel (Taxotere™). *Ann. Oncol.* **4** 610-11.

18. Schiller, H.H., Storer, B., Tutsch, K. *et al.* (1994) Phase I trial of 3-hour infusion of paclitaxel with or without granulocyte colony-stimulating factor in patients with advanced cancer. *J. Clin. Oncol.* **12,** 241-8.

19. Schwartsman, G., Scaletsky, A., Gottfridson, C. *et al.* (1994) Clinical toxicity of taxol given as a one-hour intravenous (IV) infusion in patients with solid tumors. *Ann. Oncol.* **5,** 187.

20. Sarosy, G., Kohn, E., Stone, D.A. *et al.* (1992) Phase I study of taxol and granulocyte colony stimulating factor in patients with refractory ovarian cancer. *J. Clin. Oncol.* **11,** 1165-70.

21. Piccart, M.J., Gore, M.E., ten Bokkel Huinink, W.M. *et al.* (1995) Docetaxel (Taxotere, RP56976, NSC 628503): an active new drug for the treatment of advanced epithelial ovarian cancer. *J. Natl. Cancer Inst.* **87,** 676-81.

22. Gore, M.E., Fryatt, I., Wiltshaw, E. *et al.* (1990) Treatment of relapsed carcinoma of the ovary with cisplatin or carboplatin following initial treatment with these compounds. *Gynecol. Oncol.* **36,** 207-11.

23. Markman, M., Rothman, R., Hakes, T. *et al.* (1991) Second-line platinum therapy in patients with ovarian cancer previously treated with cisplatin. *J. Clin. Oncol.* **9,** 389-93.

24. Blackledge, G., Lawton, F., Redmen, C. *et al.* (1989) Response of patients in phase II studies of chemotherapy in ovarian cancer: implications for patient treatment and the design of phase II trials. *Brit. J. Cancer.* **59,** 650-3.

25. Trimble, E.L., Adams, J.D., Vena, D. *et al.* (1993) Paclitaxel for platinum-refractory ovarian cancer: results from the first 1,000 patients registered to National Cancer Institute Treatment Referral Centre 9103. *J. Clin. Oncol.* **11,** 2405-10.

26. Aravantinos, G., Skarlos, D., Kosmidis P. *et al.* (1994) Taxol in platinum pretreated ovarian cancer patients (preliminary results) *Ann. Oncol.* **5(Suppl 8),** 102.

27. Uziely, B., Groshen, S., Jeffers, S. *et al.* (1994) Paclitaxel (Taxol) in heavily pretreated ovarian cancer: antitumour activity and complications. *Ann. Oncol.* **5,** 827-33.

28. Seewaldt, V.L., Greer, B.E., Cain, J.M. *et al.* (1994) Paclitaxel (Taxol) treatment for refractory ovarian cancer: phase II clinical trial. *Am. J. Obstet. Gynecol.* **170,** 1666-71.

29. Gore, M.E., Levy, V., Rustin, G. *et al.* (1995) Paclitaxel (Taxol) in relapsed and refractory ovarian cancer: the UK & Eire experience. *Brit. J. Cancer.* in press.

30. Markman, M., Hakes, T., Reichman, B. *et al.* (1993) Memorial Sloane Kettering experience with National Cancer Institute treatment referral center protocol 9103: Taxol in refractory ovarian cancer. *Proc. Am. Soc. Clin. Oncol.* **12,** 851.

31. Athanassiou, A., Pectasides, D., Varthalitis, I. *et al.* (1994) Taxol Patients with Cis /Carbo platin-refractory ovarian carcinoma. *Proc. Am. Soc. Clin. Oncol.* **13,** 870.

32. Thigpen, J.T., Blessing, J.A., Ball, H. *et al.*

(1994) Phase II trial of paclitaxel in patients with progressive ovarian carcinoma after platinum-based chemotherapy: a Gynecologic Oncology Group study. *J. Clin. Oncol.* **12**, 1748-53.

33. Einzig, A.I., Wiernik, P.H., Sasloff, J. *et al.* (1992) Phase II study and long-term follow-up of patients treated with Taxol for advanced ovarian adenocarcinoma. *J. Clin. Oncol.* **10**, 1748-53.

34. Kavanagh, J.J., Kudelka, A.P., Edwards, C.L. *et al.* (1993) A randomized crossover trial of parenteral hydroxyurea vs. high dose Taxol in cisplatin/carboplatin resistant epithelial ovarian cancer. *Proc. Am. Soc. Clin. Oncol* **12**, 822.

35. Kohn, E.C., Sarosy, G., Bicher, A. *et al.* (1994) Dose intense taxol: high response rate in patients with platinum-resistant recurrent ovarian cancer. *J. Natl. Cancer Inst.* **86**, 18-24.

36. McGuire, W.P., Rowinsky, E.K., Rosenshein, N.B. *et al.* (1989) Taxol: a unique anti-neoplastic agent with significant activity in advanced ovarian epithelial neoplasms. *Ann. Intern. Med.* **111**, 273-9.

37. Gore, M.E., Preston, N., Hill, C. *et al.* (1995) Platinum-Taxol noncross-resistance in epithelial ovarian cancer: The Royal Marsden experience. *Br. J. Cancer* in press.

38. Gore, M.E., Rustin, G., Slevin, M. *et al.* (1995) Single agent Paclitaxel in previously untreated patients with Stage IV epithelial ovarian cancer. *Proc. Am. Soc. Clin. Oncol.* **14**, 747.

39. McGuire, W.P., Hoskins, W.J., Brady, M.F. *et al.* (1995) Taxol and cisplatin improves outcome in advanced ovarian cancer as compared to cytoxan and cisplatin. *Proc. Am. Soc. Clin. Oncol.* **14**, 771.

40. Wasserheit, C., Alter, R., Speyer, H. *et al.* (1994) Phase II trial of paclitaxel and cisplatin (DDP) in women with metastatic breast cancer. *Proc. Am. Soc. Clin. Oncol.* **13**, 204.

41. Paul, D.M., Johnson, D.H., Hande, K.R. *et al.* (1994) Carboplatin and Taxol: A well tolerated regimen for advaced non-small cell lung cancer. *Proc. Am. Soc. Clin. Oncol.* **13**, 1181.

42. Belani, C.P., Egorin, M.J., Hiponia, D. *et al.* (1994) Phase I pharmacokinetic and pharmaco-dynamic study of taxol and carboplatin plus filagrastin support in metastatic non-small cell lung cancer. *Ann. Oncol.* **5**, (Suppl 5), 487.

43. Israel, V.K., Zaretsky S. and Natale, R.B. (1994) Phase I/II trial of combination carboplatin and taxol in advanced non-small cell lung cancer (NSCLC). *Proc. Am. Soc. Clin. Oncol.* **13**, 1175.

44. Ozols, R.F., Kilpatrick, D., O'Dwyer, P. *et al.* (1993) Phase I and pharmacokinetic study of taxol and carboplatin in previously untreated patents with advanced epithelial ovarian cancer : A pilot study of the Gynecologic Oncology Group. *Proc. Am. Soc. Clin. Oncol.* **12**, 824.

45. Kennedy, J.J., Armstrong, D., Donehower, R. *et al.* (1994) The haematologic toxicity of the taxol/cytoxan doublet is sequence-dependent. *Proc. Am. Soc. Clin. Oncol.* **13**, 342.

46. Pagani, O., Sessa, C., Goldhirsch, A. *et al.* (1994) Taxol and cyclophosphamide in patients with advanced breast cancer: A dose-finding study with the addition of G-CSF. *Proc. Am. Soc. Clin. Oncol.* **13**, 45.

47. Holmes, F.A., Newman, R.A., Madden, T. *et al.* (1994) Schedule dependent pharmaco-kinetics in a phase I trial of taxol and doxorubicin as initial chemotherapy for metastatic breast cancer. *Ann. Oncol.* **5**, (Suppl 5), 489.

Chapter 16

Docetaxel in platinum-pretreated patients

Martine J. PICCART, Gordon J.S. RUSTIN, Martin E. GORE, Wim TEN BOKKEL

HUININK, Allan VAN OOSTEROM, Maria VAN DER BURG, Anne NELSTROP,

Jean SELLESLAGS, Annet TE VELDE, Jantien WANDERS and Stanley B. KAYE

on behalf of the EORTC Early Clinical Trials Group.

16.1 INTRODUCTION

Paclitaxel (Taxol®, Bristol-Myers Squibb) is a cytotoxic drug with a unique mechanism of action [1] and a well characterized toxicity profile [2-4]. It is currently registered in the U.S. and Europe for use in ovarian cancer after failure of previous chemotherapy including platinum compounds [5-8].

Docetaxel (Taxotere®, Rhône-Poulenc Rorer) is the first semi-synthetic taxoid compound to have entered clinical trials. The main features of its preclinical development, in comparison with paclitaxel, were a doubling in potency in promoting the assembly of micro-tubules and inhibiting the disassembly process to tubulin, with consequently greater *in vitro* cytotoxic potency against murine and human cancer cell lines, and a superior *in vivo* antitumour activity against B16 melanoma [9-10]. Docetaxel showed at least equivalent cytotoxicity to paclitaxel against fresh ovarian cancers obtained at surgery and cloned *in vitro* [11]. When evaluated in nude mice bearing human ovarian carcinoma xenografts, docetaxel and paclitaxel were found to induce long-term tumour free survivors [12-14]. The occasional observation of a lack of cross resistance between the two taxoids [15] has been of interest. The drug formulations of docetaxel and paclitaxel differ. Docetaxel is formulated in polysorbate 80, while paclitaxel is formulated in Cremophor-EL.

Among several schedules of docetaxel investigated in phase I clinical trials, the one-hour schedule compatible with outpatient administration and associated with the highest delivered dose-intensity, was selected for phase II testing at the recommended dose of $100mg/m^2$ every three weeks. Antitumour activity in ovarian cancer patients has been quite consistently found in the phase I trials of docetaxel [16-19] and has stimulated the conduct of the present phase II trial by the EORTC Early Clinical Trial Group.

16.1.1 PATIENT SELECTION

The target population for this study, which started in May 1992 and closed in June 1994, consisted of patients prospectively stratified for disease progression within 0 to 4 months (group I), 4 to 12 months (group II), or more than 12 months (group III) of the end of a platinum-based chemotherapy regimen, where cisplatin and/or carboplatin were to be given at minimum dosages of 75 and $300mg/m^2$

153

respectively, if the regimen contained no more than two drugs. Entry criteria included histologically or cytologically verified epithelial ovarian cancer (borderline tumours excluded), a maximum of two prior chemotherapy regimens with a platinum drug included in the last one as a minimum, presence of at least one target lesion bidimensionally measurable, documented disease progression or, in case of stable disease, at least four prior platinum-based chemotherapy cycles, a WHO performance status of 0 to 2, adequate bone-marrow, renal and hepatic functions. Patients were not eligible for the study if they suffered symptomatic peripheral neuropathy of at least grade 2 by NCI-CTC criteria, if they had been previously exposed to paclitaxel or had received haematopoietic growth factor or autologous bone marrow support. All patients gave informed consent according to each Institution's policy and the protocol had to be approved by the local institutional review board before study activation.

16.1.2 DRUG PREPARATION.

Docetaxel was supplied by Rhône-Poulenc Rorer as a sterile solution containing 40mg/ml in 2ml vials in polysorbate 80 (Tween 80®). Each vial was reconstituted with 6ml of 5% dextrose or 0.9% saline, yielding a concentration of 10mg/ml.

The solution was immediately shaken for 20 seconds using a mixer and then further diluted in 5% dextrose or 0.9% saline to a concentration no more than 1mg/ml.

16.2 EXPERIMENTAL DESIGN AND TREATMENT PLAN

Patients were scheduled to receive docetaxel as outpatients or inpatients (depending on the investigator's choice) at the dose of 100mg/m², given as a one hour infusion every three weeks until progressive disease or unacceptable toxicity. Prophylactic regimens against nausea, vomiting or hypersensitivity reactions were

only given if these symptoms occurred within the first cycles of therapy. Because of the growing evidence that steroid premedication could ameliorate docetaxel-induced fluid retention, the last 16 patients in group III received a prophylactic regimen consisting in Methylprednisolone 32mg orally, 12 and 3 hours before docetaxel administration and continued twice daily for two consecutive days after docetaxel with an antihistamine only before the infusion.

Dose reductions by 25% were allowed only for prolonged (*i.e.* ≥ 7 days) or complicated (*i.e.* occurrence of fever ≥ 38.5°C requiring parenteral antibiotics) grade 4 neutropenia, grade 4 thrombocytopenia, for grade ≥ 2 skin or neurotoxicity or for other grade ≥ 3 toxicities, except for anaemia, alopecia and vomiting. Patients were carefully monitored during the study and at four weeks after the last dose according to the following schedule of investigations: complete blood counts weekly, history, complete physical examination, biochemistry including liver tests, CA125, EKG, every three weeks and measurements of target lesions by the appropriate technique (X-ray, echography, CT Scan and/or physical examination) every six weeks. The toxicity was graded according to the NCI common toxicity criteria.

The best overall response to treatment with docetaxel was defined as the best response designation recorded from the start of treatment until disease progression. Standard WHO criteria were used for definition of complete or partial response, no change or progressive disease, with the provision that an elevated CA125 in serum had to normalize for a patient to qualify for a complete response. No change was only accepted as 'best response' if it was measured at least six weeks (two cycles) after treatment start.

After removal from the study, patients were treated at the investigator's discretion and were followed every three months until death. If

Table 16.1 ECTG docetaxel ovarian cancer phase II trial patient characteristics

	Number
Entered	144
Eligible	132
Median age (range)	53 (30-75)
Median WHO PS (range)	1 (0-2)
Median time since diagnosis in months	17 (3-224)
Serous histology (percentage)	77 (58%)
Prior exposure to:	
cisplatin (percentage)	62 (47%)
median cumulative dose (range) in mg/m^2	420 (89-900)
carboplatin (percentage)	99 (75%)
median cumulative dose (range) in mg/m^2	2100 (300-6250)
two chemotherapy regimens (percentage)	35 (27%)
alkylating agents (percentage)	91 (69%)
anthracyclines and/or etoposide	16
hormones	5
radiotherapy	10
Progressive disease while on platinum (percentage)	35 (27%)
Target lesion(s) evaluated only by clinical exam (percentage)	11 (8%)

responding patients went off study for toxicity and received further therapy, they were censored for duration of response at the time they started another treatment.

6.2.1 STATISTICAL CONSIDERATIONS

A two-staged design was used for patients accrual [20] assuming that docetaxel was of no further interest in groups I, II and III if the true tumour response rates were less that 5%, 10% and 20% respectively (null hypothesis) and that it would be of considerable interest if the true response rates were equal to or greater than 20%, 30% and 40% respectively (alternative hypothesis). Early termination of the study was required after entry of the first 15 patients in case less than two objective responses would be documented. If such poor results were not observed, accrual could be extended up to a total of 40–45 patients per group. The significance level (*i.e.* the probability of rejecting

the null hypothesis when it is true) of this procedure was 0.06 for group I, 0.03 for group II and 0.03 for group III. The power (*i.e.* the probability of detecting a truly active drug) was 0.87, 0.84 and 0.80 for groups I, II and III respectively.

16.3 RESULTS

Among 144 patients entered into the trial, 12 were found to be ineligible for the following reasons: administration of three prior chemotherapy regimens (2 patients), no platinum in the last regimen (3 patients), inadequate prior platinum treatment, *i.e.* entry in the phase II trial with stable disease after one or two platinum courses only (3 patients), wrong histology (1 patient), two primaries (1 patient), inadequate target lesions (2 patients). The characteristics of the 132 eligible patients are outlined in Table 16.1. Of these, 42 patients started docetaxel within 4 months of their last.

155

Table 16.2 Non-haematological toxicity* of docetaxel in 132 evaluable patients

Toxicity		Number of patients with toxicity	Percent
Hair loss		113	86
Fatigue		112	85
Skin reactions	any	92	70
	≥ grade 3	8	6
Nausea		78	59
Vomiting	any	64	48
	≥ grade 3	11	8
Stomatitis (all grade 1 or 2)		63	48
Diarrhoea	any	64	48
	≥ grade 3	12	9
Neurosensory	any	68	52
	grade 3	4	3
Oedema	any	66	50
	severe	12	9
Pleural effusions		15	11
Hypersensitivity reactions	any	42	32
	≥ grade 3	10	8
Phlebitis at infusion site		37	28
Conjunctivitis (all grade 1 or 2)		28	21
Myalgia (all grade 1 or 2)		20	15
Arthralgia (all grade 1)		6	5

* By NCI-CTC criteria except for oedema

platinum course, 48 within 4–12 months and 42 after 12 months. Prior exposure to carboplatin was more frequent than prior cisplatin exposure (75% *versus* 47% of all patients respectively) and 27% of the patient population received two prior chemotherapy regimens.

Of note, as many as 27% of the patients showed disease progression while receiving platinum chemotherapy and, therefore, could be considered as truly 'refractory'. More than 50% of the patients had poorly differentiated serous cystadenocarcinoma according to their local pathology review. Most patients (92%) were evaluated by means other than clinical examination

16.3.1 TOXICITY OF DOCETAXEL

At the dose selected for this phase II study, myelosuppression, and especially neutropenia was significant but manageable and short-lasting. Among 132 eligible patients receiving 669 courses of docetaxel, 120 (91%) experienced grade 3 or 4 neutropenia, 113 anaemia and 21 thrombocytopenia. Only nine patients (7%) required hospitalization for the management of febrile neutropenia with antibiotics and one patient died from septic shock while neutropenic: she was the only 'toxic death' encountered.

A wide range of non-haematological side

effects were also observed, some of them being expected on the basis of the paclitaxel experience but some others being 'new' (Table 16.2). Alopecia was almost universal (113 patients) and fatigue was a frequent complaint (112 patients). Docetaxel induced a variety of mild to moderate skin changes in 92 patients (70%), which mainly consisted of erythema, pruritus, nail changes (onycholysis), dry skin, desquamation, maculae, swelling and onycholysis. A majority of the patients experienced a combination of these side effects, all of them being reversible during or shortly after treatment interruption. Only eight patients (6%) were reported as having experienced a grade 3 or 4 skin toxicity.

Gastrointestinal side effects were mild to moderate and included nausea in 78 patients and vomiting in 64 patients, stomatitis in 63 and diarrhoea in 64. Neurotoxicity was reported in 68 patients: it was never severe and consisted mainly of sensory neuropathy. Conjunctivitis (grade ≤ 2) was a complaint of 28 patients. Drug-induced phlebitis at the infusion site, myalgia and arthralgia were observed in 37, 20 and 6 patients, respectively. Twenty-nine patients experienced some form of hypersensitivity reaction; only ten patients, however, were considered as having experienced life-threatening events consisting of either respiratory distress, severe hypotension or angioedema, or a combination of those. No cardiac toxicity was observed.

Of concern, were the docetaxel-induced pleural effusions (15 patients) and peripheral oedema (66 patients) reported in this study. These side effects, which were never a life-threatening condition and had an insidious onset, were of a chronic, cumulative nature and only slowly reversible after stopping the drug. Diuretics were not found to be of great help.

16.3.2 DOCETAXEL DOSE-INTENSITY AND CUMULATIVE DOSE

A total of 47 patients needed a dose reduction of docetaxel from 100 to 75mg/m^2. A further dose reduction to 55mg/m^2 was necessary in six of them.

Among 669 administrations of docetaxel, 159 (24%) were dose reduced and 53 (8%) were given with at least three days delay. The reasons for dose reduction in 159 cycles were haematological toxicity in 77, non-haematological in 52, both side effects in 17, non drug-related in 2 and unclear in 12. Toxicity was rarely responsible for cycle delay: only 53 cycles (8%) were delayed for more than three days including 14 for non-haematological side effects. As a result, the median docetaxel dose-intensity given to patients receiving at least three courses of treatment was the intended dose-intensity of 33.3mg/m^2/week.

Toxic effects had more impact on treatment duration, and therefore on cumulative dose: 31 patients (23%) discontinued therapy because of toxicity and three refused to continue on treatment. The median cumulative dose of docetaxel given in this trial was 755mg with a range of 143 to 2380mg.

16.3.3 DOCETAXEL ANTITUMOUR ACTIVITY

The antitumour activity of docetaxel has been evaluated by imaging techniques (CT scan, ultrasound) in the majority of the patients, with only 8% being followed by clinical examination alone. In addition, CA125 was drawn every three weeks in almost all patients, allowing a comparison between response rate according to the standard WHO criteria and CA125 response rate according to the criteria of Rustin (see chapter 13). All 'objective' responses assessed by radiology were externally reviewed by independent experienced radiologists unaware of the clinical outcome. Serial CA125 levels from the 132 patients were provided to Dr. Rustin without information on the WHO response status. Table 16.3 describes the final response assessment according to WHO and the proportion of patients inevaluable for various reasons shown. With all patients included in the denominator (intent to treat analysis) the objective response rate is 24% (95% CI = 16–32%). There is a proportional increase of the response rate as a function of the platinum-free interval with a response rate of 17% (95% CI = 5–35%) in group I, 23% (95% CI = 12–42%) in group II and 33% (95% CI = 18–49%) in group III. In evaluable patients, the corresponding figures are 20% in group I, 28% in group II and 36% in group III. Among 34 patients entered in groups I and II, whose tumour progressed on the most recent platinum therapy, the response rate is 24% (95% CI = 8–39%). Median duration of response (calculated from the start of docetaxel) is 7.4 months for all partial responses recorded in the trial, with a range of 2.9–17.4 months; the three complete responses lasted 3, 3 and 3+ months, respectively, from the date complete response was documented. The median progression-free survival for the entire patient population is 4.2 months (Figure 16.1) and the median survival is 11.4 months (Figure 16.2).

Table 16.3 Antitumour activity of docetaxel

	Number
Eligible patients	132
Evaluable patients	116
- complete response	3
- partial response	29
- no change	48
- progressive disease	31
- failure because of early death	5
Not evaluable	16
- CT scan disqualified	7
- unreliable response assessment	4
- early interruption of treatment	5
Response rate	
- evaluable patients (95% CI)	28% (20–35)
- all eligible patients (95% CI)	24% (16–32)

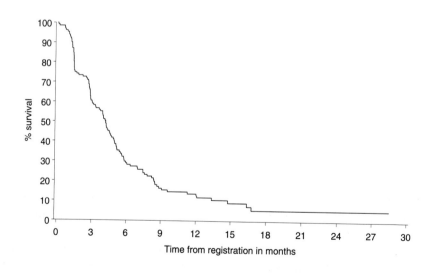

Figure 16.1 ECTG Taxotere ovarian cancer phase II trial - progression-free survival.

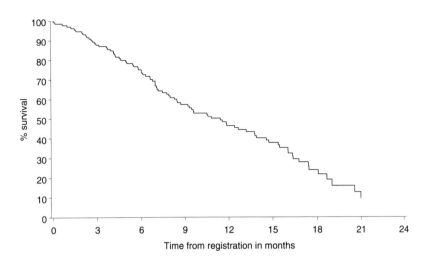

Figure 16.2 ECTG Taxotere ovarian cancer phase II trial - overall survival.

Table 16.4 CA125 response *versus* clinical response

Clinical evaluation	CA125 evaluation			Total clin. evaluation
	Response	*No response*	*Not evaluable*	
Response	23	7	2	32
N.C.	12	33	3	48
P.D.	2	18	11	31
Early death	-	3	3	5
Not evaluable - CT scan	6	1	-	7
Not evaluable - other	2	3	4	9
Total CA125 evaluation	45	64	23	132

Table 16.4 compares clinical and CA125 response evaluations in the 132 eligible patients: 116 patients were evaluable according to WHO response criteria and 109 according to CA125 response criteria. Only two patients who were considered as having progressive disease on CT scan were classified as 'responders' according to CA125. While twelve patients recorded as 'stable disease' by WHO criteria were considered as CA125 responders, seven WHO responders were classified as CA125 non-responders. Overall, 45 of 109 evaluable patients (41%, 95% CI = 32–51%) had a CA125 response and 32 of 116 evaluable patients (28%, 95% CI = 20–35%) had a WHO response (Table 16.5).

159

Table 16.5 CA125 response *versus* clinical response

	CA 125 data	Clinical data
Evaluable	109	116
Response in evaluable patients	45/109 = 41%	32/116= 28%
95 % CI	(32–51)	(20–35)

16.4 DISCUSSION

The search for new active drugs in epithelial ovarian cancer is critical and agents showing a lack of cross-resistance with platinum compounds are urgently needed: indeed, when platinum-based regimens fail, the likelihood of obtaining a response with additional chemotherapy is low and depends on the 'platinum-free interval' – the shorter the interval, the lower the probability of response [21].

Paclitaxel is the first milestone in the search for new drugs following the platinum era: when given as a three hour or 24hour infusion at doses of 135 to 250mg/m^2, response rates of 17–36% have been documented in ovarian cancer patients failing platinum [5-7,22,23]. As the next logical step, paclitaxel has been moved to the first-line therapy of advanced epithelial ovarian cancer, where, combined with cisplatin, it results in a 5 and 12 month increase in progression free and overall survival respectively, when compared with the cyclophosphamide-cisplatin regimen in a randomized clinical trial by the GOG [24].

Our large phase II experience with docetaxel shows that this new taxoid compound is also active in cancer patients with advanced epithelial ovarian cancer having failed one or two platinum-based chemotherapy regimens.

Three additional ovarian cancer phase II trials of docetaxel have been performed which report encouraging response rates in the range of 35% [25-28].

As far as toxicity is concerned, despite the high incidence of severe neutropenia, myelosuppressive complications such as febrile neutropenia and septic deaths were uncommon (7% and 0.8% of patients respectively). In addition, although fluid retention was observed in about half of the patients, the severity was mild to moderate in the majority of them (41%) and treatment discontinuation due to oedema occurred in only 10%, indicating that this cumulative side-effect was manageable. It is important to remember that the vast majority of the patients treated in the present trial did not receive steroid premedication: ongoing phase II/III trials of docetaxel, using premedication regimens point to a favourable impact of 3–5 day steroids on the onset and the severity of docetaxel-induced fluid retention [29-30].

A great deal of energy was involved in the 'objective' documentation of response through the use of computerized tomography, in the present study. Ovarian cancer is a disease notoriously difficult to assess by clinical examination and by imaging techniques; in addition, the whole peritoneal cavity is 'at risk', implying the need for abdominal and pelvic ultrasound, CT scan or NMR.

Given that standard WHO response criteria require maintenance of 'objective response' for at least one month, a minimum of three imaging tests are needed in the course of the phase II trial: one at baseline, one at the time of response and one four weeks later. The cost of these procedures is high (Table 16.6) and their acceptance by patients is usually poor. The limitations of this radiological assessment of the patient's response to therapy is evidenced by the practice of performing second look surgery to determine whether or not there is residual disease in the peritoneal cavity. Both ultrasound and CT scans are insufficiently

Table 16.6 CA125 *versus* CT scan costs

	One test	*≥ Three tests*
CA125	11Ecu	32Ecu
Abdominal. CT Scan	146Ecu	438Ecu
Pelvis CT Scan	146Ecu	438Ecu

sensitive in detecting small tumour implants or tumour seeding along the peritoneal surface. Disease in other areas such as the liver, can be easily assessed by ultrasound, while disease in the para-aortic lymph nodes, omentum and subdiaphragmatic regions is best detected by CT scan [30-39].

Agreement between experienced radiologists was not impressive in the conduct of our trial, as indicated by the need in some instances to ask for a third opinion during the external review process. When informed about the final decision of the review panel, the responsible clinician eventually was upset and remained strongly convinced that his patient had benefited from treatment contrary to the 'official' nonresponse category assigned to his patient. This cumbersome experience stimulated a parallel analysis of the results of this phase II trial through the use of CA125 serial measurements [40,41].

An analysis of serial CA125 levels from a large number of patients with advanced ovarian cancer enrolled in clinical trials and for whom a standard response status was available has allowed new response definitions according to CA125, which are easy to use and appear to be both sensitive and specific (chapter 13). There needs to be a minimal number of three CA125 measurements, the cost of which is far below the one of imaging techniques (Table 16.6). With the use of these CA125 definitions, docetaxel was identified as an active agent for epithelial ovarian cancer: the overall response

rate was 40%, slightly higher than the WHO response rate of 28%.

ACKNOWLEDGEMENTS

This trial was supported by a grant from Rhône-Poulenc Rorer.

The authors are grateful to the following EORTC-ECTG investigators who contributed to the study: R. Paridaens (Leuven), T. Wagener (Nijmegen), N. Pavlidis (Ioannina), U. Bruntsch (Nürnberg), M. Calvert (Newcastle), A. Clavel (Lyon), S. Kaplan (Basel), A. Sulkes (Tel Aviv), M. Marty (Paris), T. Cerny (Bern), H. J. Schmoll (Hannover), J. Smyth (Edinburgh) and E. Robinson (Haifa).

The authors would like to thank M. Bayssas and N. Le Bail, M.D. (Rhône-Poulenc Rorer) for collaboration in the design of the protocol, and A. Denis (Inst. Jules Bordet) for excellent secretarial work.

REFERENCES

1. Schiff, P.B., Fant, J. and Horwitz, S.B. (1979) Promotion of microtubule assembly *in vitro* by taxol. *Nature* **22**, 665-7.
2. Rowinsky, E.K., Cazenave, L.A. and Donehower, R.C. (1990 Taxol: a novel investigational antimicrotubule agent. *J. Natl. Cancer Inst.* **82**, 1247-59.
3. New, P., Barohn, R., Gales, T., *et al.* (1991) Taxol neuropathy after long-term administration. *Proc. Am. Assoc. Cancer Res.* **32**, 1226.
4. Rowinsky, E.K., McGuire, W.P., Guarnieri, T. *et al.* (1991) Cardiac disturbances during the administration of taxol. *J. Clin. Oncol.* **9**, 1704-12.
5. McGuire, W.P., Rowinsky, E.K., Rosenshein, N.B. *et al.* (1989) Taxol, a unique anti-neoplastic agent with significant activity in advanced ovarian epithelial neoplasms. *Ann. Intern. Med.* **111**, 273-9.
6. Thigpen, J.T., Blessing, J.A., Ball, H. *et al.* (1994) Phase II trial of paclitaxel in patients

with progressive ovarian carcinoma after platinum-based chemotherapy, A Gynecologic Oncology Group Study. *J. Clin. Oncol.* **12**, 1748-53.

7. Einzig, A.I., Wiernik, P.H., Sasloff, J. *et al.* (1992) Phase II study and long-term follow-up of patients treated with Taxol for advanced ovarian adenocarcinoma. *J. Clin. Oncol.* **10**, 1748-53.

8. Sarosy, G., Kohn, E., Link, C. *et al.* (1992) Taxol dose intensification in patients with recurrent ovarian cancer. *Proc. Am. Soc. Clin. Oncol.* **11**, 716.

9. Piccart, M.J. (1993) Taxotere, A second generation taxoid compound. *ASCO Educational Book*, (29th Annual Meeting, May 16-18), pp-25-32.

10. Piccart, M. (1993) Taxol® and Taxotere®, New drugs of interest in the treatment of advanced ovarian cancer. In, 'Ovarian Cancer 3' (eds F. Sharp, W.P. Mason, A.D. Blackett, and J.S. Berek) Chapman & Hall Medical, London, pp-215-223

11. Kelland, L.R. and Abel, G. (1992) Comparative *in vitro* cytotoxicity of taxol and Taxotere against cisplatin-sensitive and -resistant human ovarian carcinoma cell lines. *Cancer Chemother. Pharmacol.* **30**, 444-50.

12. Untch, M., Untch, A., Sevin, B.U. *et al.* (1994) Comparison of paclitaxel and docetaxel (Taxotere) in gynecological and breast cancer cell lines with the ATP-cell viability assay. *Anticancer drugs* **5**, 24-30.

13. Harrison, S.D., Dykes, D.J., Shepherd, R.V. and Bissery, M.C. (1992) Response of human tumour xenografts to Taxotere. *Proc. Am. Assoc. Cancer. Res.* **33**, 526.

14. Boven, E., Venema-Gaberscek, E., Erkelens, C.A.M. *et al.* (1993) Antitumor activity of Taxotere (RP 56976, NSC 628503), a new taxol analog, in experimental ovarian cancer. *Ann. Oncol.* **4**, 321-4.

15. Ringel, I. and Horwitz, S.B. (1991) Studies with RP 56976 (Taxotere), a semi-synthetic analog of taxol. *J. Natl. Cancer Inst.* **83**, 288-91.

16. Tomiak, E., Piccart, M.J., Kerger, J. *et al.* (1994) Phase I study of Taxotere (RP 56976 NSC 628503) administered as a one hour intravenous infusion on a weekly basis. *J. Clin. Oncol.* **12**, 1458-67.

17. Extra, J.M., Rousseau, F., Bruno, R. *et al.* (1992) Phase I and pharmacokinetic study of Taxotere (RP 56976; NSC 628503) given as a short I.V. infusion, every 21 days. *Cancer Res.* **53**, 1037-42.

18. Pazdur, R., Newman, R.A., Newman, B.M *et al.* (1992) Phase I trial of Taxotere, five-day schedule. *J. Natl. Cancer Inst.* **84**, 1781-8.

19. Burris, H., Irvin, R., Kuhn, J., *et al.* (1993) Phase I clinical trial of Taxotere administered as either a 2-hour or 6-hour intravenous infusion. *J. Clin. Oncol.* **11**, 950-8.

20. Fleming, T. (1982) One sample multiple testing procedure for phase II clinical trials. *Biometrics* **38**, 143-151.

21. Markman, M., Rothman, R., Hakes, T. *et al.* (1991) Second-line platinum therapy in patients with ovarian cancer previously treated with cisplatin. *J. Clin. Oncol.* **9**, 389-93.

22. Trimble, E.L., Adams, J.D., Vena, D. *et al.* (1993) Paclitaxel for platinum-refractory ovarian cancer, results from the first 1,000 patients registered to National Cancer Institute Treatment Referral Center 9103. *J. Clin. Oncol.* **11**, 2405-10.

23. Eisenhauer, E.A., ten Bokkel Huinink, W.W., Swenerton, K.D. *et al.* (1994) European-Canadian Randomized Trial of Taxol in relapsed ovarian cancer, High vs low dose and long vs short infusion. *J. Clin. Oncol.* **12**, 2654-66.

24. McGuire, W.P., Hoskins, W.J., Brady, M.F. *et al.* (1995) Taxol and Cisplatin (TP)improves outcome in advanced ovarian cancer (AOC) as compared to cytoxan and cisplatin (CP). *Proc. Am. Soc. Clin. Oncol.* **14**, 275.

25. Piccart, M.J., Gore, M., ten Bokkel Huinink, W. *et al.* (1995) Docetaxel, an active new drug for treatment of advanced epithelial ovarian cancer. *J. Natl. Cancer Inst.* 87, 676-81.

26. Aapro, M.S., Pujade-Lauraine, E., Lhommé, C. *et al.* (1994) EORTC Clinical Screening Group , Phase II study of Taxotere[R] (Docetaxel) in ovarian cancer. *Proc 8th NCI-EORTC Symposium on new drugs in cancer therapy* 202, 508.

27. Kavanagh, J., Kudelka, A., Freedman, R. *et al.* (1994) Taxotere (Docetaxel), activity in platin refractory ovarian cancer and amelioration of toxicity. *Proc. Am. Soc. Clin. Oncol.* 13, 237.

28. Francis, P., Hakes, T., Schneider, J. *et al.* (1994) Phase II study of docetaxel (Taxotere[®]) in advanced platinum-refractory ovarian cancer (CA). *Proc. Am. Soc. Clin. Oncol.* 13, 260.

29. Schrijvers, D., Wanders, J., Dirix, L. *et al.* (1993 Coping with toxicities of docetaxel (Taxotere[TM]). *Ann. Oncol.* 4, 610-611.

30. Piccart, M.J., Klijn, J., Mauriac, L. *et al.* (1994) Weekly docetaxel with or without prophylactic steroids as 2nd line treatment for metastatic breast cancer , a randomized trial of the EORTC Breast Cancer Study Group. *Ann. Oncol.* 5, 27.

31. Khan, O., Cosgrove D.O., Fried, A.M. and Savage, P.E. (1986) Ovarian carcinoma follow-up, US *versus* laparotomy. *Radiology* 159, 111.

32. Kerr-Wilson, R.H.J. Shingleton, H.M., Orr, J.W. and Hatch, K.D. (1984) The use of ultrasound and computed tomography scanning in the management of gynecology cancer patients. *Gynecol. Oncol.* 18, 54-61.

33. Wicks, J.D., Mettler, F.A., Hilgers, R.D. and Ampuero, F. (1984) Correlation of ultrasound and pathological findings in patients with epithelial carcinoma of the ovary. *J. Clin. Ultrasound* 12, 397-402.

34. Sonnendecker, E.W.W. and Butterworth, A.M. (1985) Comparison between ultrasound and histopathological evaluation in ovarian cancer patients with complete clinical remission. *J. Clin. Ultrasound* 13, 5-9.

35. Sommer, F.G., Walsh J.W., Schartz P.E. *et al.* (1982) Evaluation of gynecologic pelvic masses by ultrasound and computed tomography. *J. Reprod. Med.* 27, 45-50.

36. Levitt, R.G., Sagel, S.S. and Stanley, R.J. (1978) Detection of neoplastic involvement of the mesentery and omentum by computed tomography. *AJR* 131, 835-8.

37. Bernardino, M.E., Jing, B.S. and Wallace, S. (1979) Computed tomography diagnosis of mesenteric masses. *AJR* 132, 33-6.

38. Whitley, N., Brenner, D., Francis, A. *et al.* (1981) Use of the computed tomographic whole body scan to stage and follow patients with advanced ovarian carcinoma. *Invest. Radiol.* 16, 479-86.

39. Johnson, R.J., Blackledge, G., Eddleston, B. and Crowther, D. (1983) Abdomino-pelvic computed tomography in the management of ovarian carcinoma. *Radiology* 146, 447-52.

40. Bast, R.C. Jr, Feeney, M., Lazarus, H. *et al.* (1981) Reactivity of a monoclonal antibody with human ovarian carcinoma. *J. Clin. Invest.*, 68, 1331-7.

41. Bast, R.C., Klug, T.L., St-John, E. *et al.* (1983) A radioimmunoassay using a monoclonal antibody to monitor to course of epithelial ovarian cancer . *N. Engl. J. Med.* 309, 883-7.

Chapter 17

Carboplatin and paclitaxel combination chemotherapy

Robert F. OZOLS and Michael A. BOOKMAN

17.1 INTRODUCTION

Most patients with advanced ovarian cancer present with widespread intra-abdominal disease at the time of diagnosis. The standard treatment approach to these patients has been surgery, both to stage the patient and to remove as much tumour as feasible, followed by chemotherapy [1]. Ovarian cancer is a drug sensitive tumour with a wide variety of agents having individual activity. In addition, numerous combination chemotherapy regimens have been evaluated in clinical trials in the last two decades. However, there has not been a general consensus regarding what constitutes optimal chemotherapy. It has been generally accepted, until recently, that the most active agent was a platinum compound and that combinations which included a platinum compound were superior to single agent platinum [2]. Controversy has persisted regarding whether carboplatin can replace cisplatin in all chemotherapy regimens and what additional drugs should be combined with a platinum compound to produce optimal results [3]. More recently, the taxanes have been shown to be particularly active agents in previously treated patients with advanced ovarian cancer [4]. There has, however, been only one randomized trial in previously untreated patients with advanced

ovarian cancer which has compared a traditional platinum based regimen versus a combination of paclitaxel together with cisplatin [5]. The results of this trial have demonstrated that paclitaxel chemotherapy was superior to the old standard regimen and, in the United States, the largest co-operative group conducting clinical trials in gynaecological cancer, the Gynecologic Oncology Group (GOG), has accepted that the new standard chemotherapy should be paclitaxel plus cisplatin. Numerous questions remain about how paclitaxel should be used best in previously untreated patients with advanced ovarian cancer and it is the purpose of this review to summarize the current status of clinical trials in ovarian cancer which are addressing the role of paclitaxel based chemotherapy.

17.2 DEVELOPMENT OF PACLITAXEL

Two taxanes are currently undergoing clinical evaluation throughout the world, paclitaxel and docetaxel. Paclitaxel has already been approved for use by the Food and Drug Administration (FDA) in the United States for previously treated patients with ovarian cancer and breast cancer. Initial phase I trials of this agent were hampered by hypersensitivity reactions [4]. In these trials, paclitaxel was administered in a short

165

infusion. In an effort to overcome hypersensitivity reactions, the length of the infusion was increased to 24h and patients were premedicated with steroids, cimetidine, and diphenhydramine. Several phase II studies demonstrated that not only did this premedic-ation and the increased length of infusion essentially eliminate hyper-sensitivity reactions as a clinical problem, paclitaxel also was associated with a response rate of 30–40% in previously treated patients with advanced disease [5-8]. Even in patients who were considered to be platinum resistant, defined as having disease progression while on cisplatin, or with a duration of remission that lasted less than six months, paclitaxel was reported to have a response rate of 25–30%. In these initial trials, paclitaxel was administered at a dose of 110–250mg/m^2 [9]. The latter dose required G-CSF administration to deal with neutropenia. It is of note that the investigators from the National Cancer Institute in Bethesda, Maryland as well as from the MD Anderson Cancer Center in Texas reported a response rate of 48% in previously-treated ovarian cancer patients when the drug was administered at the highest dose together with G-CSF [10,11]. Other toxicities associated with paclitaxel included alopecia, peripheral neuropathy (which is dose limiting) and myalgias. While myelosuppression was observed, this was primarily manifested as neutropenia with little effect upon platelets.

Once it was determined that a 24h infusion of paclitaxel could be safely administered with premedication, a subsequent trial was performed to determine whether premedication would actually permit a more convenient and less costly three h infusion. European-Canadian investigators randomized previously treated patients in a two-by-two bifactorial design to receive either paclitaxel by a 24h infusion or

a three h infusion and also to receive to different doses of the drug, 175mg/m^2 and 135mg/m^2 [12]. All patients received standard premedication. Hypersensitivity reactions were infrequent (1.5%) and were not affected by either dose or schedule of administration. In this study, 382 patients were evaluable for response. There was a slightly higher response rate at the 175mg/m^2 dose (20%) *versus* the 135mg/m^2 dose (15%). Progression free survival was significantly longer in the high dose group (19 weeks *versus* 14 weeks). Response rates were similar for patients receiving the 24h and three h infusions (19% *vs.* 16%). It is of particular note that in this trial significantly less neutropenia was observed in the short infusions of paclitaxel. There was zero incidence of febrile neutropenia in patients receiving the three h infusion compared to a 12% rate of febrile neutropenia in patients treated with a longer infusion. Consequently, based upon this trial a three h infusion at 175mg/m^2 of paclitaxel became the accepted dose and schedule for patients with recurrent ovarian cancer [9]. Because of the markedly decreased neutropenia associated with the three h infusion without any apparent decrease in efficacy, this schedule of administration has also been utilized in recent clinical trials of paclitaxel combinations whereas the earlier combinations of paclitaxel with platinum compounds utilized the 24h infusion.

The two largest phase II trials of paclitaxel were conducted by the Gynecologic Oncology Group and by the National Cancer Institute. In the GOG trial, 49 patients were treated with a dose of paclitaxel at 175mg/m^2 over a 24h infusion every three weeks [8]. In the 43 patients who were assessable for response, there were eight complete and eight partial responses (37%), the median progression free interval was 4.2 months and median survival was 16 months. In the

Table 17.1 GOG Protocol 111: Cisplatin plus cyclophosphamide *vs.* cisplatin plus paclitaxel
Patients: previously untreated suboptimal stage III and stage IV epithelial ovarian cancer

Results	Cisplatin plus cyclophosphamide	Cisplatin plus paclitaxel
Response rate	63%	77%
Clinical complete response	33%	54%
PCR or microscopic positive	25%	41%
Median time to progression	13 months	18 months
Median survival	23 months	37 months

Reference [5,14]

group of patients who were platinum resistant, there were five complete (18%) and four partial (15%) responses. In the group of patients who were considered platinum sensitive, *i.e.* they had responded to cisplatin and progressed after six months without treatment, there was an overall response rate of 44% which included three complete (19%) and four partial (25%) responses. Subsequently, the NCI made paclitaxel available to over 1000 women with previously treated ovarian cancer who were treated at comprehensive cancer centres throughout the United States [6]. In this study, paclitaxel was administered at the dose of 135mg/m^2 by 24h infusion every three weeks. The objective response rate was 22% (4% complete responses and 18% partial responses). The median time to progression was 7.1 months in responding patients and 4.5 months for the entire group. Median survival for all patients on study was 8.8 months.

17.3 PACLITAXEL PLUS CISPLATIN IN PREVIOUSLY UNTREATED PATIENTS WITH ADVANCED DISEASE

Based on the activity shown in the phase II trials, a phase I trial was performed by Rowinsky *et al.* combining paclitaxel and cisplatin [13]. In this trial there was increased toxicity when cisplatin was

administered prior to paclitaxel. In a sequence of a 24h infusion followed by cisplatin, both drugs could be administered at full therapeutic doses with acceptable toxicity. It was this schedule that was used in the GOG prospective randomized trial of cisplatin plus cyclophosphamide *versus* cisplatin plus paclitaxel, (Table 17.1) [5,14]. Patients eligible for this trial had suboptimal stage III and IV disease with a good performance status and no prior chemotherapy. Approximately 400 patients were randomized in this nationwide trial. All patients received six cycles of chemotherapy at which point they were clinically reassessed and those who were clinically without disease underwent a second look laparotomy. No dose reductions of cisplatin were allowed on this study. Paclitaxel was initially administered at a dose of 135mg/m^2 and dose reduction to 110mg/m^2 was allowed for grade 4 neutropenia. The two groups were well balanced for known prognostic factors. There was an increase in neutropenia fever and alopecia in the patients treated with paclitaxel although there was no increase in documented septic events with the paclitaxel combination. Based upon the parameters of response shown in Table 17.1, and the marked improvement in median survival (37 months compared to 23 months), the GOG accepted paclitaxel plus cisplatin to be the new standard regimen for patients with advanced ovarian cancer.

Table 17.2 summarizes other recent GOG trials which have been completed in previously untreated patients with advanced stage disease by the GOG [15,16]. In GOG protocol 114, optimal stage III patients, defined as patients having no residual nodule greater than 1cm disease after cytoreductive surgery, were randomized to standard cisplatin plus paclitaxel or a to a higher dose regimen which consisted of two cycles of carboplatin dosed to an AUC of nine followed by six cycles of intraperitoneal cisplatin and intravenous paclitaxel [15]. No results are currently available from this trial. Similarly, while GOG protocol 132 has been completed, there are no results available from this trial which followed GOG 111 and randomized patients with bulky stage III and IV ovarian cancer to receive either single agent cisplatin, single agent paclitaxel, or a combination of the two drugs [16]. There

Table 17.2 GOG trials of paclitaxel and platinum compounds

Optimal Stage III (GOG 114)

Regimen I: Cisplatin   75mg/m^2 plus paclitaxel 135mg/m^2
Regimen II: 2   cycles   of   carboplatin (AUC = 9) followed by 6 cycles of 100mg/m^2 cisplatin IP and 135 mg/m^2 paclitaxel IV

Suboptimal Stage III and IV (GOG 132)

Regimen I: Cisplatin 100mg/m^2
Regimen II: Paclitaxel 200mg/m^2
Regimen III: Cisplatin   75mg/m^2 plus paclitaxel 135mg/m^2

---

was a cross-over design to permit patients to receive the other agent at the time of progression or if they had an incomplete response to the initial chemotherapeutic regimen.

17.4 CARBOPLATIN PLUS PACLITAXEL

Investigators at the Fox Chase Cancer Center coordinated a phase I and phase II study for the GOG of paclitaxel together with carboplatin in previously untreated patients with advanced ovarian cancer [17,18]. The purpose of this study was to determine the optimum doses and schedules of carboplatin together with paclitaxel. The rationale for this combination was developed from previous clinical studies. There were several studies including two large North American clinical trials which were prospectively performed comparing carboplatin together with cyclophosphamide *versus* cisplatin-plus-cyclophosphamide [19,20]. These two trials in patients with previously untreated advanced ovarian cancer demonstrated that the combination of carboplatin plus cyclophosphamide was significantly less toxic than the cisplatin regimen primarily because of a lower incidence of nausea and vomiting, nephrotoxicity and neurotoxicity. In the 800 patients entered on these two prospective trials, there was no significant difference in overall survival. Carboplatin dose escalation has been limited by development of thrombocytopenia.

Carboplatin undergoes extensive urinary excretion during the first 24hs after administration. Consequently blood levels and area under the curve (AUC) are dependent upon renal function, specifically glomerular filtration rate (GFR) [21]. Calvert *et al.* [22] developed a formula that has taken into account individual variations in GFR to help select the optimum dose of carboplatin for clinical trials [23]. It was postulated that using AUC dosing carboplatin could be combined at full therapeutic doses with paclitaxel. It was also felt that this could be a less toxic regimen due to a decrease in neuropathy since the combination of cisplatin plus paclitaxel could potentially be limited by the development of peripheral neuropathy which is associated with both agents. Carboplatin is essentially devoid of neuro-toxicity. Furthermore, the combination of carboplatin plus paclitaxel could theoretically be administered completely as an outpatient regimen minimizing cost and improving quality of life.

The clinical trial of paclitaxel plus carboplatin was a three part study (Table 17.3). In the first part, patients were treated at a fixed dose of paclitaxel (135mg/m^2 by 24h infusion) and groups of patients received different doses of carboplatin dosed to AUCs of 5, 7.5 and 10. In an effort to maintain dose intensity, cycles were administered on a 21 day schedule. In part two of this study, patients received a fixed dose of carboplatin at an AUC of 7.5, which was determined to be the maximum tolerated dose (MTD) in part one and the paclitaxel dose was

Table 17.3 GOG 9202: Carboplatin plus paclitaxel

Part One	Paclitaxel: 135mg/m^2 by 24h infusion Carboplatin: Groups of patients dosed to AUC of 5.0, 7.5, 10.0
Part Two	Paclitaxel: 175mg/m^2 and 225mg/m^2 by 24 h infusion Carboplatin: Initial dose fixed at AUC of 7.5
Part Three	Paclitaxel: 175mg/m^2 and 225mg/m^2 by 3h infusion Carboplatin: Initial dose fixed at AUC = 7.5

Reference [17,18]

increased to 175mg/m^2 and to 225mg/m^2 by 24h infusions in separate groups of patients. All patients received G-CSF in this part of the study. However, G-CSF was not able to completely decrease the chronic neutropenia that developed in some patients and this led to dose reductions and dose delays [17,18]. The third part of the study was based upon the European-Canadian trial in which paclitaxel was administered in a three h infusion [12]. Groups of patients received paclitaxel at 175mg/m^2 and 225mg/m^2 by three h infusion with carboplatin dosed to an AUC of 7.5. At the lower dose of paclitaxel in this part of the study, G-CSF was not used.

The results of this study have recently been updated by Bookman *et al.* [18]. Thirty five patients were entered at a median age of 54 (range 40–70) and an excellent performance status (range 0–2). Almost 200 cycles of this combination were administered with 30 patients receiving the full six cycles. Six of the patients were removed due to progressive disease, however, no patients were removed from this study due to toxicity or death. It is of particular note that less than 2% of the cycles had grade four thrombocytopenia or fever with neutropenia. The dose and schedule selected for further evaluation was paclitaxel at 175mg/m^2 by a three h infusion together with carboplatin at an AUC of 7.5. In this combination, the majority (64%) of the cycles could be administered on schedule. Among 24 patients with measurable disease, there were 16 clinical complete remissions (67%). Survival data is preliminary but the median survival has not yet been reached and will be greater than 60 weeks. This study demonstrated that using the three h infusion of paclitaxel full doses could be administered together with full doses of carboplatin without the necessity for G-CSF and that cycles could be administered on a dose intense 21 day schedule.

17.5 CURRENT GOG TRIALS IN OVARIAN CANCER

Prognosis for patients with advanced ovarian cancer is dependent upon multiple factors, particularly the stage of disease and the volume of the residual tumour following cytoreductive surgery. Consequently the GOG separates its clinical trials for specific patient populations: patients with early stage disease with poor prognostic features, patients with suboptimal stage III and IV disease, and patient with optimal stage III disease. Table 17.4 summarizes the current clinical trials which are being performed by the GOG in these clinical categories of patients. While questions remain regarding the efficacy of any form of therapy in patients with early stage poor prognosis ovarian cancer, the question being asked by the GOG is whether three cycles of carboplatin plus paclitaxel produces equivalent results compared to six cycles of the same combination. Survival in this group of patients is superior to that for patients with advanced disease with 60–70% of patients experiencing long term disease free survival. The goal of treatment in this group of patients is to decrease toxicity while at the same time further improving the results of therapy. In patients with optimal stage III disease, the five year survival rates are approximately 3–40% and it appears that platinum compounds have made their greatest impact in this group of patients. The GOG is evaluating both the schedule of paclitaxel administration and a choice of platinum compounds in these prognostically favourable patients with advanced disease.

The standard chemotherapeutic arm will consist of cisplatin (7 mg/m^2) plus paclitaxel (135mg/m^2) by a 24h infusion. There will be two experimental arms in this study. One experimental arm will have the same dose of cisplatin but paclitaxel will now

Table 17.4 Current and proposed GOG trials

Early Stage Ovarian Cancer

Eligibility: Stage II and stage Ic (stage Ia and Ib with poorly differentiated histology, tumour excrescences, ruptured capsule, ascites or positive peritoneal washings)

Randomization: 3 *vs.* 6 cycles of carboplatin dosed to an AUC of 7.5 plus paclitaxel 175mg/m^2 by 3h infusion

Optimal Stage III

Randomization:
  Regimen I: Cisplatin 75mg/m^2 plus paclitaxel 120mg/m^2 by 24h infusion
  Regimen II: Cisplatin 75mg/m^2 plus paclitaxel 120mg/m^2 by 96h infusion
  Regimen III: Carboplatin (AUC = 7.5) plus paclitaxel 175mg/m^2 by 3h infusion

Suboptimal Stage III and IV

Randomization:
  Regimen I: Six cycles of cisplatin 75mg/m^2 plus paclitaxel 135mg/m^2 by 24h infusion
  Regimen II: Three cycles of cisplatin 75mg/m^2 plus paclitaxel 135mg/m^2 by 24h infusion followed by interval debulking surgery and three more cycles of same chemotherapy

be administered at a dose of 120mg/m^2 by 96h infusion [24]. The other experimental arm consists of the carboplatin-paclitaxel combination as described above. All patients will receive six cycles of treatment and surgical reassessment is not mandatory in this trial. This trial has opened for accrual in the second quarter of 1995 and it is estimated that approximately 1000 patients will be required with accrual over the next three to four years.

The primary question being addressed in patients with suboptimal stage III and IV disease is whether interval debulking surgery impacts upon overall survival of patients who were not able to successfully undergo initial surgical debulking. This study is based upon a prior EORTC trial in which patients who were similarly not able to be initially debulked were randomized to receive either three cycles of cisplatin plus cyclophosphamide followed by intervention debulking surgery and three more cycles of the same chemotherapy or to six cycles of chemotherapy with the same drugs without any interval debulking surgery [25]. There was an improvement in the EORTC trial in both disease free survival and overall survival for patients who underwent interval debulking surgery. The GOG study will use paclitaxel plus a cisplatin regimen but otherwise will have the same basic study design. It can be seen, therefore, from Table 17.4 that the GOG has now accepted that paclitaxel be considered as part of the primary chemotherapy regimen for all patients with ovarian cancer. Clinical trials are in progress to address important issues with regard to doses and schedule and whether there is an advantage for the combination of paclitaxel plus carboplatin compared to paclitaxel plus cisplatin.

17.6 PACLITAXEL ISSUES IN OVARIAN CANCER

Paclitaxel plus a platinum compound has now been accepted to be standard therapy by the GOG. However, many issues remain regarding how best to use paclitaxel in this disease. Other combinations of paclitaxel are being developed including the combination of cisplatin, cyclophosphamide and paclitaxel by investigators at the NCI [26]. Furthermore, paclitaxel does not have cumulative toxicity and studies are being planned in which more than six cycles of paclitaxel will be administered. The dose of paclitaxel also remains an area of investigation. The GOG has almost completed a prospective randomized trial in previously treated patients with advanced ovarian cancer who were randomized to one of three different doses of paclitaxel, $135mg/m^2$, $175mg/m^2$, and $225mg/m^2$. The lower dose has been dropped due to problems in patient accrual once the drug became commercially available. Further exploration of the importance of dose intensity is being performed with high dose chemotherapy regimens which require haematological support [27]. It should be emphasized that currently there is no evidence that doses which require either peripheral stem cell transfusions or autologous bone marrow transplantation have been shown to improve survival in any subset of patients with advanced ovarian cancer. While many phase I and phase II studies have been performed with high dose therapy, most of these studies were in patients with drug resistant and/or bulky disease, subsets of patients in whom high dose chemotherapy is unlikely to be beneficial. High dose chemotherapy should be explored in patients who have both a drug sensitive tumour and small volume disease. The GOG will be conducting a pilot study in previously untreated patients with small volume disease who will receive multiple cycles of high dose chemotherapy together with peripheral blood stem cell transfusions. The drug combinations remain to be determined but will include both paclitaxel and high dose carboplatin. The goals of this pilot study will be to define the safety of such an approach and to establish the doses which can be used in a larger trial to compare multiple cycles of high dose therapy versus standard therapy in previously untreated patients with optimal advanced ovarian cancer.

Similarly, the role of intraperitoneal therapy in ovarian cancer still has not been established. Paclitaxel has pharmacological advantages which make it an attractive candidate for further investigation [28]. The GOG will be performing clinical trials to determine the efficacy and toxicity of such an approach in patients with small volume residual disease following induction chemotherapy.

17.7 CONCLUSIONS

In the United States, there is now a new standard of care for patients with advanced ovarian cancer. Paclitaxel together with a platinum compound has been accepted by the GOG as well as other investigators to be the preferred regimen following surgery in patients with advanced disease. However, numerous questions still remain as how best to use this agent including optimization of dose and schedule, number of cycles, and relative efficacy of different platinum-paclitaxel combinations.

REFERENCES

1. Ozols, R.F. (1992) Ovarian cancer, part II: Treatment. *Curr. Prob. Cancer* 16, 65-126.
2. Advanced Ovarian Trialists Group (1991) Chemotherapy in advanced ovarian cancer: An overview of randomised clinical trials. *BMJ* 303, 884-93.
3. Vermorken, J.B., ten Bokkel Huinink W.W., Eisenhauer, E.A. *et al.* (1993) Carboplatin versus cisplatin. *Ann. Oncol.* 4 (suppl 4), 41-8.
4. Donehower, R.C. and Rowinsky, E.K. (1994) Paclitaxel. In: *Principles & practice of oncology* (PPO updates, Volume 8, No. 10.) J.B. Lippincott Co.,Philadelphia
5. McGuire, W.P., Hoskins, W.J., Brady, M.F. *et al.* (1993) A phase III trial comparing cisplatin/Cytoxan (PC) and cisplatin/Taxol (PT) in advanced ovarian cancer (AOC) (Abstract). *Proc. Am. Soc. Clin. Oncol.* 12, 255.
6. Trimble, E.L., Adams, J.D., Vena, D. *et al.* (1993) Paclitaxel for platinum-refractory ovarian cancer: Results from the first 1,000 patients registered to National Cancer Institute Treatment Referral Center 9103. *J. Clin. Oncol.* 11, 2405-10.
7. Einzig, A.I., Wiernik, P.H., Sasloff, J. *et al.* (1992) Phase II study and long-term follow-up of patients treated with Taxol for advanced ovarian adenocarcinoma. *J. Clin. Oncol.* 10, 1748-53.
8. Thigpen, J.T., Blessing, J.A., Ball, H. *et al.* (1994) Phase II trial of paclitaxel in patients with progressive ovarian carcinoma after platinum-based chemotherapy: A Gynecologic Oncology Group study. *J. Clin. Oncol.* 12, 1748-53.
9. Arbuck, S.G. (1994) Paclitaxel: What schedule? What dose? *J. Clin. Oncol.* 12, 233-6.
10. Kohn, E.C., Sarosy, G., Bicher, A. *et al.* (1994) Dose-intense taxol: High response rate in patients with platinum-resistant recurrent ovarian cancer. *J. Natl. Cancer Inst.* 86, 18-24.
11. Kavanagh, J.J., Kudelka, A.P., Edwards, C.L. *et al.* (1993) A randomized cross-over trial of parenteral hydroxyurea vs high dose taxol in cisplatin/carboplatin resistant epithelial ovarian cancer. *Proc. Am. Soc. Clin. Oncol.* 12, 259.
12. Eisenhauer, E.A., ten Bokkel Huinink, W.W., Swenerton, K.D. *et al.* (1994) European-Canadian randomized trial of paclitaxel in relapsed ovarian cancer: High-dose versus low-dose and long versus short infusion. *J. Clin. Oncol.* 12, 2654-66.
13. Rowinsky, E.K., Gilbert, M.R., McGuire, W.P. *et al.* (1991) Sequences of Taxol and Cisplatin: A phase I and pharmacologic

study. *J. Clin. Oncol.* **9**, 1692-703.

14. McGuire, W.P., Hoskins, W.J., Brady, M.F. *et al.* (1995) Taxol and cisplatin improves outcome in advanced ovarian cancer compared to Cytoxan and cisplatin. *Proc. Am. Soc. Clin. Oncol.* (in press).

15. Markman, M., Principle Investigator. Gynecologic Oncology Group Protocol 114.

16. Muggia, F., Principle Investigator. Gynecologic Oncology Group Protocol 132.

17. Ozols, R.F., Kilpatrick, D., O'Dwyer, P. *et al.* (1993) Phase I and pharmacokinetic study of Taxol (T) and carboplatin (C) in previously untreated patients (PTS) with advanced epithelial ovarian cancer (OC): A pilot study of the Gynecology Oncology Group. (Abstract). *Proc. Am. Soc. Clin. Oncol.* **12**, 259.

18. Bookman, M.A., McGuire ,W.P., Kilpatrick, D. *et al.* (1995) Phase-I Gynecologic Oncology Group (GOG) study of 3-H and 24-H paclitaxel with carboplatin as initial therapy for advanced epithelial ovarian cancer (OvCa). *Proc. Am. Soc. Clin. Oncol.*, (in press).

19. Swenerton, K., Jeffrey, J., Stuart, G. *et al.* (1992) Cisplatin-cyclophosphamide versus carboplatin-cyclophosphamide in advanced ovarian cancer: A randomized phase III study of the National Cancer Institute of Canada Clinical Trials Group. *J. Clin. Oncol.* **10**, 718-26.

20. Alberts, D.S., Green, S., Hannigan, E.V. *et al.* (1992) Improved therapeutic index of carboplatin plus cyclophosphamide versus cisplatin plus cyclophosphamide: Final report by the Southwest Oncology Group of a phase III randomized trial in stages III and IV ovarian cancer. *J. Clin. Oncol.* **10**, 706-17.

21. Egorin, M.J., Van Echo, D.A., Olman, E.A. *et al.* (1985) Prospective validation of a pharmacologically based dosing scheme for the cis-diamminedichloroplatinum (II) analogue diammine cyclobutane-dicarboxylatoplatinum. *Cancer Res.* **45**, 6502-6.

22. Calvert, A.H., Newell, D.R., Gumbrell, L.A. *et al.* (1989) Carboplatin dosage: Prospective evaluation of a simple formula based on renal function. *J. Clin. Oncol.* **7**, 1748-56.

23. Jodrell, D.I., Egorin, M.J., Canetta, R.M. *et al.* (1992) Relationships between carboplatin exposure and tumor response and toxicity in patients with ovarian cancer. *J. Clin. Oncol.* **10**, 520-8.

24. Wilson, W.H., Berg, S.L., Bryant, G. *et al.* (1994) Paclitaxel in doxorubicin-refractory or mitoxantrone-refractory breast cancer: A phase I/II trial of 96h infusion. *J. Clin. Oncol.* **12**, 1621-29.

25. van der Burg, M.E.L., van Lent, M., Kohierska, A. *et al.* (1993) Intervention debulking surgery (IDS) does improve survival in advanced epithelial ovarian cancer (EOC): An EORTC Gynecologic Cancer Cooperative Group (GCCG) Study. *Proc. Am. Soc. Clin. Oncol.* **12**, 258.

26. Kohn, E., Reed, E., Link, C. *et al.* (1993) A pilot study of Taxol, cisplatin, cyclophosphamide and GCSF in newly diagnosed stage III/IV ovarian cancer patients. *Proc. Am. Soc. Clin. Oncol.* **12**, 257.

27. Schilder, R.J. (1993) High-dose chemotherapy with autologous hematopoietic cell support in gynecologic malignancies, In: *Principles and Practice of Gynecologic Oncology Updates* (Volume 1, No. 3) J.B. Lippincott Co., Philadelphia

28. Markman, M., Rowinsky, E., Hakes, T. *et al.* (1992) Phase I trial of intraperitoneal Taxol: A Gynecologic Oncology Group Study. *J. Clin. Oncol.* **10**, 1485-91.

Chapter 18

Palliation of nausea and vomiting

John WELSH

18.1 INTRODUCTION

Nausea and vomiting is a common distressing symptom experienced by about 60% of patients with cancer who are not receiving chemotherapy [1]. The definition, incidence, physiology, causes and treatment of nausea and vomiting are discussed here. Over the past decade or so there has been a vast improvement in the ability to control chemotherapy and radiotherapy induced nausea and vomiting. In a large part this is due to the use of high dose metoclopramide [2] and the clinical availability of 5HT3 antagonists [3,4]. Many antiemetics have been studied. However, a relatively neglected area of study is that involving the patient with advanced cancer who is nauseated, retching or vomiting from other causes. Palliative medicine – an old art but a newly conceived speciality – addresses control of this debilitating symptom which on its own can have major negative effects on the quality of a patient's life. This chapter specifically examines nausea and vomiting not related to chemotherapy or radiotherapy.

18.2 NAUSEA, RETCHING AND VOMITING

Nausea is generally a persistent 'queasy' feeling, which may be present without vomiting. The definition of nausea is 'a desire to vomit'. Nausea is not invariably linked to vomiting and may be harder to control.

Retching can occur before or after vomiting and can be both exhausting and painful for the frail patient. Vomiting occurs as the stomach relaxes and the abdominal muscles contract powerfully. The consequences of poor control of this symptom are reduced fluid and food intake, dehydration and electrolyte imbalance, lowered morale, increased weakness and stress on the carers.

18.2.1 INCIDENCE

In patients with cancer the overall incidence of vomiting is 62%, not including emesis secondary to chemotherapy. The prevalence rate is 40% in the last six weeks of life [1]. Perhaps due to the high incidence of nausea and vomiting associated with ovarian cancer the incidence is higher in females than males. The incidence of bowel obstruction appears to increase in line with advanced stage [5], and the patients presenting with more advanced disease may develop obstruction more rapidly [6].

18.2.2 PHYSIOLOGY

The areas of the body chiefly involved in control of nausea and vomiting are the chemoreceptor trigger zone (CRTZ), the area postrema, the gastrointestinal tract and the vomiting centre. The CRTZ is located outwith the blood barrier in the region of the nucleus tractus solitarius (NTS) and the vomiting centre is found in the medulla oblongata on the floor of the fourth ventricle. The vomiting centre is

175

stimulated by events in the cerebral cortex, the CRTZ, the vestibular apparatus and afferent nerves in the gastrointestinal system. Receptors are found in the submucous plexus of the gut which respond to distension or toxins and via the vagus nerve and the sympathetic dorsal root ganglion impulses are carried to the NTS and the area postrema. Local gastrointestinal disorders are first detected in the gut and then relayed chiefly via the vagus nerve, to the chemoreceptor trigger zone. Systemic, metabolic or drug related nausea and vomiting is initially noted within the chemoreceptor trigger zone through contact with the cerebrospinal fluid or the circulation. The final common pathway whatever the source of vomiting is through the vomiting centre.

With a greater understanding of neural chemical control, the emetic pathway and of gut motility at both a central and peripheral level, progress has been made towards a more logical approach to the control of emesis. Different receptors are involved in the emetic pathway and the location of these receptors is now better defined [7]. Receptors found in the vomiting centre are chiefly cholinergic (acetylcholine transmitter), histaminic and dopaminergic. The CRTZ has a predominance of dopaminergic and histamine receptors. In the cerebral cortex the receptors involved in the emetic pathway are cholinergic and histaminic.

The vestibular apparatus is primarily involved through histaminergic and cholinergic responsive receptors. The upper gastrointestinal system contains 5HT3, cholinergic and histamine receptors. There may be 5HT3 receptors in the area postrema. The knowledge of the distribution of these receptors greatly aids in the rational prescription of antiemetics.

18.3 CAUSES OF NAUSEA AND VOMITING

These may be single or multiple. The cause may be secondary to the cancer; hyper-calcaemia, diabetes mellitus, uraemia, secondary hypoadrenalism, hepatic metastases or raised intracranial pressure. Raised intracranial pressure as a source of vomiting is generally readily recognized. Nausea and vomiting may of course be iatrogenic caused by one of the many medications prescribed to advanced cancer patients (mean being six medications) [8].

There may be vestibular damage by the cancer or a non-cancer related defect of this apparatus. Infection especially in the elderly or very young, intractable cough and psychological factors may all produce nausea and vomiting.

Another cause of this symptom may be intestinal obstruction. This may be direct occlusion due perhaps to an annular carcinoma, a large polyp or maybe extrinsic compression. The obstruction may be caused by adhesions, single or multiple or by severe constipation. Intestinal obstruction is more likely in pelvic cancers. Overall 5.5–25% ovarian cancers will obstruct [6,9–11] and 5–24% colorectal cancers will obstruct [12,13]. Considering only those with terminal ovarian cancer, one may expect 42% to develop symptoms of bowel obstruction [7]. Non-metastatic manifestations of malignancy may induce an atonic bowel secondary to an autonomic neuropathy or myenteric dystrophy. Gastroparesis may be induced by drugs, the commonest being the opioids, drugs which are widely used in palliative medicine.

18.4 PRINCIPLES OF DIAGNOSIS AND TREATMENT

After an appropriate detailed history which includes current medication, a careful examination including rectal examination should be done. Thereafter, any appropriate necessary investigations should be carried out. The object is to define the cause of the nausea/vomiting, to define the anatomical site(s) involved in initiating the emetic process

Table 18.1 Relative blocking affinity of some useful antiemetics

Antiemetic	5HT3	Dopamine	Acetylcholine	Histamine
Cyclizine			Mild	Strong
Hyoscine			Strong	
Metoclopramide	Moderate (at high dose)	Strong		
Domperidone	None	Strong		
Haloperidol		Strong		
Ondansetron	Strong			
Phenothiazines		Strong	Mild	Moderate

Affinity for receptor: mild: moderate: strong

Table 18.2 Logical choice of antiemetic in relation to receptor distribution and site of insult in emetic pathway

Emetic pathway	Receptor predominance (i.e. stimulation induces vomiting)	Appropriate antiemetic
Vomiting centre	Histamine Acetylcholine Dopamine	Cyclizine Hyoscine
Chemoreceptor Trigger Zone	Dopamine 5HT3	Haloperidol Metoclopramide Domperidone Trifluoperazine Ondansetron
Vestibular Apparatus	Histamine Acetylcholine	Cyclizine
Cortex	Acetylcholine Histamine	Cyclizine Hyoscine Benzodiazepines
Upper gastro-intestinal tract	5HT3 Dopaminergic	Ondansetron Metoclopramide Domperidone
Other postulated neuro transmitters: γ-aminobutyric acid Cholecystokinin Endogenous opioids		Miscellaneous: Steroids

and to prescribe the antiemetic which has the greatest antagonism for the receptors found at that site. The relative affinity of common antiemetics is shown in Table 18.1 and receptor distribution and the more effective antiemetics at that site are shown in Table 18.2.

Once chosen, the dose of antiemetic must be increased to its maximum before acceptance that it is not functioning. If side effects are intolerable, combining two antiemetics with sensibly complementary but different sites of action may allow lower doses of each to be prescribed and obviate toxicity. Routes used to deliver these drugs are sub-lingual, oral, rectal, and subcutaneous. The intramuscular route is to be avoided, if possible, in all patients, especially the emaciated. In severe nausea and vomiting the subcutaneous (SC) route can be particularly effective and cyclizine, hyoscine (butylbromide if little sedation required, hydrobromide if more sedation desired), metoclopramide, haloperidol and metho-trimeprazine can all be administered by the SC route.

Intestinal obstruction is a common cause of nausea and vomiting [8] and its onset in ovarian cancer may be insidious. Once diagnosed, surgery must be the first line of treatment considered. However, if the patient is too ill due to the advanced nature of their cancer, has multiple levels of obstruction or massive ascites, or has perhaps had operations previously and does not wish another, surgery may not be the best course. Medical management is possible [8]. This consists of antiemetics and analgesia if required administered subcutaneously *via* a syringe driver. Haloperidol is probably the first choice drug but metoclopramide is used by many palliative medicine specialists. If colic is a problem hyoscine may be added to the subcutaneous infusion. Hyoscine is also an antiemetic and reduces intestinal secretions. If vomiting persists then octreotide (a synthetic analogue of somatostatin) may be useful [14–

16]. Octreotide has a 12h duration of action [17], and can be given subcutaneously twice daily or preferably in a continuous infusion. The dose ranges from 200–800µg per 24h. Although it is expensive it is effective but it is not an antiemetic [18]. In proximal bowel obstructions, control of vomiting may not be successful and in this case a venting gastrostomy may greatly ease the patient's suffering.

18.5 CONCLUSIONS

Non-chemotherapy or radiotherapy related nausea and vomiting must be actively targeted in cancer patients. An accurate diagnosis must be made. Depending upon the type of receptor in the emetic pathway being stimulated, the antiemetic with the greatest antagonism for that particular receptor must be chosen and used to its maximum dose if tolerated. The most suitable route of administration must be used. Careful and regular review of response must be made and if symptoms are not alleviated a reappraisal of the cause must ensue and alteration in antiemetic be made accordingly. Persistence can be rewarded by success.

REFERENCES

1. Reuben, D.B. and Mar V. (1983) Nausea and vomiting in terminal cancer patients. *Arch. Intern. Med.* **146**, 2021-3.
2. Gralla, R.J., Itri L.M., *et al.* (1981) Antiemetic efficacy of high dose metoclopramide. *N. Engl. J. Med.* **305**, 905-9.
3. Leader article (1987) 5HT3 receptor antagonist, A new class of antiemetics. *Lancet* **8548**, 1470-1.
4. Priestman, T.J. (1989) Clinical studies with ondansetron in the control of radiation-induced emesis. *Eur. J. Cancer Clin. Oncol.* **25**, 29-33.
5. Tunca, J.C., Buchler, D.A., Mack, E.A. *et al.*, (1981) The management of ovarian cancer-caused bowel obstruction. *Gynecol. Oncol.*

12, 186-92.

6. Beattie, G.J., Leonard, R.C.F. and Smyth J. (1989) Bowel obstruction in ovarian carcinoma, a retrospective study and review of the literature. *Pall. Med.* **3**, 275-80.

7. Sykes, N. (1990) The management of nausea and vomiting. *The Practitioner.* **234**, 286-90.

8. Leishman, J.G., McGovery, E.M., McKay, S., *et al.* (1995) An audit of the pharmaceutical care provided to terminally ill patients in the hospice and community. *Clinical Resource and Audit Group*, Scotland.

9. Baines, M., Oliver, D.J. and Carter, R.L. (1985) Medical management of intestinal obstruction in patients with advanced malignant disease. *Lancet* **11**, 990-3.

10. Lund, B., Hansen, M., Lundvall, F. *et al.* (1989) Intestinal obstruction in patients with advanced carcinoma of the ovaries treated with combination chemotherapy. *Surg. Gynecol. Obstet.* **169**, 213-8.

11. Castaldo, T.W., Petrilli, E.S., Ballon, S.C. *et al.*, (1981) Intestinal operations in patients with ovarian carcinoma. *Am. J. Obstet. Gynecol.* **139**, 80-4.

12. Solomon, H.J., Atkinson, K.H. and Coppleson, J.V.M. (1983) Bowel complications in the management of ovarian cancer. *Aust. NZ. J. Obstet. Gynaecol.* **23**, 65-8.

13. Philips, R.K.S., Hittinger, R., Fry, J.S., *et al.*, (1985) Malignant large bowel obstruction. *Br. J. Surg.* **72**, 296-302.

14. Kyllonen, L.E.J. (1987) Obstruction and perforation complicating colorectal carcinoma. *Acta. Chir. Scand.* **153**, 607-14.

15. Mercadante, S., Spoldi, E., Carceni, A. *et al.* (1993) Octreotide in relieving gastrointestinal symptoms due to bowel obstruction. *Pall. Med.* **7**, 295-9.

16. Ripamonti, C. (1994) Malignant bowel obstruction in advanced and terminal cancer patients. *Eur. J. Pall. Care* **1**, 16-9.

17. Riley, J. and Fallon, M. (1994) Octreotide in terminal malignant obstruction of the gastrointestinal tract. *Eur. J. Pall. Care* **1**, 23-5.

18. Fallon, M. (1994) The physiology of somatostatin and its synthetic analogue, octreotide. *Eur. J. Pall. Care* **1**, 20-2.

Part Three

Optimizing Treatment

III - Survival Analysis

Chapter 19

Location of treatment: impact on survival

Elizabeth J. JUNOR, David J. HOLE and Charles R. GILLIS

19.1 INTRODUCTION

It is a common supposition that all advances and improvements in survival from cancer are the result of laboratory research and clinical trials. However, the results from these kinds of research must be implemented at patient level before overall survival rates improve. The influence of the organization and delivery of treatment is less well understood.

Several prognostic factors, such as age, disease stage, histological type and degree of differentiation, performance status and ascites have been identified which influence survival of patients with ovarian cancer [1–4]. The volume of residual disease postoperatively [5] is also recognized as having prognostic significance and clinical trials of chemotherapy have identified platinum [6] and taxol [7] as the agents most capable of producing improved survival in patients with ovarian cancer.

Data exist to show that participation in clinical trials [8–11] and referral to specialist centres confers survival advantage on patients with certain types of cancer. These benefits have been shown in childhood cancers [12], teratoma [13], and breast cancer [14]. In ovarian cancer the presence of a gynaecological oncologist at the time of operation has a significant influence on survival [15].

In the west of Scotland (population 2.8 million), 3-year survival for patients under 55 years of age diagnosed between 1975 and 1988 improved by 14%. Patients aged 55-64 showed

a survival improvement of 6%. Those patients treated in teaching hospitals survived longer than those treated elsewhere [16]. The difference in survival between patients treated in teaching hospitals increased with time which prompted a study to determine the treatment factors which influenced survival in patients with ovarian cancer at a population level.

19.2 PATIENTS AND METHODS

A detailed study of all cases of ovarian cancer diagnosed in Scotland in 1987 was performed. 533 patients were registered to the Scottish Cancer Registration Scheme in 1987. 34 patients were excluded because of incorrect pathology or year of diagnosis and the case records for a further 20 patients could not be traced. Information with regard to presentation, investigation, management and basic biological features were extracted from the case records of the remaining 479 patients. Detailed information on the specialty of the clinician who operated, subsequent management and in particular the presence or absence of multidisciplinary team management was recorded. Five years of follow up were included for each patient. Retrospective FIGO staging was determined by one individual using a combination of operation notes, pathology reports and available investigations at the time of presentation.

For the analysis, patients receiving platinum chemotherapy (either cisplatinum or

183

Table 19.1 Patient characteristics and unadjusted survival for ovarian cancer patients diagnosed in Scotland in 1987

Characteristics		Number (%) of cases	Percentage surviving		
			1 year	3 years	5 years
All patients		479	54	30	24
Stage:	I	119(26.3)	92	77	66
	II	49(10.8)	61	41	33
	III	212(46.9)	46	15	8
	IV	72(15.9)	31	4	0
	Not known	27	4	0	0
Age group	<45	39(8.1)	82	67	56
	45-54	85(17.7)	67	40	29
	55-64	133(27.8)	61	32	24
	65-74	129(26.9)	51	26	20
	75+	93(19.4)	25	12	9
Degree of differentiation	Well	40(12.5)	70	60	55
	Moderate	78(24.3)	60	35	28
	Poor	203(63.2)	50	22	14
	Not known	158	53	32	26
Presence of ascites	No	354(76.0)	60	36	29
	Yes	112(24.0)	35	12	6
	Not known	13	69	46	23
Histological type	Borderline	12(2.6)	100	92	83
	Germ cell	5(1.1)	100	80	80
	Mucinous	71(15.3)	72	52	46
	Serous	123(26.5)	65	34	25
	Endometrioid	34(7.3)	59	44	35
	Mesonephroid	19(4.1)	47	37	32
	Granulosa cell	7(1.5)	100	57	57
	Adenocarcinoma	176(37.9)	38	13	7
	Mixed mesodermal	12(2.6)	25	8	0
	Miscellaneous	5(1.1)	60	40	0
	Not Known	15	13	0	0
Mode of admission	Elective	303(66.2)	60	34	26
	Emergency	155(33.8)	44	25	21
	Not known	21	38	24	14

carboplatin) with or without other agents constituted the 'platinum group', those receiving an alkylating agent alone, the 'alkylating agent group', and a third group the 'no chemotherapy group', those patients receiving hormones or no anti-tumour agents. A joint clinic was defined as one in which gynaecologists and oncologists agreed the most appropriate management throughout the postoperative period.

The effect of clinical management on survival was examined taking account of prognostic features by use of Cox's proportional hazard model [17]. A model looking at the organizational component of patient management was constructed featuring the specialty of the first hospital doctor to see the patient, the specialty of the person performing the operation, attendance at a joint clinic, participation in a clinical trial and the teaching status of the treating hospital. This was called the 'referral model'. A 'treatment model' incorporating the two treatment related factors, volume of residual disease and platinum chemotherapy, was also constructed.

19.3 RESULTS

Table 19.1 shows the results of the Cox's proportional hazard analysis relating the risk of death to the five significant prognostic factors. Poor pathological type ($p<0.001$), increasing age ($p<0.001$), late stage of disease ($p<0.001$), poorer histological differentiation ($p<0.01$), older age ($p<0.001$) and the presence of ascites ($p<0.01$) significantly increased the risk of death. Survival was improved when the patient was initially seen by a gynaecologist as opposed to a surgeon or physician ($p<0.05$) In addition if the initial laparotomy was performed by a gynaecologist and not a general surgeon the chance of death was decreased ($p<0.05$). The final significant feature relating to referral was management by a multidisciplinary team at a joint clinic ($p<0.001$). Time to presentation, time to referral, time to laparotomy and other factors

were examined and found not to relate significantly to survival.

Examination of the treatment model revealed two factors which significantly improved survival. These were residual disease less than 2cm ($p<0.001$) and receiving platinum chemotherapy ($p<0.05$). Adjustment for the five prognostic factors age, stage, degree of differentiation, histology and presence of ascites was performed and these effects were still apparent and of significance. Categories of patients who were unlikely to have been considered for platinum chemotherapy in 1987 (those over 75 years of age and/or patients with stage Ia or Ib disease) were excluded from a subsequent analysis and the use of platinum was still associated with improved survival ($p<0.01$).

231 patients (48.2%) were seen initially by a gynaecologist, 167 (34.9%) by a surgeon and 65 (13.6%) by a physician. The 5-year survival for those patients seen initially by a gynaecologist was 35% compared with 16% for those seen by a either a general surgeon or physician. After adjustment for age and stage this difference reduced to 21% from 27%.

The 5-year survival rate for those patients operated on by gynaecologists was 28% compared with 14% by non-gynaecologists. After adjustment for age and stage this difference reduced to 19% from 27%. Of the 432 patients (90.2%) who underwent laparotomy, 367 were performed by gynaecologists and the remainder (65) by non-gynaecological surgeons. Patients operated on by surgeons were older (50.8% were aged 65 and over compared with 40.9% for gynaecologists) and had more advanced disease (72.3% were stage III or IV compared with 57.5% for gynaecologists).

Both in early ($p<0.01$) and late ($p<0.01$) stage disease optimal debulking was more often achieved when the operation was performed by a gynaecologist even after adjustment for the other four prognostic features. Table 19.2

Table 19.2 Relationship between the likelihood of disease <2cm remaining after operation,the five prognostic factors and the specialty of the person performing the primary operation

Factor	Number of cases[a]	Relative[b] probability	95% confidence interval
Stage:			
I	101	14.6	7.1 - 30.1
II	48	5.6	2.5 - 12.3
III	195	1	Baseline
IV	55	0.5	0.2 - 1.1
Not known	5		
		Test for trend t = 8.02 (p<0.001)	
Age:			
<45	38	2.5	0.8 - 8.2
45-64	197	1	Baseline
65+	169	0.5	0.3 - 0.9
		Test for trend t = 3.44 (p<0.001)	
Degree of differentiation:			
Well	36	1.3	0.5 - 3.4
Moderate	72	1.1	0.5 - 2.4
Poor	182	1	Baseline
Not known	114	0.7	0.3 - 1.3
		Test for trend t = 1.05 (NS)	
Pathological type:			
Good	16	3.9	0.4 - 42.8
Moderate	236	1	Baseline
Poor	152	0.5	0.3 - 0.9
		Test for trend t = 3.05 (p<0.01)	
Presence of ascites:			
No	304	1	Baseline
Yes	88	0.7	0.4 - 1.4
Who performed operation?			
Gynaecologist	346	1	Baseline
Surgeon	57	0.2*	0.1 - 0.6

[a] Excluding 47 patients who had no operation and 28 patients with no statement on the extent of residual disease.
[b] Probability that patient with characteristic given will have residual disease of <2cm after operation relative to that of a patient with baseline characeristic. Adjusted for other prognostic factors.
[c] Insufficient cases to allow estimation.
* p<0.01

shows the relationship between the extent of residual disease postoperatively, the specialty of the person performing the operation and the five prognostic factors.

The number of patients operated on by any individual was examined. Table 19.3 shows the relationship between survival and the number of patients operated on by an individual, both before and after adjustment for prognostic variables. It can be seen that there is a trend for better survival in patients who have had their laparotomy performed by individuals who more frequently treat patients with ovarian cancer.

In all 130 patients (27.1%) were referred postoperatively to a multidisciplinary joint clinic. Patients referred to these joint clinics were younger than those not so referred. 98 of 257 patients under 65 years of age (38%) were referred compared with 32 of 222 aged over 65 years (14%).

When examining the prescription of platinum chemotherapy it was found that age and stage of disease were the major influences. Of those patients younger than 65 years of age, 50.2% were prescribed platinum as opposed to only 20.2% of those patients between 65 and 74 years. Table 19.4 shows the factors influencing the likelihood of being treated with platinum. Patients over 75 years of age and those staged Ia or Ib were excluded from the analysis. Even after adjustment for age, stage, histology, degree of differentiation, presence of ascites and volume of residual disease patients attending a multidisciplinary combined clinic were twice as likely to be prescribed platinum chemotherapy than those not attending such a clinic (p<0.01). Restricting analysis to only those patients who received some form of chemotherapy, patients attending a joint clinic were still almost twice as likely (relative probability=1.90; p<0.07) to receive platinum. Drug dose was not analysed.

19.4 DISCUSSION

The five prognostic factors identified in this study are those well recognized and reported

Table 19. 3 Relationship between survival and the number of patients operated on by an individual

Operations per year	Patients numbers	5 year survival (unadjusted)	RHR unadjusted	adjusted
1	159	16%	1	1
2-4	225	27%	0.73**	0.94
>5	72	33%	0.54***	0.74+

Adjusted = adjusted for prognostic factors age, stage, histology, degree of
  differentiation and ascites.
+ = P<0.1 ** P<0.01 *** = P<0.001
RHR = Relative Hazard Ratio

frequently. Being seen initially by a gynae-cologist, being operated on by a gynaecologist, having debulking surgery to <2cm, receiving platinum chemotherapy and being managed in a multidisciplinary joint clinic all lead to significantly improved survival. The advantage of debulking surgery has been known for some time [5] and the place of platinum chemotherapy has been highlighted in an overview of chemotherapy in ovarian cancer carried out by the Advanced Ovarian Cancer Trials Group [6].

Three main management factors influence the overall outcome of any disease process - making the diagnosis, deciding on the most effective treatment and implementing treatment. Paradoxically more than 50% of patients were first seen by surgeons or physicians. Surgeons most frequently performed only a biopsy and were unlikely to perform a total hysterectomy and bilateral oophorectomy and their patients were therefore less likely to have less than 2cm of residual disease remaining. It is recognized that some tumours may be easier to debulk than others due to their inherent characteristics but it is unlikely that this could explain the 5-fold difference in the likelihood of tumour debulking associated with the specialty of the person performing the operation.

A highly significant improvement in survival was conferred by management in a multidisciplinary joint clinic (p<0.001). The increased prescription of platinum chemo-therapy at these clinics could have been an explanation for this feature but even after adjustment for the effect of platinum there still remained some unexplained component of multidisciplinary management in a specialist clinic. It may be that the clinicians working in a multidisciplinary clinic may be more likely to have a particular interest in gynaecological malignancy or it may be that several heads are better than one when considering the optimal management for patients with ovarian cancer. The part played by specialist nurses and other non-medical staff cannot be ignored when seeking explanations for the beneficial effect of joint clinics.

There was no statistically significant benefit to being treated in a teaching hospital. After adjusting for the prognostic factors age, stage, degree of differentiation, histology and presence of ascites, the relative hazard ratio for non-teaching compared to teaching hospitals is 1.19 using Cox's proportional hazard model. This hazard ratio is similar in size to that found in a larger study of 3000 cases diagnosed between 1975 and 1988 [16] which produced a relative hazard ratio of 1.13 and was statistically

Table 19.4 Relationship between the likelihood of receiving platinum, the five presenting prognostic factors, extent of residual disease and attendance at a joint clinic (excluding patients aged 75 years and over or stage Ia,Ib)

Factor	Number of cases	Relative probabilities	95% confidence interval
Stage			
I	56	0.14	0.05 - 0.34
II	42	0.36	0.15 - 0.88
III	164	1	Baseline
IV	58	1.40	0.69 - 2.88
NK	13	0.21	0.06 - 0.73
	Test for trend t = 3.98, p<0.001		
Age			
<45	29	1.54	0.55 - 4.34
45-64	191	1	Baseline
65-74	113	0.20	0.11 - 0.35
	Test for trend t = 4.45, p<0.001		
Degree of differentiation			
Well	21	1.23	0.39 - 3.90
Moderate	52	0.69	0.33 - 1.44
Poor	162	1	Baseline
NK	98	0.43	0.23 - 0.79
	Test for trend t = 0.40, p = NS		
Pathological type			
Good	7	0.32	0.04 - 2.45
Moderate	184	1	Baseline
Poor	142	0.52	0.30 - 0.92
	Test for trend t = 1.3,0 p = NS		
Presence of ascites			
Yes	76	1	Baseline
No	246	1.29	0.69 - 2.41
Extent of residual disease			
<2cm	177	1	Baseline
>2cm	122	1.64	0.84 - 3.22
Attendance at a joint clinic			
Yes	102	2.02*	1.13 - 3.60
No	231	1	Baseline

* p<0.05
NK=not known

significant. The non-significant finding in this study we believe is due to insufficient numbers of patients to detect such a difference rather than the absence of a true effect. Likewise the effect of the number of patients operated on by an individual is not statistically significant after adjustment for prognostic factors but we believe that this is a function of insufficient number of cases to detect the difference. A larger number of patients would be required to clarify the effect with statistical significance.

19.5 CONCLUSIONS

This population-based study suggests that patients with ovarian cancer have improved survival if they follow a management path with individuals being initially assessed by a gynaecologist and having a laparotomy carried out by a gynaecologist who performs maximum debulking surgery. Subsequent management by a multidisciplinary team including gynaecologists and oncologists with the prescription of platinum chemotherapy also improves survival. Gynaecologists who have a special interest in gynaecological malignancy and therefore perform operations on a larger number of patients with ovarian cancer are advantageous in the management of patients with this disease. Improved survival from ovarian cancer in a total population should be attainable if well recognized and proven methods of treatment are available to all patients.

ACKNOWLEDGEMENTS

We thank the British Journal of Cancer for permission to reproduce elements of previously-published work.

REFERENCES

1. Einhorn N., Nilsson B. and Sjovall K. (1985) Factors influencing survival in carcinoma of the ovary: study from a well defined Swedish population. *Cancer* 55, 2019-25.
2. Hogberg T., Carstensen J. and Simonsen E.

(1993) Treatment results and prognostic factors in a population-based study of epithelial ovarian cancer. *Gynecol. Oncol.* **48,** 38-49.

3. Marsoni S., Torri V., Valsecchi M.G. *et al.* (1990) Prognostic factors in advanced epithelial ovarian cancer. Gruppo Interregionale Cooperativo di Oncologia Ginecologica (GICOG) *Brit. J. Cancer* **62,** 444-50.

4. Omura G.A., Brady M.F., Homsley H.D. *et al.* (1991) Long-term follow-up and prognostic factor analysis in advanced ovarian carcinoma. The Gynecologic Oncology Group experience. *J. Clin. Oncol.* **9,** 1138-50.

5. Griffiths C.T. (1975) Surgical resection of tumour bulk in the primary treatment of ovarian carcinoma. Symposium on ovarian carcinoma. *Monogr. Natl. Cancer Inst.* **42,** 101-4.

6. Advanced Ovarian Cancer Trialists Group (1991) Chemotherapy in advanced ovarian cancer: an overview of randomised trials. *BMJ* **303,** 884-93.

7. McGuire W.P., Hoskins W.J., Brady M.F. *et al.* (1993) A phase III Trial comparing cisplatin/cytoxan and cisplatin/taxol in advanced ovarian cancer. For the Gynecologic Oncology Group (GOG). *American Society of Clinical Oncology,* Orlando FL.

8. Lennox E.L., Draper G.J., Sanders B.M. (1975) Retinoblastoma: a study of natural history and prognosis of 268 cases. *BMJ* **3,** 731-4.

9. Davis S., Wright P.W., Schulman S.F. *et al.* (1985) Participants in prospective randomised trials for resected non-small cell lung cancer have improved survival compared with non participants in such trials. *Cancer* **56,** 1710-8.

10. Karjaleinen S. and Palva I. (1989) Do treatment protocols improve end results? A study of survival of patients with multiple myeloma in Finland. *BMJ* **299,** 1069-72.

11. Stiller C.A. and Draper G.J. (1989) Treatment centre size, entry to trials, and survival in acute lymphoblastic leukaemia. *Arch. Dis. Child.* **64,** 657-61.

12. Stiller C.A. (1988) Centralisation of treatment and survival rates for cancer. *Arch.Dis.Child.* **63,** 23-30.

13. Harding M.J., Paul J., Gillis C. and Kaye S.B. (1993) Management of malignant teratoma. Does referral to a specialist unit matter? *Lancet* **341,** 999-1002.

14. Karjaleinen S. (1990) Geographical variation in cancer patient survival in Finland: chance, confounding or effect of treatment? *J. Epidemiol .Comm. Health* **44,** 210-4.

15. Eisenkop S.M., Spirtos N.M., Montag T.W. *et al.* (1992) The impact of subspecialist training on the management of advanced ovarian cancer. *Gynecol. Oncol.* **47,** 203-9.

16. Gillis C.R., Hole D.J., Still R.M. *et al.* (1991) Medical audit, cancer registration and survival in ovarian cancer. *Lancet* **337,** 611-2.

17. Cox DR. (1972) Regression models and life-tables (with discussion). *J. Roy. Statist. Soc.* **B34,** 187-220.

Chapter 20

Neural networks for survival prediction

Marc M.H.J. THEEUWEN, Hilbert J. KAPPEN and Jan P. NEIJT

20.1 INTRODUCTION

One of the leading issues in the treatment of cancer is the identification of patients with a good or poor prognosis. The assessment of prognosis is valuable in the planning of treatment for individual patients and for the stratification of patients in clinical trials. Quantitative methods for analysis of prognostic information are important to the optimal use of this knowledge. We employed a new quantitative method to define the prognosis of cancer patients: an artificial neural network.

20.2 NEURAL NETWORKS

Neural networks are powerful algorithms that can be used to learn relations in a database, and which can predict output parameters on novel data. At present neural networks are rapidly making their way into various areas of the biomedical sciences. They are being applied to pattern recognition or decision making in diverse fields including nucleic acid sequence analysis, quantitative cytology, diagnostic imaging [1] breast cancer research [2,3] and cancer drug development [4].

The fundamental building blocks in neural networks are 'units' which can be likened to neurones, and weighted connections which can be likened to synapses. The networks have a variable number of input units (encoding the patient characteristics) and one or more output units (encoding the classes to which this patient belongs).

Between the inputs and outputs of the network, commonly one hidden layer of neurones is placed whose number of units can vary. Each hidden unit is connected to all in- and outputs. In addition, there are direct links between input and output units. The more hidden units, the more complex the patterns that can be learned. With a set of patients whose survival duration is known, we can train the network and learn to predict survival. During the learning process the weighting factors in the links change [5]. For the networks considered, here the output encodes the probability of membership to one of two possible classes such as alive or dead.

20.2.1 SURVIVAL AS A CLASSIFICATION PROBLEM

Recently new classes of neural networks, Boltzmann Perceptrons have been developed that allow a probabilistic interpretation of the output [6]. We used these Boltzmann Perceptrons with fast learning rules [7,8]. In the first stage the Boltzmann Perceptrons are trained with a part of the data. The remaining part is not presented during training. The criterion that is minimized during training, and that is used for evaluating the quality of the network solution is the Kullback divergence between the probability that is observed in reality and the probability given by the network. This criterion is an accurate measure for the predictive value of the model, and better embedded in information theory than for instance the percentage of correctly classified patients. In the absence of censoring, for a set of P patients, labelled $\mu = 1,......,P$ the Kullback divergence reduces to the log-likelihood:

$$K = -\frac{1}{P}\sum_{\mu=1}^{P}\log(p(y^{\mu}|\vec{x}^{\mu}))$$

where $p(y|\vec{x})$ denotes the probability that a patient with characteristics $\vec{x}$ belongs to class $y = \pm 1$. When all patients are classified correctly, $p(y^{\mu}|\vec{x}^{\mu}) = 1$ for all patients and thus $K = 0$. Worst case behaviour is obtained, when there is no relation between patient characteristics and survival. In that case $p(y^{\mu}|\vec{x}^{\mu})$ is independent of $\vec{x}^{\mu}$ and

$$K_0 = -\frac{P_+}{P}\log\left(\frac{P_+}{P}\right) - \frac{P_-}{P}\log\left(\frac{P_-}{P}\right)$$

(1)

with $P_{+,-}$ denoting the number of patients in the two classes, and $P_+ + P_- = P$ the total number of patients. A solution that significantly differs from K_0 on the test set indicates that there are patient characteristics that have prognostic impact.

After training, the networks can be used for prediction of survival in the following way: a network with one output can be trained to predict whether a patient will survive longer or shorter than Y years with $Y = 1, 2,......$. Thus, a number of neural networks are trained, each specializing in survival for a specific number of years. The advantages of this approach are that:
1. No assumption is made about the overall shape of the survival distribution. This is also one of the appealing properties of proportional hazard models.
2. No assumption is made about the way in which the characteristics influence the survival distribution. This is different from proportional hazard models, where the patient characteristics are assumed to multiply the hazard.
3. By inspection of the solutions found by the different networks, the influence of patient characteristics on short-term and long-term survival can be obtained.

20.2.2 GENERALIZATION PERFORMANCE

For the method discussed here, the general problem exists of overfitting on the data. It is quite easy to improve the prediction of the network on a training set by choosing a more complex network. However this will not necessarily improve the results on an independent set of test data. In fact, the performance on the test data is the only relevant criterion. This is called the generalization performance. To evaluate the generalization performance we have trained the networks on 80% of the data and tested on the remaining 20%. This division into training set and test set was done at random. The experiment was repeated ten times to make sure that the result is not dependent on the particular choice of training and test set.

The generalization performance of a network can be improved by introducing a complexity reducing term on the weights. The most well known example is called 'weight decay', and amounts to adding a term $\lambda \sum_i w_i^2$ to the cost function w_i are the different weight values in the network. This term will favour solutions with small weights. These solutions are 'smoother' than solutions with large weights. It can therefore be expected that a certain amount of weight decay (controlled by λ) will improve generalization.

A disadvantage of weight decay is that it penalizes large weights more than small weights. As a result, solutions with many small weights will be favoured over solutions with one large weight. This makes the interpretation of the neural network more difficult. For this reason we have experimented with another complexity reducing term, which favours solutions with as few as possible weights on. We defined the next complexity reducing term:

$$S = -\sum_i^N p_i \log(p_i); p_i = \frac{w_i^2}{\sum_j^N w_j^2}$$

S is called the entropy of the probability distribution p_i, $i = 1,\ldots, N$. The entropy is maximal for broad distributions, with all $p_i = 1/N$, and is minimal for peaked distributions, with $p_i = \delta_{ik}$ for some k. When k out of N weights have an equally significant contribution, and the remaining weights have no significance, $S = \log k$. The term λS can be added to the cost function, to obtain solutions with as few as possible non-zero weights.

20.3 INITIAL EXPERIMENTS AND RESULTS

20.3.1 METHODS

For our initial experiments we used the data of two Dutch studies, initiated in 1979 and 1981, respectively. The first study compared a combination of hexamethylmelamine, cyclophosphamide, methotrexate, and 5-fluorouracil (Hexa-CAF) with cyclopho-sphamide and hexa-methylmelamine alternating with doxorubicin and a five day course of cisplatin (CHAP-5) in 186 patients

with advanced epithelial ovarian carcinoma [9]. In the second study, initiated in 1981, 191 eligible patients were enrolled and treated with either CHAP-5 or cyclophosphamide and cisplatin (CP) both administered intravenously on a single day at 3-week intervals [10]. Protocol entry criteria, pre-treatment staging, histology grading, the randomization procedure, assessment and definitions of tumour response, evaluation and statistical methods were the same in both studies.

We used four Boltzmann Perceptrons to predict survival and progression-free survival after Y years, with $Y = 1, 2, 4, 8$. For 1, 2, 4 and 8 year prediction, respectively 1, 4, 5 and 6 censored patients were encountered, which were excluded from this analysis. The characteristics that were used for this study included: residual tumour size, FIGO stage, Karnofsky index, place of diagnosis, age, haemoglobin, leukocytes, thrombocytes, Broders' grade, hospital experience, weight, length, cell type and serum creatinine. Missing values for several characteristics were filled in with the average value for that characteristic. For each classification task we determined the optimal number of hidden units and λ for both weight decay and entropy term. This was done by generating ten random test sets consisting of 20% of the patients. The training and test sets were constructed in a way that they contained the same ratio of long- and short-survivors as in the original data set.

20.3.2 NETWORK ARCHITECTURE

For both survival and progression-free survival it was found that the addition of hidden units improved the performance on the training set significantly, but did not improve the performance on the independent test set.

As could be expected the weight decay criterion improved the generalization of the network. Similar results were found with the entropy term. However, the expected effect that solutions could be obtained with less patients characteristics was not found. We therefore decided to use the standard weight decay in further experiments.

20.3.3 SURVIVAL PREDICTION

The results for survival and progression-free survival are given in Table 20.1 and Table 20.2. For each year the optimal value of the Kullback divergence on independent test data is given, averaged over the ten runs together with the variation. For comparison the Kullback divergence K_0, Equation (1), that could be obtained if there was no relation between the patient characteristics and survival or progression-free survival is presented.

As shown in the tables, the predictive power of the method as expressed by the Kullback value, is better than the no relation assumption between patient characteristics and survival. The difference between the

Table 20.1 Optimal generalization results for survival prediction with the Boltzmann Perceptron on 377 patients. Results are shown without hidden units and a standard weight decay (λ). For each year, the optimal generalization is presented, expressed in terms of the Kullback divergence as well as percentage of patients predicted correct. For comparison, the K_0 and percentage predicted correct without any relation between patient characteristics and survival is presented. The greater the distance between the Kullback and K_0, the greater is the predictive power of the network

Years	Kullback	K_0	Percent correct	No relation	λ
1	0.517 ± 0.013	0.556	75.8 ± 0.9	75.3	1.0
2	0.630 ± 0.020	0.693	65.7 ± 4.4	50.1	0.8
4	0.536 ± 0.017	0.616	73.6 ± 3.2	69.4	0.5
8	0.435 ± 0.029	0.488	82.2 ± 1.3	80.9	0.5

Table 20.2 Optimal generalization results of the Boltzmann Perceptron for prediction of progression-free survival

Years	Kullback	K_0	Percent correct	No relation	λ
1	0.629 ± 0.019	0.683	64.4 ± 3.8	57.2	0.8
2	0.602 ± 0.031	0.666	69.5 ± 3.5	61.7	0.5
4	0.444 ± 0.021	0.510	80.1 ± 0.6	79.3	0.5
8	0.348 ± 0.025	0.390	87.7 ± 0.0	86.8	0.5

Kullback value and K_0 is always around 0.05, independent of the number of years. This indicates that the patient characteristics fed into the network have important impact on both short- and long-term survival. When the percentage of correctly classified patients is taken as a criterion, the difference between the model predictions and 'no relation' is not as consistent. This is because the Kullback value is directly calculated from the probabilities, whereas the 'percent correct' value is obtained by truncating the probabilities to binary values 'correct' and 'false' and then summed. Thus, the situation may arise that a Kullback value significantly lower than K_0 is found, without a significantly better prediction percentage (for instance at one year survival).

20.4 DISCUSSION

During extensive simulations with different numbers of hidden units we found that the non-linear relations present in the Dutch database could be successfully fitted by neural networks. However, the best generalization results were obtained with a network without hidden units. This indicates that there are probably not sufficient data in the Dutch database to extract a non-linear relationship from noise.

At present there are several arguments for the use of neural networks instead of the conventional statistical methods such as Cox regression analysis. An advantage of neural networks is that the influence of a large number of potentially relevant patient and treatment characteristics can be assessed in one network. Neural networks easily can reveal time dependencies in the predictiveness of patient characteristics by not assuming the proportionality of the hazard. This is especially important in the analysis of cancer data where a given prognostic factor may have a major impact early during treatment but have no influence on long-term survival. Neural networks may also have an advantage above conventional statistics when the relationship between a prognostic factor and outcome is non-linear and when the prognostic factors are dependent of each other [11].

Once methods for using neural networks for survival analysis have further improved, we expect that the method will outperform the standard statistical methods like the Cox regression analysis. Further research is needed on how to take into account censored data and how to compute confidence levels. Interpretation of the neural network architecture to discover the relative importance and significance of patient characteristics over time is currently being developed on a larger database.

REFERENCES

1. Erler, B.S., Hsu, L., Truong, H.M. *et al.* (1994) Methods in laboratory investigation: image analysis and diagnostic classification of hepatocellular carcinoma using neural networks and multivariate discriminant functions. *Lab. Invest.* **71**, 446-51.
2. Floyd, C.E., Jr., Lo, J.Y., Yun, A.J. *et al.* (1994) Prediction of breast cancer malignancy using an artificial neural network. *Cancer* **74**, 2944-8.
3. De Laurentiis, M. and Ravdin, P.M. (1994) Survival analysis of censored data, neural network analysis detection of complex interactions between variables. *Breast Cancer Res. Treat.* **32**, 113-8.
4. Weinstein, J.N., Kohn, K.W., Grever, M.R. *et al.* (1992) Neural computing in cancer drug development, prediction mechanism of action. *Science* **258**, 447-51.
5. Hinton, G.E. How neural networks learn from experience. (1992) *Sci. Am.* **267**, 145-51.
6. Kappen, H.J. (1994) Using Boltzmann machines for probability estimation, a

general framework for neural network learning. In *Proc. Pattern Recognition in Practice IV* (eds E.S. Gelsema and L.N. Kanal) Elsevier, Amsterdam, pp. 299-312.

7. Ackley, D., Hinton, G. and Sejnowski, T. A. (1985) Learning algorithm for Boltzmann machines. *Cogn. Sci.* **9**, 147-69.

8. Kappen, H.J. (1994) Using Boltzmann machines for probability estimation. In *Proc. ICANN '93* (eds H.J. Kappen, and S. Gielen), Springer Verlag, London, pp. 521-6.

9. Neijt, J.P., ten Bokkel Huinink, W.W., Van der Burg, M.E.L. *et al.* (1984) Randomised trial comparing two combination chemotherapy regimens (Hexa-CAF *vs.* CHAP-5) in advanced ovarian carcinoma. *Lancet* **2**, 594-600.

10. Neijt, J.P., ten Bokkel Huinink, W.W., Van der Burg, M.E.L. *et al.* (1987) Randomized trial comparing two combination chemotherapy regimens (CHAP-5 vs. CP) in advanced ovarian carcinoma. *J. Clin. Oncol.* **5**, 1157-68.

11. De Laurentiis, M. and Ravdin, P.M. (1994) A technique for using neural network analysis to perform survival analysis of censored data. *Cancer Lett.* **77**, 127-38.

Part Four

New Treatment Approaches

Chapter 21

New strategies for prevention and treatment

Robert C. BAST, Jr., Cinda M. BOYER, Robert M. DABLE, Feng-Ji XU,

Yin-Hua YU and Andrew BERCHUCK

21.1 NOVEL APPROACHES TO THE PREVENTION OF EPITHELIAL OVARIAN CANCER

More than 90% of ovarian cancers in adults are thought to arise from a single layer of epithelial cells that covers the ovarian surface or lines inclusion cysts. Transformation of this epithelium requires multiple genetic changes that downregulate tumour suppressor genes, activate oncogenes and interfere with normal regulation by growth factors. Proliferation is an apparent requisite for these changes. Ovarian surface epithelial cells are generally quiescent, but can proliferate to repair the defects that are created by ovulation.

Epidemiological studies indicate that factors which increase the total number of ovulatory cycles increase the risk of ovarian cancer, these include early or late menopause, nulliparity and the use of fertility stimulating drugs. Conversely, factors that suppress ovulation decrease the risk of ovarian cancer in later life. Multiple pregnancies, prolonged lactation, and the use of oral contraceptives have all been associated with a lower incidence of ovarian cancer.

21.1.1 THE POTENTIAL ROLE OF TGF-β IN CHEMOPREVENTION

Following ovulation, a variety of factors control the proliferation of ovarian cancer cells including autocrine growth factors produced by the cells themselves and paracrine growth factors produced by the underlying stroma and follicular fluid. Most of the growth factors studied to date have stimulated proliferation of ovarian epithelium, including TGF-α, EGF, TNF, IL-1, and IL-6 [1]. One inhibitory factor that has been well characterized is transforming growth factor beta (TGF-β). Proliferation of normal ovarian epithelial cells can be regularly inhibited by TGF-β and the normal epithelium expresses TGF-β1 and TGF-β2 [2]. Expression of TGF-β is lost in approximately 40% of ovarian cancers, but cells taken directly from ascites fluid can still be inhibited by exogenous TGF-β in 95% of cases [3]. Consequently, a significant fraction of ovarian cancers have lost the potential for autocrine, but not for paracrine growth inhibition by TGF-β. Importantly, TGF-β can induce apoptosis in a fraction of ovarian cell lines and in tumour cells taken directly from patients [4]. Apoptosis was observed in three of ten ascites tumour cell cultures, but

199

in none of seven cultures of normal epithelial cells. Consequently, ovarian cancer cells appear to acquire susceptibility to apoptosis during malignant transformation. TGF-β may participate in a surveillance mechanism that could eliminate cells as they undergo transformation.

21.1.2 THE POTENTIAL ROLE OF RETINOIC ACID DERIVATIVES IN CHEMOPREVENTION

Factors that regulate TGF-β expression in the normal ovary are not well understood. In other settings, retinoids have induced TGF-β expression. Different retinoic acid derivatives, including 9-cis-retinoic acid, 4-hydroxy-phenylretinamide (4-HPR), and all-trans-retinoic acid (ATRA) can inhibit thymidine incorporation by a fraction of ovarian cancer cell lines [5]. Growth inhibition by these retinoic acid derivatives in ovarian cancer cells has not, however, been associated with increased expression of TGF-β. In one ovarian cancer cell line, the addition of both TGF-β and ATRA produced synergistic inhibition of thymidine incorporation [5].

When ovarian cancer cells were studied directly from ascites fluid, two patterns of growth inhibition were observed in the presence of TGF-β and/or ATRA. With a majority of specimens, TGF-β alone produced nearly maximal inhibition of thymidine incorporation. In a significant minority of specimens, TGF-β and ATRA each produced partial inhibition of thymidine incorporation, but completely suppressed thymidine incorporation when used in combination. Among 12 preparations of tumour cells from different individuals, seven were inhibited by TGF-β, two by retinoic acid, and all twelve by the combination [5].

If TGF-β does eliminate ovarian epithelial cells as they undergo transformation, agents such as retinoids that induce TGF-β in ovarian stroma may prove of value for chemoprevention. In this regard, retinoic acid derivatives can induce TGF-β in many tissues. In one study performed at the National Cancer Institute of Milan between 1987 and 1992, fenretinide (4-HPR) was given daily to women at risk of developing a second primary breast cancer [6]. During the trial, six cases of ovarian cancer were observed in the control group, but none among those women taking fenretinide. This difference proved highly significant upon statistical analysis.

Although the chemoprevention activity of fenretinide observation requires confirmation, retinoic acid derivatives may have a role in preventing ovarian cancer. In the future, models for spontaneous transformation of ovarian surface epithelium, as well as models to understand interactions of ovarian stroma and epithelium will be helpful in developing chemopreventive strategies. In addition, if clinical trials are to be performed with limited numbers of subjects, individuals at increased risk of ovarian cancer must be identified. The ability of oral contraceptives to prevent ovarian cancer should be tested prospectively in clinical trials.

21.2 NOVEL APPROACHES TO THE TREATMENT OF EPITHELIAL OVARIAN CANCER

21.2.1 MOLECULAR TARGETS FOR THERAPY

A number of molecular alterations have been observed in ovarian cancer that could provide targets for treatment of established disease. Ovarian cancer cells retain expression of the epidermal growth factor receptor in 70% of cases, overexpress HER-2/neu (c-erbB2) in 30%, and exhibit novel expression of fms in more than 50% [7-9]. All of these receptors can participate in autocrine or paracrine growth stimulation.

Inhibitors of the epidermal growth factor receptor, HER-2/neu and fms might downregulate proliferation of cells in which autocrine or paracrine loops had been established. Paracrine growth stimulation can also occur through macrophage derived cytokines such as tumour necrosis factor [10], interleukin-1 [10] and interleukin-6 [11], as well as the ovarian cancer activating factor (OCAF), a novel phosphatidic acid derivative found in ascites fluid [12]. Superagonists and antagonists for each of these factors might influence growth of ovarian cancer. Inhibitors of their receptors deserve further attention. Although the ras gene is mutated in only a minority of ovarian cancers, the ras protein appears to be physiologically activated in a majority of ovarian cancer cell lines. Consequently, inhibitors of ras might also be useful.

Overexpression of PTP1B has been observed in more than 90% of ovarian cancers [13] and modulation of its expression might also impact on ovarian cancer growth. Given the 50% incidence of p53 mutation in advanced ovarian cancer [14], agents that restore p53 function might slow proliferation of ovarian cancer cells. Recent experiments with gene transfer support this approach [15].

21.2.2 ANTIBODY MEDIATED INHIBITION OF TUMOUR CELLS THAT OVEREXPRESS ERBB2

The erbB2 gene product has already been used as a target for immunological intervention. In 70% of ovarian cancers there is approximately the same level of expression of erbB2 that is found in normal epithelial cells. In 30% of ovarian cancers, erbB2 is overexpressed and often amplified [8,16]. In some, but not all studies, erbB2 overexpression has been associated with a poor prognosis [8]. To date studies have not taken into account the co-ordinate expression of erbB2, erbB3, erbB4, and the ligand heregulin. Regardless of its prognostic value, overexpression of erbB2 could provide a target for therapy in almost one third of patients.

Over the last several years a number of monoclonal antibodies have been developed against the extracellular domain of the erbB2 protein (p185). Through cross blocking experiments, multiple epitopes have been mapped [17]. Monoclonal antibodies to 7 of 11 epitopes on the extracellular domain of p185 inhibit anchorage independent growth of tumour cells. Growth inhibition depends upon the density of p185 determinants, but not upon the isotype of the antibody. Inhibition of anchorage independent growth correlates with the autophosphorylation of p185. Antibodies that inhibit growth also decrease intracellular levels of the lipid second messenger diacylglycerol (DAG) [18].

Heregulin is a ligand which binds to erbB3 and erbB4 receptors alone or in combination with p185. The cloning and expression of heregulin has permitted comparison of the activities of anti-p185 antibodies with those of the ligand. Both the antibodies and the ligand inhibit anchorage independent growth of tumour cells that overexpess p185. Heregulin stimulates growth in tumours cells with low levels of p185 expression, whereas these particular antibodies do not. Both heregulin and anti-p185 antibodies increase autophosphorylation of p185, but only the antibodies decrease intracellular DAG levels [19]. Both antibodies and ligands stimulate invasion of matrigel membranes. Heregulin also increases CD44, ICAM, and MMP-9 expression in cells that overexpress p185 [20]. Consequently, increased invasiveness, rather than increased proliferation may contribute to the worse prognosis of tumours that overexpress erbB2.

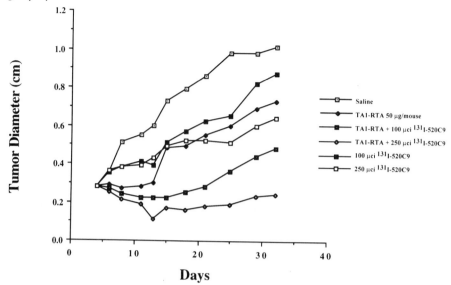

Figure 21.1 Growth of human ovarian carcinoma (SKOv3-clone 18) heterografts after treatment with TAI-RTA immunization, [131]I-520C9 radionuclide conjugate or a combination of the two agents.

21.2.3 COMBINED ANTITUMOUR ACTIVITY OF RADIONUCLIDE CONJUGATES AND IMMUNOTOXINS

Unconjugated antibodies can inhibit growth of approximately 90% of clonogenic cancer cells *in vitro*. Despite this relatively modest activity *in vitro*, clinical responses have been observed in recent studies using anti-p185 antibodies alone or in combination with cisplatin [21]. Greater antitumour activity might be obtained by linking monoclonal antibodies to radionuclides or to toxins. Immunotoxins have been prepared by conjugating murine monoclonal antibodies against p185 with the *A* chain of ricin. After binding to p185 on the cell surface, immunotoxin conjugates are internalized into endosomes. The ricin *A* chain is translocated to the cytoplasmic compartment where it inhibits ribosomal protein synthesis.

Immunotoxins have been prepared from monoclonal antibodies against a number of different epitopes on p185. The optimal conjugate is capable of inhibiting 99.99% of clonogenic units. Susceptibility of tumour cells to immunotoxins depends critically upon the density p185 determinants. In tumour cell lines with 104 determinants, immunotoxins produced less than 90% inhibition of clonogenic tumour cell growth, whereas in lines with 106 determinants, immunotoxins could inhibit clonogenic growth by 99.99%. This suggests that there might be a substantial therapeutic index *in vivo*.

Immunotoxins against p185 have been evaluated in nude mouse heterograft models. The TA1-RTA immunotoxin produced transient growth inhibition of the SKOv3-clone18 human ovarian cancer subline that overexpressed p185, but did not cure heterograft recipients. De Santes *et al.*, observed only transient inhibition of erbB2 transfected murine tumour transplants using anti-p185 antibodies conjugated with [131]I [22].

Antibodies against seven different epitopes on p185 have been compared for their ability to deliver ^{131}I to tumour heterografts. Approximately 18% uptake of ^{131}I was obtained with the [131]I-520C9 antibody conjugate [23]. At a maximally-tolerated dose of 400 μCi, [131]I-520C9 produced transient inhibition of SKOv3-clone18, but also failed to cure graft recipients.

Studies in cell culture suggest that radionuclide conjugates and immunotoxins can produce synergistic toxicity for tumour cells that overexpress p185 [23]. Isobolographic analysis of limiting dilution assays demonstrated synergistic cytotoxicity between external beam irradiation and anti-p185 immunotoxins. Mechanistic studies suggested that treatment with immunotoxin completely suppressed replication repair, reflected by unscheduled incorporation of radiolabeled thymidine. Preliminary studies *in vivo* (Figure 21.1) suggest that at least additive antitumour activity can be obtained with anti-p185 radionuclide conjugates and immunotoxins. Long term survivors (>120 days) have been observed following use of both types of conjugates in combination.

Whether these immunological approaches will prove useful in the clinic remains to be determined. In the future, small molecules that inhibit oncogenes, replace tumour suppressor function and modulate growth factor activity should almost certainly impact on the prevention and treatment of ovarian cancer.

REFERENCES

1. Bast, R.C. Jr., Jacobs, I. and Berchuck, A. (1992) Editorial: Malignant trans-formation of ovarian epithelium. *J. Natl. Cancer Inst.* **84**, 556-8.
2. Berchuck, A., Rodriguez, G., Olt, G.J. *et al.* (1992) Regulation of growth of normal ovarian epithelial cells and ovarian cancer cell lines by transforming growth factor-β. *Am. J. Obstet. Gynecol.* **166**, 676-84.
3. Hurteau, J., Rodriguez, G.C., Whitaker, R.S. *et al.* (1994) Transforming growth factor-β inhibits proliferation of human ovarian cancer cells obtained from ascites. *Cancer* **74**, 93-9.
4. Havrilesky, L.J., Hurteau, J.A., Whitaker, R.S. *et al.* (1995) Regulation of apoptosis in normal and malignant ovarian epithelial cells by transforming growth factor-β. *Cancer Res.* **55**, 944-8.
5. Dabal, R., Boyer, C.M., Berchuck, A. *et al.* (1995) Synergistic inhibition of ovarian cancer cell proliferation by TGF and retinoic acid (RA) derivatives. *Proc. Am. Assoc. Cancer Res.* **36**, 635.
6. De Palo, G., Veronesi, U., Camerini, T. *et al.* (1995) Can fenretinide protect women against ovarian cancer? *J. Natl. Cancer Inst.* **87**, 146-7.
7. Berchuck, A., Rodriguez, G.C., Kamel, A. *et al.* (1991) Epidermal growth factor receptor expression in normal ovarian epithelium and ovarian cancer. I. Correlation of receptor expression with prognostic factors in patients with ovarian cancer. *Am. J. Obstet. Gynecol.* **164**, 669-74.
8. Berchuck, A., Kamel, A., Whitaker, R. *et al.* (1990) Overexpression of HER-2/neu is associated with poor survival in advanced epithelial ovarian cancer. *Cancer Res.* **50**, 4087-91.
9. Kacinski, B.M., Carter, D., Mittal, K. *et al.* (1990) Ovarian aenocarcinomas express fms-complementary transcripts and fms antigen, often with coexpression of CSF-1. *Am. J. Pathol.* **137**, 135-47.
10. Wu, S., Boyer, C.M., Whitaker, R. *et al.* . (1993) Tumor necrosis factor-alpha (TNF-α) as an autocrine and paracrine growth factor for ovarian cancer, Monokine induction of tumor cell proliferation and TNF-α expression. *Cancer Res.* **53**, 1939-44.
11. Watson, J.M., Sensintaffar, J.L., Berek, J.S. and Martinez-Maza, O. (1990). Constitutive production of interleukin 6

by ovarian cancer cell lines and by primary ovarian tumor cultures. *Cancer Res.* **50**, 6959-65.

12. Mills, G.B., Hashimoto, S., Hurteau, J.A. *et al.* (1988). A putative new growth factor in ascitic fluid from ovarian cancer patients, identification, characterization and mech-anism of action. *Cancer Res.* **48**, 1066-71.

13. Wiener, J.R., Hurteau, J.A., Kerns, B.-J.M. *et al.* (1994) Overexpression of the tyrosine phosphatase PTP1B is associated with human ovarian carcinomas. *Am. J. Obstet. Gynecol.* **170**, 1177-83.

14. Berchuck, A., Kohler, M.F., Marks, J.R. *et al.* (1994) The p53 tumorsuppressor gene frequently is altered in gynecologic cancers. *Am. J. Obstet. Gynecol.* **170**, 246-52.

15. Santoso, J.T., Tang, D., Lane, S.B. *et al.* (1995). Adenovirus-based p53 gene therapy in ovarian cancer. *Gynecol. Oncol.* **59**, 171-8.

16. Slamon, D.J., Godolphin, W., Jones, L.A. *et al.* (1989). Studies of the HER-2/neu proto-oncogene in human breast and ovarian cancer. *Science* **244**, 707-12.

17. Xu, F.J., Lupu, R., Rodriguez, G.C. *et al.* (1993) Antibody induced growth inhibition ismediated through immunochemically and functionally distinct epitopes on the extracellular domain of the c-erbB2 (HER-2/neu) gene product p185. *Int. J. Cancer* **53**, 401-8.

18. Boente, M.P., Berchuck, A., Whitaker, R.S. *et al.* (1995) Suppression of diacylglycerol levels by antibodies reactive with the c-erbB2 (HER-2/neu) gene product p185erbB2 in breast and ovarian cancer cell lines. *Submitted for publication.*

19. Bae, D.S., Xu, F.-J., Mills, G. and Bast. R.C. Jr. (1995) Heregulin and antibodies against p185c-erbB2 (p185) activate distinct signaling pathways. *Proc. Am. Assoc. Cancer Res.* **36**, 55 (A#328).

20. Xu, F.J., Rodriguez, G., Bae, D.S. *et al.* (1994) Heregulin and anti-p185c-erbB2 antibodies inhibit proliferation, increase invasiveness and enhance tyrosine autophosphorylation of breast cancer cells that overexpress p185c-erbB2. *Proc. Am. Assoc. Cancer Res.* **35**, 38 (A#225).

21. Pegram, M., Lipton, A., Pietras, R. *et al.* . (1995) Phase II trial of intravenous recombinant humanized anti-p185 HER-2 monoclonal antibody (rhuMAb HER-2) plus cisplatin in patients with HER-2/NEU overexpressing metastatic breast cancer. *Proc. Am. Soc. Clin. Oncol.* **14**, 106.

22. De Santes, K., Slamon, D., Anderson, S.K. *et al.* (1992) Radiolabeled antibody targeting of the HER-2/neu oncoprotein. *Cancer Res.* **52**, 1916-23.

23. Xu, F.-J., Leadon, S.A., O'Briant, K. *et al.* (1995) Synergistic cytotoxicity is produced with ionizing radiation and anti-p185c-erbB2 immunotoxins in cells that overexpress p185c-erbB2. *Proc. Am. Assoc. Cancer Res.* **36**, 484 (A#2885).

Chapter 22

Cellular responses to DNA damage and cisplatin resistance

Robert BROWN

22.1 INTRODUCTION

Cis-diamminedichloroplatinum II (cisplatin) and other platinum coordination complexes have been shown to be highly effective anticancer drugs [1], widely used in the treatment of ovarian, testicular, and head and neck carcinomas [2]. Certain malignancies such as germ cell tumours are exquisitely sensitive to cisplatin with cure being achieved in most cases [3]. However, in the majority of tumour types responses when they occur are not durable in the long term and recurrence usually occurs with non-responsive tumour. At present the mechanisms underlying the differences in sensitivity or resistance of tumours to cisplatin therapy are not fully understood. A large number of studies are consistent with DNA as the crucial target for the cytotoxic action of cisplatin. Many of the studies on cisplatin resistance have focused on the cellular pharmacology prior to DNA damage and have been reviewed extensively [4-7]. Such studies have implicated mechanisms of cisplatin resistance that include decreased cellular accumulation of cisplatin, increased levels of intracellular metallothioneins and increased levels of glutathione (GSH) or of glutathione-S-transferase activity. However, recently, the importance of biological responses after DNA damage has become apparent [8-10]. Such responses that will

affect drug sensitivity include DNA repair, cell cycle checkpoints and cell death. How these responses interact to affect drug sensitivity is crucial to our understanding of why certain agents such as cisplatin are effective anticancer drugs and how drug resistance can occur. In addition it remains unclear how DNA damage is coupled to biochemical pathways leading to these interlinked cellular responses.

If such post-DNA damage mechanisms prove to be relevant types of mechanism for clinical resistance of tumours, this will have important implications in the design of new anti-tumour drugs or overcoming drug resistance. Thus, while analogues or resistance modulators which can increase levels of initial DNA damage will be important for overcoming pharmacological resistance, they will not overcome post-DNA biological resistance and therefore will not improve long-term survival. Novel approaches will need to be developed to overcome such post-DNA-damage resistance mechanisms or which utilize biochemical changes in resistant tumours as chemo-therapeutic targets.

22.2 DNA AS THE THERAPEUTIC TARGET FOR CISPLATIN

The vast majority of evidence supports DNA as being the critical target for the cytotoxicity of cisplatin [1,11]. The major DNA adducts formed when cisplatin binds to DNA are intrastrand cross-links between N-7 atoms of adjacent purines; d(GpG) and d(ApG) 1,2 intrastrand cross-links representing respectively 65% and 25% of the total adducts [11]. Minor lesions include intrastrand cross-links between purine residues separated by one base, interstrand cross-links between two purine residues on opposite strands, monofunctional adducts on purine residues and DNA-protein cross-links. Identifying the crucial chemotherapeutic lesion induced by cisplatin is complicated by the fact that, theoretically, one unrepaired lesion in the DNA of a cell could be cytotoxic. Therefore rare lesions which have a high biological effectiveness due to the nature of the damage induced may be crucial for cytotoxicity, but will be difficult to identify.

The presence of large bulky adducts in DNA modified by cisplatin leads to structural alterations in the conformation of DNA. The 1,2 intrastrand cross-links unwind the duplex by 13° and cause a 34° kink in the direction of the major groove [12]. Cisplatin adducts in DNA have also been shown to cause local melting of the DNA producing short single-stranded regions near the adduct [13]. The presence of cisplatin DNA adducts or subsequent changes in DNA topology will affect the ability of the DNA to be used as a template for processes such as DNA replication. Blocking DNA replication may generate DNA strand breaks which are important signals for apoptosis [14] and may explain the apparent necessity for cellular proliferation in thymocytes for cisplatin induced apoptosis [15].

22.3 CISPLATIN-INDUCED CELL CYCLE ARRESTS AND RESISTANCE

Multiple cell-cycle perturbations have been observed in tumour cells treated with cisplatin [16,17]. One of the earliest effects is a reduction in the rate of DNA synthesis and

a consequent slow-down in the traverse of cells through S-phase. Subsequently there is a dose-dependent arrest in G2 [16-19]. It has been suggested that the G2 arrest is a prerequisite for cell death and that essential events occur during G2 which are required for death to occur by apoptosis [8].

The G1 arrest induced in mammalian cells by DNA damaging agents such as ionizing radiation and topoisomerase inhibitors has been shown to be dependent on functional activity of the tumour suppressor gene TP53 [20,21]. Cisplatin can induce increased levels of p53 protein in ovarian cells [22] and increased mRNA levels of genes whose transcription is mediated by p53 (such as the cell cycle kinase inhibitor WAF1/CIP1 [23]). However, a cisplatin-induced G1 arrest has not been observed in the majority of cell cycle studies on cisplatin treatment of mammalian cells [16,17]. These studies have been done on rodent and human lines that do not have demonstrable wild type p53 functional activity. Work from our laboratory has shown that human ovarian cells, which possess wild-type TP53 and a functional ionizing radiation induced G1 arrest, do arrest at G1 after exposure to cisplatin [22]. Furthermore, this cisplatin G1 arrest is lost after transfection of these cells with a dominant negative mutant of p53, which is known to abrogate an ionizing radiation induced arrest [24].

Ovarian tumour cell lines which have been selected for resistance to cisplatin have been shown to have increased constitutive levels of p53 protein [22]. This increase in p53 protein levels occurs concomitantly with a loss of a cisplatin and radiation induced G1 arrest suggesting that these resistant lines have lost p53 function. Furthermore gain of wild-type p53 function in human non-small cell lung tumour cells that have a homozygous deletion of p53, increases the sensitivity of these cells to cisplatin [25]. A regain of p53 function may also explain why cisplatin resistant cells transfected with mutant p53 become more sensitive to cisplatin [22]. As will shortly be described these observation may solely be explained by the requirement for p53 function in cisplatin-induced apoptosis. However it is also possible that arrest in the cell cycle make the cells permissive for entry into an apoptotic programme.

22.4 CISPLATIN RESISTANCE AND APOPTOSIS

Cisplatin has been shown to be capable of inducing apoptosis in a wide variety of cell systems [18,26,27]. As previously mentioned, it has been suggested that the cell cycle G2 arrest is a prerequisite for cell death and that essential events occur during G2 which are required for death to occur by apoptosis [28]. The mechanisms controlling the decision to enter apoptosis at G2 are still to be elucidated. However it has been shown that cisplatin fails to induce apoptosis in quiescent thymocytes, but does so in proliferating thymocytes [15]. Quiescent thymocytes are normally very sensitive to a wide variety of DNA damaging agents which induce apoptosis [29]. These observations suggest that cisplatin-induced apoptosis requires proliferation, in thymocytes at least. It is presently not clear whether the dependence of cisplatin-induced apoptosis on proliferation is due to; (a) cisplatin adducts being converted by DNA replication to a signal, such as DNA double-strand breaks, required for apoptotic response pathways in the cells, or (b) the entry into apoptosis requiring passage of the cells through particular phases of the cell cycle (for instance cells at the G1 phase of the cell cycle have been suggested to be particularly sensitive to cisplatin [30]).

A number of genes and gene products have now been implicated to have a role in apoptosis induced by DNA damaging agents. It has been shown that cells from

mice, with the p53 gene genetically inactivated, acquire resistance to apoptosis induced by a variety of DNA damaging agents, including ionizing radiation and topoisomerase II inhibitors [21,31]. Recently we have shown that cisplatin induced apoptosis is also abrogated in cell from p53-null mice [Jones, Brown and Dive, unpublished]. Furthermore human ovarian cell line models with dysfunctional p53 have a reduced apoptotic response [22,24 and McIlwrath and Brown, unpublished].

Increased expression of the proto-oncogene bcl2 protects cells from the cytocidal effects of a variety of toxic agents including chemotherapeutic drugs [32]. Furthermore, increased bcl2 expression abrogates an increased sensitivity to cytotoxic agents elicited by expression of c-myc proto-oncogene [33]. Bcl2 is one of a growing family of related proteins that can either inhibit apoptosis or antagonize the anti-apoptotic response. This latter response is mediated by proteins such as bax which can heterodimerize with bcl2 and thereby antagonize the anti-apoptotic response of the latter [34]. No doubt the next few years will see a further explosion in the identification of genes potentially involved either in the sensing, decision-making or executioner steps of DNA damage-induced apoptosis. An interesting development in this context is the gene suppressor element approach that is being used to isolate apparently recessively acting genes involved in drug resistance [35]. Preliminary reports have described the identification of gene sequences that can operate in an antisense or dominant negative manner to confer resistance to cisplatin [36].

22.5 REPAIR OF CISPLATIN INDUCED DNA DAMAGE

It is possible that one of the reasons cisplatin is an effective chemotherapeutic drug is because the DNA damage induced in tumour cells by cisplatin is not repaired and that

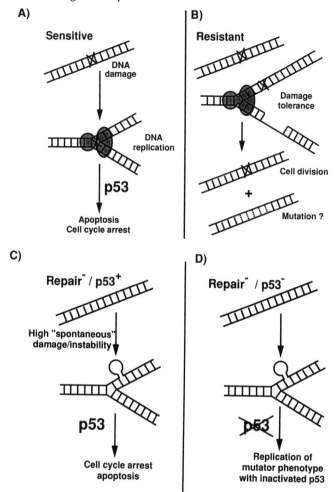

Figure 22.1 Hypothetical model for the acquisition of drug resistance by selection for cells with increased replication bypass of DNA damage.

(a) In certain cell types cell proliferation is required to couple cisplatin-induced DNA damage to an apoptotic response [15]. This may be due to DNA replication being blocked or aberrant replication producing DNA double strand breaks a lesion known to be important for the induction of p53-dependent apoptosis [14]. Expression of functional p53 is required for cisplatin induced apoptosis [22,24 and Jones, Brown and Dive, unpublished].

(b) Cells able to undergo adduct bypass will tolerate the DNA damage and will be selected for by the drug. This replicative adduct bypass may be due to inactivation of proteins involved in maintaining the fidelity of DNA replication such as mismatch repair proteins. This will lead to a mutator phenotype in the cells selected.

(c) Cells deficient in mismatch repair will produce high levels of mutations and spontaneous damage in the genome. In cells expressing wild type functional p53 this may lead to cells undergoing cell cycle arrest and apoptosis.

(d) Cells with abrogated p53 function may be selected for during growth leading to selection for cells with inactivated mismatch repair and which have inactivated p53.

208

adduct persistence eventually leads to cell death [37]. Adduct persistence could occur if the DNA damage is not recognized by cellular DNA repair enzymes or if the induced damage is complex and irreparable. Using an *in vitro* DNA repair synthesis assay it has been shown that extracts from mammalian cells can repair damage induced by cisplatin [38]. However, the major adducts, the 1,2 intrastrand cross-link, are not repaired as efficiently as minor cisplatin-DNA adducts or other types of cross-linking DNA damage such as UV-induced pyrimidine-dimers [39].

Increased tolerance of platinum-DNA adducts also appears to play a significant role in platinum resistance of human tumour cells *in vitro* [40-42]. This has been suggested to be due to enhanced replicative bypass, defined as the ability of the replicative complex of a cell to synthesize DNA past the site of DNA damage. It is proposed that bypassing DNA damage during S-phase allows a cell to survive into G2 where it can then potentially arrest the cell cycle and repair the damaged sites before proceeding into mitosis. Enhanced replicative bypass of platinum-DNA adducts is observed in cisplatin-resistant human ovarian cell lines [42]. This ability of the cell to bypass lesions may be due to alteration in specific proteins involved in the replication complex. It is also possible that increased replication bypass could be due to alterations in cisplatin-damage recognition proteins, although changes in such proteins have not been observed in the cell lines with increased platinum-adduct tolerance [43,44]. If adducts are tolerated through several cell cycles, this will mean that normal biological responses to the damage, such as cell cycle checkpoints or apoptosis, will have to be suppressed. We have observed in cisplatin resistant ovarian cell lines increased mutation of repetitive DNA sequences, so-called microsatellite instability [45]. Thus these cells appear to generate replication errors (RER+ phenotype) probably due to deficiency in mismatch repair [46]. This deficiency in mismatch repair may allow increased bypass of DNA damage such as platinum adducts in DNA (Figure 22.1).

22.6 CLINICAL RELEVANCE OF POST-DNA DAMAGE MECHANISMS OF RESISTANCE

At present the evidence for post-DNA damage mechanisms of resistance operating in patients' tumours is circumstantial. Altered expression of p53 has been shown to be prognostic in a variety of tumour types [47-49], however so far there is no clear correlation between response to treatment and p53 status. Preliminary studies have suggested that the presence of p53 mutations may be associated with clinical resistance to carboplatin in ovarian cancer [50]. It is also worth noting that tumour types that are considered intrinsically sensitive to chemotherapy, such as testicular carcinoma and neuroblastoma, generally have wild-type p53 gene sequence and function [51,52].

One limitation of these types of studies is that p53 function can be inactivated by a number of mechanisms other than p53 gene mutation [53]. Therefore in such clinical studies it would be useful to relate response to a measure of p53 function, such as the presence of a damage inducible G1 arrest. Similarly measuring levels of bcl2 expression in tumours may not be very informative concerning the ability of these cells to undergo apoptosis. Bcl2 is only one member of a family of anti-apoptotic genes which interact with the bax-like gene family [32]. Again a means of directly measuring apoptosis in cells would be useful, such as the types of assays that detect the DNA cleavage generated during apoptosis [54].

22.7 CONCLUSIONS

Over the last few years experimental models using mice and human cell lines have shown the potential importance for drug resistance of events occurring after cisplatin induces damage in DNA. An important challenge in the near future will be to assess the relevance of these mechanisms in patients' tumours in relation to response to cisplatin-based chemotherapy. Although measurement of expression of specific proteins such as p53 and BCL2 will provide relevant information, these proteins are only components of an entire cellular response pathway leading to cell death or survival. Therefore, it will be important to attempt to measure the function of the entire pathway using cellular response end-points such as apoptosis or cell cycle arrest.

Until recently the main approach to increasing the efficacy of a given drug and to overcoming resistance has either been to synthesize new analogues or use drugs which modulate the amount of active drug reaching the intracellular target. However, these approaches will not overcome cellular biological resistance due to post-DNA damage mechanisms. As our understanding of the mechanisms of cell death and cell cycle arrest increases, novel approaches to overcome resistance may become possible. If increased mutation at microsatellite loci are present in resistant tumours, this may provide a tumour selective target which could be used in the design of new chemotherapeutic agents. Thus microsatellite mutations will represent the occurrence of high levels of mismatched DNA sequences occurring in the tumour cells. Mismatch repair proteins are known to bind to such DNA damage and may provide insight into possible small molecules that can target tumour cells with an RER+ phenotype.

REFERENCES

1. Rosenberg, B. (1985) Fundamental studies with cisplatin. *Cancer* **5**, 2303-16.
2. Loehrer, P.J. and Einhorn, L.H. (1984) Diagnosis and treatment, drugs five years later. *Ann. Intern. Med.* **100**, 704-13.
3. Peckham, M. (1988) Testicular Cancer. *Rev. Oncol.* **1**, 439-53.
4. Andrews, P.A. and Howell, S.B. (1990) Cellular pharmacology of cisplatin, perspectives on mechanisms of acquired resistance. *Cancer Cells* **2**, 35-43.
5. Perez, R.P., Hamilton, T.C. and Ozols, R.F.(1990) Resistance to alkylating agents and cisplatin, insights from ovarian carcinoma systems. *Pharm. Therap.* **48**, 19-27.
6. Timmer-Bosscha, H., Mulder, N.H. and De Vries, E.G.E. (1992) Modulation of cis-diamminedichloroplatinum(II) resistance, a review. *Br. J. Cancer* **66**, 227-38.
7. Gately, D.P. and Howell, S.B. (1993) Cellular accumulation of the anticancer agent cisplatin, a review. *Br. J. Cancer* **67**, 1171-6.
8. Eastman, A.(1990) Activation of programmed cell death by anticancer agents, cisplatin as a model system. *Cancer Cells*, **2**, 275-80.
9. Dive, C. and Hickman, J.A. (1991) Drug-target interactions, only the first step in the commitment to a programmed cell death?. *Br. J. Cancer* **64**, 192-6.
10. Brown, R. (1993) p53, a target for new anticancer drugs or a target for old drugs?. *Ann. Oncol.* **4**, 623-9.
11. Sherman, S.E. and Lippard, S.J. (1987) Structural aspects of platinum anticancer drug interactions with DNA. *Chem. Rev.* **87**, 1153-81.
12. Anin, M. and Leng, M. (1990) Distortions induced in double-stranded oligo-

nucleotides by the binding of cis- or trans-diammine-dichloroplatinum (II) to the d(GTG) sequence. *Nucleic Acids Res.* **18**, 4395-400.

13. Bellon, S.F., Coleman, J.H. and Lippard, S.J. (1991) DNA unwinding produced by site-specific intrastrand cross-links of the antitumour drug cis-diammine-dichloroplatinum (II). *Biochemistry* **30**, 8026-35.

14. Nelson, W.G. and Kastan, M.B. (1994) DNA strand breaks, the DNA template alterations that trigger p53-dependent-DNA damage response pathways. *Mol. Cell. Biol.* **14**, 1815-23.

15. Evans, D.L., Tilby, M. and Dive, C. (1994) Differential sensitivity to the induction of apoptosis by cisplatin in proliferating and quiescent immature rat thymocytes is independent of the level of drug accumulation and DNA adduct formation. *Cancer Res.* **54**, 1596-603.

16. Ormerod, M.G., Orr, R.M. and Peacock, J.H. (1994) The role of apoptosis in cell killing by cisplatin, a flow cytometric study. *Br. J. Cancer* **69**, 93-100.

17. Demarcq, C., Bastian, G. and Remvikos, Y. (1992) BrdUrd/DNA flow cytometry analysis demonstrates cis-diammine-dichloroplatinum (II)-induced multiple cell-cycle modifications on human lung carcinoma cells. *Cytometry* **13**, 416-22.

18. Sorenson, C.M., Barry, M.A., and Eastman, A. (1990) Analysis of events associated with cell cycle arrest at G2 phase and cell death induced by cisplatin. *J. Natl. Cancer Inst.*, **82**, 749-755

19. Sorenson, C.M. and Eastman, A. (1988) Mechanisms of cis-diammine-dichloro-platinum (II)-induced cytotoxicity, role of G2 arrest and DNA double-strand breaks. *Cancer Res.* **48**, 4484-8.

20. Kuerbitz, S.J., Plunkett, B.S., Walsh, W.V. and Kastan, M.B. (1992) Wild-type p53 is a cell cycle checkpoint determinant following irradiation. *Proc. Natl. Acad.*

Sci. USA **89**, 7491-5.

21. Lowe, S.W., Ruley, H.E., Jacks, T. and Housman, D.E. (1993) p53-dependent apoptosis modulates the cytotoxicity of anticancer agents. *Cell* **74**, 957-67.

22. Brown, R., Clugston, C., Burns, P. *et al.* (1993) Increased accumulation of p53 in cisplatin-resistant ovarian cell lines. *Int. J. Cancer* **55**, 1-7.

23. El-Deiry, W.S., Tokino, T., Velculescu, V.E. *et al.* (1993) WAF-1, a potential mediator of p53 tumour suppression. *Cell* **75**, 817-25.

24. McIlwrath, A.J., Vasey, P.A., Ross, G.M. and Brown, R. (1994) Cell cycle arrests and radiosensitivity of human tumour cell lines, dependence on wild-type p53 for radiosensitivity. *Cancer Res.* **54**, 3718-22.

25. Fujiwara, T., Grimm, E.A., Mukhapadhyay, T. *et al.* (1994) Induction of chemosensitivity in human lung cancer cells *in vivo* by adenovirus-mediated transfer of the wild-type p53 gene. *Cancer Res.* **54**, 2287-91.

26. Gorczyca, W., Gong, J., Ardelt, B. *et al.* (1993) The cell cycle related differences in susceptibility of HL-60 cells to apoptosis induced by various antitumour agents. *Cancer Res.* **53**, 3186-92.

27. Evans, D.L. and Dive, C. (1993) Effects of cisplatin on the induction of apoptosis in proliferating heparoma cells and non-proliferating immature thymocytes. *Cancer Res.* **53**, 2133-9.

28. Hickman, J.A. (1992) Apoptosis induced by anticancer agents. *Cancer Metast. Rev.* **11**, 121-39.

29. Wyllie, A.H. (1993) Apoptosis. *Br. J. Cancer*, **67**, 205-8.

30. Roberts, J.J. and Fraval, H.N. (1980) Repair of cisplatinum diammine-dichloroplatinum (II) -induced DNA damage and cell sensitivity. In, *Cisplatin: current status and new developments.* (eds. A.W. Prestayko, S.T. Crooke and S.K.

Carter), Academic Press, New York. pp. 57-77.

31. Clarke, A.R., Purdie, C.A., Harrison, D.J. et al. (1993) Thymocyte apoptosis induced by p53-dependent and independent pathways. *Nature* 362, 849-52.

32. Reed, J.C. (1994) Bcl-2 and the regulation of programmed cell death. *J. Cell Biol.* 124, 1-6.

33. Fanidi, A., Harrington, E.A., and Evan, G.I. (1992) Cooperative interaction between c-myc and bcl-2 proto-oncogenes. *Nature* 359, 554-6.

34. Oltvai, Z.N., Milliman, C.L. and Korsmeyer, S.J. (1993) Bcl-2 heterodimerizes *in vivo* with a conserved homolog, BAX, that accelerates programed cell death. *Cell* 74, 609-19.

35. Gudkov, A.V., Kazarov, A.R., Thimmapaya, R. et al. (1994) Cloning mammalian genes by expression selection of genetic suppressor elements, association of kinesin with drug resistance and cell immortalization. *Proc. Natl. Acad. Sci. USA* 91, 3744-8.

36. Kirschling, D.J., Gudkov, A.V. and Roninson, I.B. (1994) Identification of genes responsible for cisplatin sensitivity in human cells. *Proc. Am. Assoc. Cancer Res.* 35, 438.

37. Ciccarelli, R.B., Solomon, M.J., Varshavsky, A., and Lippard, S.J. (1985) *In vivo* effects of cis- and trans-diammine-dichloroplatinum (II) on SV40 chromosomes. *Biochemistry* 24, 7533-40.

38. Hansson, J. and Wood, R.D. (1989) Repair synthesis by human cell extracts in DNA damaged by cis-and trans-diammine-dichloroplatinum(II). *Nucleic Acids Res.* 17, 8073-91.

39. Szymkowski, D.E., Yarema, K., Essigmann, J.M. et al. (1992) An intrastrand d(GpG) platinum cross-link in duplex M13 DNA is refractory to repair by human cell extracts. *Proc. Natl. Acad.*

Sci. USA 89, 10772-6.

40. Parker, R.J., Eastman, A., Bostick-Bruton, F., and Reed, E. (1991) Acquired cisplatin resistance in human ovarian cancer cells is associated with enhanced repair of cisplatin-DNA lesions and reduced drug accumulation. *J. Clin. Invest.* 87, 772-7.

41. Schmidt, W. and Chaney, S.G. (1993) Role of carrier ligand in platinum resistance of human carcinoma cell lines. *Cancer Res.* 53, 799-805.

42. Mamenta, E.L., Poma, E.E., Kaufmann, W.K. et al. (1994) Enhanced replicative bypass of platinum-DNA adducts in cisplatin-resistant human ovarian carcinoma cell lines. *Cancer Res.* 54, 3500-5.

43. Benchekroun, M.N., Parker, R., Reed, E., and Sinha, B.K. (1993) Inhibition of DNA repair and sensitization of cisplatin in human ovarian carcinoma cells by interleukin-1 alpha. *Biochem. Biophys. Res. Comm.* 195, 294-300.

44. Andrews, P.A. and Jones, J.A. (1991) Characterisation of binding proteins from ovarian carcinoma and kidney tubule cells that are specific for cisplatin modified DNA. *Cancer Comm.* 3, 93-102.

45. Anthoney, A. and Brown, R. (1995) The detection of genomic instability in drug resistant human tumour cell lines. *Proc. Am. Assoc. Cancer Res.* 36, 323.

46. Parsons, R., Li, G.M., Longley, M.J. et al. (1993) Hypermutability and mismatch repair deficiency in RER+ tumor cells. *Cell* 75, 1227-36.

47. Thor, A.D. and Yandell, D.W. (1993) Prognostic significance of p53 overexpression in node-negative breast carcinoma, preliminary studies support cautious optimism. *J. Natl. Cancer Inst.* 85, 176-7.

48. Allred, D.C., Clark, G.M., Elledge, R. et al. (1993) Association of p53 protein expression with tumor cell proliferation

rate and clinical outcome in node-negative breast cancer. *J. Natl. Cancer Inst.* **85**, 200-6.

49. Silvestrini, R., Benini, E., Daidone, M.G. *et al.* (1993) p53 as an independent prognostic marker in lymph node-negative breast cancer patients. *J. Natl. Cancer Inst.* **85**, 965-70.

50. Al-Azraqi, A., Chapman, C., Challen, C. *et al.* (1994) P53 alterations in ovarian cancer as adeterminant of response to carboplatin. *Br. J. Cancer* **69**, *Suppl. XXI*, 7.

51. Peng, H., Hogg, D., Malkin, D. *et al.* (1993) Mutations of the p53 gene do not occur in testis cancer. *Cancer Res.* **53**, 3574-8.

52. Komuro, H., Hayashi, Y., Kawamura, M. *et al.* (1993) Mutations of the p53 gene are involved in Ewing's sarcomas but not in neuroblastomas. *Cancer Res.* **53**, 5284-8.

53. Vogelstein, B. and Kinzler, K.W. (1992) p53 Function and disfunction. *Cell* **70**, 523-6.

54. Gorczyca, W., Gong, J., and Darzynkiewicz, Z. (1993) Detection of DNA strand breaks in individual apoptotic cells by the *in situ* terminal deoxynucleotidyl transferase and nick translation assays. *Cancer Res.* **53**, 1945-51.

Chapter 23

Causes of clinical drug resistance

Stanley B. KAYE

23.1 INTRODUCTION

Laboratory-based scientists sometimes find it difficult to understand the vagaries of clinical research, and nowhere is this more evident than in the field of drug resistance as it applies to cancer therapy. Perhaps the best example is the management of ovarian cancer. Here are three clinical scenarios, describing patients treated in our unit.

1. A 55 year old woman with FIGO stage IV epithelial ovarian cancer receives chemotherapy with cyclophosphamide and cisplatin and achieves a clinical complete remission which lasts for 13 months. After symptomatic relapse, treatment with carboplatin results in a further clinical response, but its duration is shorter, lasting only five months before she relapses again. Treatment with other agents (i.e. including topoisomerase I inhibitors in a Phase I trial) is ineffective and she dies three months later, three years after diagnosis.

2. A 35 year old woman with FIGO stage III epithelial ovarian cancer receives chemotherapy with cyclophosphamide and cisplatin and after three courses there is little evidence of tumour shrinkage. The serum CA125 has not fallen, and after two months she has developed symptoms of intestinal obstruction. Further surgery is carried out with palliative intent, and treatment with taxol is instituted. This results in temporary improvement, but the disease progresses four months later and she dies 11 months from diagnosis.

3. A 25 year old patient develops abdominal distension and at surgery was found to have a large ovarian cyst with ascites and multiple intra-abdominal deposits. The primary tumour was removed and proved to be an endodermal sinus (germ cell) tumour of the ovary. Chemotherapy with cisplatin, etoposide and bleomycin was given and the remaining disease disappeared completely. No further surgery was required and she has remained disease-free five years later.

These 3 cases illustrate the following points:
(a) The development of drug resistance in epithelial ovarian cancer at two stages, either after several months of remission (which is more common), or early, i.e. during initial therapy (which is uncommon).
(b) The fundamental difference between epithelial and the much rarer germ cell carcinoma of the ovary. The latter is generally curable with chemotherapy, whereas epithelial ovarian cancer is more often fatal because of the development of drug resistance.

A number of questions arise. They include:
(i) For epithelial ovarian cancer, what are the essential mechanisms which underlie its development, and do these differ according to whether resistance develops 'early' or 'late' in the course of treatment?
(ii) Why do most cases of epithelial ovarian cancer eventually develop drug resistance which proves to be fatal, whereas germ cell ovarian cancer essentially remains drug sensitive and curable?

At present the answers to these questions are unknown, but interesting observations from experimental models could give some clues. However, it is important first to consider the overall framework for drug resistance, and to recognize all the factors which can contribute. The mechanisms which underlie drug resistance in tumour cells are frequently categorized as either 'pharmacological' or 'cellular'.

23.2 PHARMACOLOGICAL FACTORS

Pharmacological factors are those which determine the extent of exposure of tumour cells to the active drug, and this is essentially a function of concentration and duration of exposure. Dose, as well as schedule, is therefore the first critical determinant of the activity of agents generally used in ovarian cancer, since it is assumed (and there are supportive data from experimental models) that within the clinically relevant dose range, cell kill will be proportional to dose. What data are there to support this from clinical studies in ovarian cancer?

Randomized clinical trials specifically addressing the issue of dose have concentrated on the most active drug, cisplatin, and results of two of these studies are particularly interesting. The first large randomized trial in the USA focused on the issue of dose-intensity (expressed as mg/m^2 per week), and compared two treatments in which the dose-intensity was doubled in one arm, but the total dose was the same for the key drug cisplatin [1]. Patients therefore received either eight cycles of cyclophosphamide, 500mg/m^2 and cisplatin 50mg/m^2, or four cycles of cyclophosphamide 1g/m^2 and cisplatin 100mg/m^2, all at three-weekly intervals. The study accrued a total of 485 patients all with bulk residual disease after initial therapy and the results indicated no significant difference in overall response (45% *vs.* 53%), or in median survival (20.7 *vs.* 23.9 months).

In Scotland, we conducted a randomized trial which was similar in that the patients received double the dose-intensity in one arm compared to the other, but was different in that they also received double the total dose of cisplatin. In our study patients therefore received six cycles of cyclophosphamide 750mg/m^2 and cisplatin either 50mg/m^2 or 100mg/m^2, all at three-weekly intervals. Another difference was that our study included patients both with bulk and minimal residual disease. In 1992, we published the first results and these showed a clear survival benefit for patients in the high dose cisplatin arm, with a doubling of the median survival from 69 to 114 weeks (p = 0.003) [2]. At that stage, accrual was closed with 179 cases on study. We have however, recently completed an updated analysis of this trial, full results of which will be summarised elsewhere. In brief, 115 patients have now died, and the median follow-up is 4.5 years. At this time the survival curves have clearly come closer together, with four year survival rates for the high dose and low dose cisplatin arms of 32.4% and 26.6% respectively. One interpretation of these data is that, despite clear evidence of an initial impact of dose through the eradication of a certain proportion of sensitive cells, eventually there is the regrowth of a population of drug resistant cells (possibly at a faster rate than previously), and these come to dominate the clinical picture.

Studies of high dose chemotherapy in ovarian cancer are clearly continuing and with the use of new methods for haemopoietic protection, it is now possible to substantially escalate doses of drugs such as carboplatin, further than is feasible with cisplatin. The impact of this approach is not yet clear, but the likelihood that dose increments alone will substantially change the outcome seems rather small.

A further factor to consider is that following the administration of a given dose of the agent(s) in question, substantial variations may apply in the extent to which the drug is metabolized. These could have clear implications for the activity of drugs used in ovarian cancer, *e.g.* cyclophosphamide, which requires hepatic activation by the cytochrome P450 enzyme system [3]. Genetic and environmental influences on this enzyme family could play an important role in the overall response to alkylating agents. For cisplatin, it has also been proposed that genetic and/or environmental factors will influence tumour response by determining a patient's innate capacity to repair DNA damage induced by the drug. Platinum-DNA adduct levels in non-tumour cells, *e.g.* buccal mucosa or leukocytes have been found to be highest in patients whose tumours respond to the drug, and it is claimed that the effect is independent of variations in drug doses [4].

23.3 CELLULAR (BIOCHEMICAL) FACTORS

Once the active cytotoxic moiety reaches the tumour cell, a number of factors appear to be important in the extent to which the cell may become resistant. For platinum, which is the most important drug type in the treatment of ovarian cancer, factors which have been identified through the study of experimental cell lines include: defective drug transport, increased cellular inactivation and enhanced DNA repair [5]. These will each be considered in detail in subsequent chapters. For taxol, which is clearly another important drug for the management of this disease, factors which have been identified in experimental models of drug resistance include mutations in the intracellular target, tubulin, and also enhanced drug efflux through the classical multidrug resistance (MDR) pathway which operates through membrane associated P-glycoprotein and which may be reversed by certain MDR modulators [6]. Disappointingly however, the elucidation of these various mechanisms from *in vitro* systems has not yet led to significant clinical

improvements, and this may well be because in the clinical situation, multiple factors are involved, several of which have presumably not been identified.

In interpreting data from experimental models, it is of course important to recognize their limitations, particularly when they involve drug resistant tumour cell lines in which the drug resistance has been derived *in vitro*. The concentrations (of drugs such as cisplatin) which have been used to derive resistant cells may far exceed those which are relevant clinically; moreover the frequent technique of continuous exposure of tumour cells *in vitro* may evoke resistance mechanisms which are quite different to those which may result from the intermittent exposure which typifies clinical treatment. In addition, the level of resistance achieved in such cell lines is often far greater than that observed in cell lines derived directly from patients with resistant tumours [7]. An alternative to an *in vitro* system is an *in vivo* model, and there are now a number of human tumour xenografts of drug resistant ovarian cancer which have been developed. Worthwhile information can indeed be obtained from these, particularly on potential means for modulation, since low levels of drug resistance which are probably more relevant clinically are generally seen [5].

Of course, experimentally-derived resistant cell lines do serve a useful function in providing initial leads regarding mechanisms, but these clearly have to be pursued in clinically-derived material. A number of cell lines have in fact been established from patients' tumours in which clinical drug resistance was clearly evident [8]. These could be expected to reflect more accurately the cellular changes which may have taken place, but even so the selection pressures which occur in deriving a cell line raise many questions about their true validity. Therefore information which can be obtained directly from biopsies taken from tumours which are clearly resistant is potentially the most valuable.

In ovarian cancer there are relatively few studies where sequential biopsies have been taken in this way, *i.e.* individual patients in whom tumour samples have been obtained and studied before and after chemotherapy; rather more information is available in patients in whom biological parameters measured at the initial (pre-treatment) biopsy have been correlated with subsequent outcome. Although these data are of interest, they offer only indirect insight into resistance mechanisms themselves. Until more information from repeat biopsies is available, it will be difficult to provide a clear answer to the question as to whether there are any differences between resistance developing 'early' or 'late', as in the two cases presented here. At present, it is assumed that the clinical differences reflect variations in the proportions of resistant and sensitive cells present at diagnosis, rather than any fundamental differences in cellular mechanism.

Whatever the clinical presentation, the limited information so far from tumour biopsies suggests that:
1. Inactivation of platinum compounds through the activity of glutathione-S-transferases is unlikely to be important [9,10].
2. Expression of P-glycoprotein occurs at higher frequency in treated patients and could contribute to resistance to certain agents, *e.g.* taxol [10].
3. The vesicular protein, lung resistance protein (LRP) could play a role in the development of resistance to a range of agents [11].
4. Functional inactivation of the p53 gene may be directly or indirectly involved in the clinical response to drugs such as the carboplatin [12].
These aspects will be developed further in subsequent chapters.

23.4 FUTURE DIRECTIONS

Firstly, it will be important in future to take every opportunity to obtain representative tumour specimens from patients at diagnosis and when clinical resistance occurs. The organization of this is now well underway in some centres, but there are a number of practical problems, including the one of heterogeneity in small tumour samples. Secondly, it will be important to broaden the scope of studies which examine cellular mechanisms, particularly as new data on the genetic basis for drug activity itself begins to emerge. For example, the clinical importance of upregulation of the jun, fos and myc oncoproteins remains to be established; recent studies have linked higher expression (of c-fos) to cisplatin resistance [13]. It seems highly likely that a number of genetic events will take place as drug resistance evolves through spontaneous mutation in tumour cells, and it will be important whenever possible to assess the clinical relevance of coordinate expression of multiple factors.

Another element underlying the current limited understanding of the nature of clinical resistance may be that until comparatively recently, investigators have concentrated mainly on events leading up to DNA damage, and the process of DNA damage itself, rather than events taking place after DNA damage has occurred.

Cytotoxic drugs in general have in common the property of damaging cellular DNA, and an attractive hypothesis, which could explain drug resistance to any DNA damaging agent, is that resistant cells survive because the key signals which switch on the process of cell death, *i.e.* apoptosis, after DNA damage are missing or mutated. Candidates for this role include the p53 gene, lack of function of which has been associated with cisplatin-resistance in ovarian cancer cell lines in our own laboratory [14]. Other genes such as bcl-2 have the opposite effect, *i.e.* will antagonize apoptosis induced by wild-type p53 [15]. As mentioned above, preliminary data from clinical material do suggest a correlation between lack of response to initial therapy (with carboplatin) and the presence of p53 mutations. This would seem to be a potentially fruitful line of future research, since it could eventually lead to a better understanding of the factors relevant to the most fundamental question in drug resistance: why are certain tumours, *e.g.* ovarian germ cell tumours, exquisitely sensitive and indeed curable?

In vitro models of germ cell tumours do exist, and the clear contrast in curability seen clinically between such tumours and other epithelial tumours treated with platinum is reflected by the differences in chemosensitivity in culture systems [16]. It is possible that germ cell tumours respond to DNA damage by engaging apoptosis through mechanisms which are only rarely seen in more chemoresistant epithelial tumours. It is also tempting to speculate that similar parallels can be drawn between various normal tissues and their response to DNA damage, *e.g.* germ cells and epithelial cells.

Clearly this is a simplistic view, but the answer to the question of why do we not yet understand what causes clinical drug resistance may lie in the observation that we do not yet understand what underlies exquisite clinical drug sensitivity. What is perhaps therefore needed is a reproducible technique, applicable in clinical material, for assessing the response of tumour cells to DNA damage in terms of the extent to which they begin the process of apoptosis. Such an assay would provide a test of function of certain candidate genes, and one major task for the future is to examine the possibility that mutations in these genes provide a unifying explanation for the development of clinical resistance to a number of different drugs. If so, this would provide a rational target for novel therapeutic manoeuvres aimed at the circumvention of drug resistance in ovarian cancer. Meantime, investigators await with interest the results from early clinical trials of resistance modulators, including glutathione depletion using buthionine sulfoximine (BSO) [17], the repair inhibitor aphidocolin [18], and the MDR-modulator PSC 833 in conjunction with taxol [19]. Hopefully, the results from these and other studies will be placed in proper perspective with a better appreciation of all the factors which underlie clinical drug resistance.

ACKNOWLEDGEMENTS

The author is grateful to Dr R. Brown for discussion of the manuscript, and to the Cancer Research Campaign for support of our work.

REFERENCES

1. McGuire, W.P., Hoskins, W.J., Brady, M.F. *et al.* (1992) A Phase II trial of dose intense versus standard dose cisplatin and cytoxan for advanced ovarian cancer. *Proc. Am. Soc. Clin. Oncol.* **11**, 226.

2. Kaye, S.B., Lewis, C.R., Paul, J. *et al.* (1992) Randomised study of two doses of cisplatin with cyclophosphamide in epithelial ovarian cancer. *Lancet,* **340**, 329-33.

3. Colvin, M. and Hilton, J. (1981) Pharmacology of cyclophosphamide and metabolites. *Cancer Treat. Rep.* **65**, 89-95.

4. Reed, E., Ozols, R.F., Tarone, R. *et al.* (1993) Platinum-DNA adducts in leucocyte DNA of a cohort of 49 patients with 24 different types of malignancies. *Cancer Res.* **53**, 3694-9.

5. Andrews, P.A. and Howell, S.B. (1990) Cellular pharmacology of cisplatin, perspectives on mechanisms of required resistance. *Cancer Cells* **2**, 35-43.

6. Jachez, B., Nordmann, R. and Loor, F. (1993) Restoration of taxol sensitivity of multidrug resistant cells by the cyclosporin SDZ PSC 833 and the cyclopeptide SDZ 280-446. *J. Natl. Cancer Inst.* **85**, 478-83.

7. Behrens, B.C., Hamilton, T.C., Masuda, H. *et al.* (1987) Characterization of a cisplatin-resistant human ovarian cancer cell line and

its use in the evaluation of platinum analogues. *Cancer Res.* **47**, 414-8.

8. Hamilton, T., Young, R. and Ozols, R.F. (1984) Experimental model systems of ovarian cancer, applications to the design and evaluation of new treatment approaches. *Semin. Oncol.*, **11**, 285-98.

9. Murphy, D., McGown, A.T., Hall, A. *et al.* (1992) Glutathione-S-transferase activity and isoenzyme distribution in ovarian tumour biopsies taken before or after cytotoxic chemotherapy. *Br. J. Cancer* **66**, 937-42.

10. Van der Zee, A.G., Hollema, H., Swurmeizer, A.J. *et al.* (1995) The value of P-glycoprotein, glutathione-S-transferase, C-erbB-2 and p53 as prognostic factors in ovarian carcinomas. *J. Clin Oncol.* in press.

11. Izquierdo, M.A., van der Zee, A., Vermorken, J. *et al.* (1994) Prognostic significance of the drug resistance associated protein LRP in advanced ovarian carcinoma. *Ann. Oncol.* **5**, 98.

12. Al-Azraqui, A., Chapman, C., Challen, C. *et al.* (1994) p53 alterations in ovarian cancer as a determinant of response to carboplatin. *Br. J. Cancer* **69**, 7.

13. Scanlon, K.J., Kashani-Sabet, M. and Sowers, L.C. (1989) Molecular basis of cisplatin resistance in human carcinomas, model systems and patients. *Anticancer Res.* **9**, 1301-12.

14. Brown, R., Clugston, C., Burns, P. *et al.* (1993) Increased accumulation of p53 protein in cisplatin-resistant ovarian cell lines. *Int. J. Cancer* **55**, 678-84.

15. Wang, Y.S., Szekely, L., Okan, I. *et al.* (1993) Wild-type p53 triggered apoptosis is inhibited by BCL-2 in a v-myc induced T-cell lymphoma line. *Oncogene* **8**, 3427-31.

16. Walker, M.C., Parris, C.N. and Masters, J.R.W. (1987) Differential sensitives of human testicular and bladder tumour cell lines to chemotherapeutic drugs. *J. Natl. Cancer Inst.* **29**, 213-6.

17. O'Dwyer, P.J., Hamilton, T.C., Young, R.C. *et al.* (1992) Depletion of glutathione in normal and malignant human cells *in vivo* by buthionine sulfoximine, clinical and biochemical results. *J. Natl. Cancer Inst.* **84**, 264-7.

18. Sessa, C., Zuchetti, M., Davoli, E. *et al.* (1991) Phase I and clinical pharmacological evaluation of aphidocolin glycinate. *J. Natl. Cancer Inst.* **83**, 1160-4.

19. Fisher, G.A., Halsey, J. Hausdorff, J. *et al.* (1994) A Phase I study of paclitaxel (taxol) in combination with SDZ PSC 833, a potent modulator of multidrug resistance (MDR). *Anticancer Drugs* **5**, Suppl. 1, 43.

Chapter 24

Drug resistance factors

Ate G.J. VAN DER ZEE and Elisabeth G.E. DE VRIES.

24.1 INTRODUCTION

Intrinsic or acquired resistance to cytotoxic drugs is the major obstacle in the management of patients with advanced-stage ovarian cancer, and is therefore, responsible for the poor outlook of these patients [1]. Studies in cultured (ovarian) tumour cells have provided insight in the diverse cell biological mechanisms that may be involved in drug resistance, such as increased expression of membrane associated drug transport glycoproteins, detoxifying cytosolic non-proteins and DNA damage repair enzymes. In the development of (ovarian) cancer, multiple and sequential changes in oncogenes and tumour suppressor genes occur. Recent studies show that these changes are not only responsible for diverse growth characteristics of malignant tumours but also for different sensitivities to cytotoxic drugs.

Despite the fact that knowledge on cell biological factors and genetic changes involved in drug resistance has developed rapidly in cultured (ovarian) tumour cells, the translation of this knowledge into the clinic is just beginning. In this chapter diverse cell biological features are described, working at different cellular levels, that have been linked to drug resistance in ovarian cancer. Their possible clinical relevance is also reviewed.

24.2 CELL MEMBRANE ASSOCIATED DRUG RESISTANCE

24.2.1 P-GP

P-glycoprotein (P-GP) is a glycoprotein acting as an efflux pump for certain classes of unrelated drugs, such as doxorubicin, epipodophyllotoxins and taxol (natural products). The overexpression of P-GP in tumour cell lines selected for resistance to a single natural product is accompanied by cross-resistance to other natural products, resulting in the so-called multidrug resistance (MDR) phenotype [2].

In several human ovarian cancer cell lines overexpression of P-GP has been found to be (in part) responsible for reduced cytotoxicity of drugs such as doxorubicin and taxol [3-6]. The range in reported frequency of P-GP expression in human ovarian cancer is wide. Depending on the methodology used for the detection of P-GP, lower (0-6%) [7,8] and higher (70-80%) [8-11] expression rates have been described.

The prognostic significance of P-GP in ovarian cancer is also disputed. In a uniformly treated (cisplatin, cyclophosphamide, doxorubicin) series of 89 patients with advanced ovarian cancer, we found positive P-GP immunostaining (15%) to be related neither to response to chemotherapy, nor to survival [12]. In a later study in a smaller series of patients with advanced stage ovarian cancer treated with mainly platinum based chemotherapy these findings were confirmed [13]. Holzmayer *et al.* found, in a small study, high expression of P-GP to be related to failure to respond to chemotherapy [10], while Arao *et al.* did not find such a relation [11]. The problem of both studies is that the clinical information is incomplete and patient selection undefined, which weakens the strength of the observations.

Induction of P-GP expression by doxorubicin or taxol containing chemotherapy has been reported in different studies and points to a role of P-GP in acquired drug resistance in ovarian cancer [8,12,14].

In a variety of malignancies attempts have been made to modulate clinical MDR by co-administration of non-cytotoxic inhibitors of P-GP, *e.g.* verapamil [15]. In ovarian cancer Ozols *et al.* were unable to demonstrate potentiation of the activity of doxorubicin by verapamil in eight patients with drug resistant tumours, which were not evaluated for P-GP expression [16]. The recent introduction of taxol in first and second line chemotherapy may increase the importance of P-GP mediated drug resistance in ovarian cancer. Consequently, efforts to modulate P-GP mediated resistance to taxol may become more clinically relevant.

24.2.2 MRP/LRP

Recently, new drug resistance associated proteins, MDR-associated Protein (MRP), and lung resistance protein (LRP) have been identified. Overexpression of MRP and/or LRP has been found in non-P-GP expressing tumour cell lines with MDR phenotype [17,18]. MRP is capable of extruding glutathione conjugates (see below) [19]. In primary ovarian cancer we found a high frequency of MRP expression (70%), but no prognostic significance with regard to

response to mainly platinum based chemotherapy or survival [20].

LRP is a major vault protein, that is primarily found in cytoplasmic vesicles and in the pores of the nuclear membrane [21]. How LRP confers drug resistance has not been elucidated yet. However, we found that positive LRP immunostaining is strongly related to response to (mainly platinum) chemotherapy, and also the strongest prognostic factor with regard to survival in uni- and multivariate analysis [13,20]. More information on the function of LRP should elucidate the background of the prognostic impact of LRP in ovarian cancer, and also provide ways to modulate its possible mechanism of drug resistance.

24.3 CYTOSOLIC (NON) PROTEIN-ASSOCIATED DRUG RESISTANCE

24.3.1 GLUTATHIONE

Glutathione is a tripeptide thiol, which has an important role in cellular detoxification of various xenobiotics, such as platinum compounds and alkylating agents [22]. How glutathione influences resistance to drugs is not completely clear. It appears that either by direct binding or conjugation of drugs to glutathione their interaction with their intracellular target is prohibited.

Glutathione synthesis requires the formation of precursors such as glutamate by the cell membrane-bound enzyme gamma-glutamyl transpeptidase (GGT) [23]. Successive actions of the cytosolic enzymes gamma-glutamylcysteine synthetase (GCS) and glutathione synthetase subsequently catalyse the synthesis of glutathione. The first glutathione synthesis step, catalysed by GCS, is rate-limiting and inhibited by buthionine sulfoximine [24].

In human ovarian cancer cell lines a strong relation has been found between levels of glutathione and glutathione synthesis enzymes (GCS, GGT) and sensitivity to platinum compounds and alkylating agents. It has been shown that resistance to these compounds can be reversed by depleting high glutathione levels in ovarian cancer cells with buthionine sulfoximine [25,26]. However, at the same time several platinum and alkylating agents resistant human ovarian cancer cell lines have been described that do not have an elevated glutathione level [27]. It still may be that glutathione elevations in platinum resistant cell lines turn out to be a rather general and non-specific response to any selection pressure [28].

Only limited data exist on glutathione levels in human ovarian cancer samples. The assessment of glutathione levels in tumour biopsies is associated with technical problems [29] and is also hampered by significant intratumour variation in glutathione levels [30,31]. In unpaired samples Britten *et al.* found higher glutathione levels in specimens from patients after chemotherapy in comparison to untreated patients [32]. Hanigan *et al.* determined GGT expression in benign and malignant human ovarian tumours. The GGT level may be a marker of the cellular capacity for glutathione synthesis, which may be an even more important parameter of detoxifying capacity than steady-state glutathione levels. Data on a possible relation of GGT expression and response to chemotherapy are not yet available [33].

24.3.2 GLUTATHIONE S-TRANSFERASES

Glutathione S-transferases (GSTs) are cytosolic proteins that function as enzymes of detoxification by catalysing the conjugation of electrophilic agents such as platinum and/or alkylating compounds to glutathione [34]. In man, cytosolic GSTs have been divided into four major classes termed alpha, mu, pi, and theta [35,36]. As these isozymes are known to have different substrate specificities, both total GST activity and GST isozyme composition may be determinants of a tumour's ability to detoxify chemotherapeutic agents [37]. In several platinum and alkylating agent-resistant human tumour cell lines, an enhanced GST content has been described [27,38]. However, in two different panels of ovarian cancer cell lines no relation was found between GST levels and resistance to platinum compounds and alkylating agents [25,26]. Gene transfection studies showed an unequivocal role for GSTs in platinum resistance, while in similar studies the most convincing evidence for a role in alkylating agent resistance was found for GST alpha [for summary, see ref. 39].

We and other groups have found that GST pi is the predominant GST isozyme in human ovarian cancer, while in most studies no relation between GST pi expression and response to chemotherapy or survival is reported [12,40-42]. However, Green *et al.* found high intensity of GST pi staining to be related to resistance to cytotoxic chemotherapy and shorter overall survival [43]. Overall it appears from *in vitro* studies and (most) data in human ovarian cancer that GST levels are not important markers of drug resistance.

24.3.3 METALLOTHIONEINS

Metallothioneins are a range of small cytosolic proteins involved in cellular heavy metal detoxification [44]. Platinum compounds have been shown to bind to metallothioneins [45]. Evidence on the role of metallothioneins in platinum resistance is weak. In most platinum resistant ovarian cancer cell lines, metallothionein levels are unchanged [27]. Transfection experiments with a metallothionein gene construct yielded inconsistent effects on cisplatin resistance [46,47]. In malignant ovarian tumours Murphy *et al.* found neither changes in metallothioneins levels by chemotherapy, nor a relation between metallothionein content and response to chemotherapy. However, the number of patients in this study was small and non-sequential biopsies were studied [48].

24.3.4 ALDEHYDE DEHYDROGENASE

Detoxification of cyclophosphamide can be mediated by aldehyde dehydrogenase (ALDH). This cytosolic enzyme catalyses the conversion of aldophosphamide (activated cyclophosphamide) to (inactive) carboxy-phosphamide [49]. Elevated levels of ALDH correlated with resistance to cyclo-phosphamide in different (non-ovarian) tumour cell lines [50,51]. In fresh biopsies of untreated human ovarian tumours (n=15) Djuric *et al.* found very low ALDH levels, while ALDH levels were slightly increased in (unpaired) tumours (n=7) after chemo-therapy [52]. No studies on ALDH levels have yet been performed in larger series of patients.

24.4 NUCLEAR PROTEIN-ASSOCIATED DRUG RESISTANCE

24.4.1 TOPOISOMERASES

Topoisomerase (Topo) I and II are nuclear enzymes involved in various DNA transactions such as replication, trans-cription, and recombination. Topo I and II targeted drugs, *e.g.* camptothecin and epipodophyllotoxins respectively, produce stabilized drug-Topo-DNA cleavable complexes, that result in cell death [53]. Apart from decreased Topo levels (providing less target for the drug), qualitative alterations in Topo I and II can result in insensitivity of the target for the drug. For the Topo II enzyme two isozymes, Topo IIà and IIá, have been described, that have different affinities to Topo II targeted drugs, such as doxorubicin and etoposide. Changes

in the ratio of Topo IIà to IIá may also be responsible for altered sensitivity of tumour cells to Topo II targeted drugs [54]. Recently an etoposide resistant human ovarian cancer cell line has been described with decreased Topo II activity [55]. Hamaguchi *et al.* showed that cross-resistance to doxorubicin in cisplatin resistant ovarian cancer cell lines was not due to alterations in Topo II expression [56].

In subsequent studies we have shown that Topo II activity is higher in human malignant ovarian tumours in comparison to benign tumours. Topo II activity varies significantly between malignant tumours. Tumours after platinum-based chemotherapy have lower Topo II activity in comparison to untreated tumours, while no differences exist in Topo I activity [57]. Topo IIà protein levels in human ovarian cancer are not regulated by DNA amplification. Different levels of Topo II in ovarian cancer may (in part) be responsible for the variable response of ovarian cancers to Topo II targeted drugs [57-59]. Based on these studies in ovarian cancer Topo I may be a promising target for newly developed campthocecin analogues in this malignancy.

24.4.2 DNA DAMAGE REPAIR ENZYMES

Several platinum-resistant ovarian cancer cell lines show increased levels of DNA repair, as determined by enhanced loss of platinum adducts and increased synthesis of DNA repair enzymes [27,60]. Repair of DNA damage caused by platinum-DNA-adducts occurs primarily by the nucleotide excision repair pathway in which a large number of enzymes are involved[61]. A variety of individual DNA repair enzymes have been linked to platinum resistance in (ovarian) tumour cell lines [62-64].

Besides increased DNA repair in the total genomic DNA preferentially repair of transcriptionally active genes has also been reported [65]. In a series of cisplatin-resistant ovarian cancer cell lines Johnson *et al.* found increased removal of platinum compounds from total genomic DNA to be associated with increased resistance. Increased repair of inter-strand cross-links in the resistant cell lines was also more apparent in actively transcribed sequences [60].

The complexity of the DNA repair mechanism offers major problems to evaluate DNA repair capacity in tumour specimens. In human ovarian cancer the levels of rate-limiting human DNA repair genes such as ERCC-1 and XPAC were found to be expressed at higher levels in clinically drug resistant tumours than in responsive tumours. However, the number of patients in these studies were small, and patient selection was not defined [64,66]. It may be questionable to link the expression of one or two of the many enzymes involved in DNA repair to clinically encountered resistance of tumours to cytotoxic drugs.

As DNA damage repair involves many proteins several opportunities are available to modulate resistance due to increased repair. Drugs such as aphidicolin, interfere at different levels in DNA repair and have been found to modulate platinum compound cytotoxicity in tumour cell lines [67]. A phase I clinical trial of aphidicolin showed that prolonged steady-state levels can be achieved at concentrations proven to be maximally inhibiting repair of platinum-induced DNA damage [68]. Recently, O'Dwyer *et al.* found in mice superior activity of the combination of aphidicolin and platinum compounds in comparison to platinum compounds alone against cisplatin-resistant human ovarian cancer [69].

Repair of DNA damage, caused by alkylating agents occurs both by DNA base repair and nucleotide excision repair. DNA base repair enzymes such as O-6-alkylguanine-DNA-alkyltransferase (ATase)

remove alkyl groups from damaged DNA [70]. In different (non-ovarian) tumour cell lines resistant to alkylating agents such as nitrosurea, ATase has been found to be overexpressed [71,72]. Transfection of ATase cDNA into ATase deficient cells conferred resistance to alkylating agents [72]. No data exist on ATase in human ovarian cancer cell lines. Lee *et al.* reported high ATase expression in human ovarian cancers in comparison to Hodgkin's lymphoma. It was suggested that the reported low efficacy of nitrosurea in ovarian cancer in comparison to high efficacy in Hodgkin's lymphoma may be due to different ATase levels in these tumours [73].

Enhanced repair of DNA damage caused by platinum compounds or alkylating agents is very frequently encountered in cultured platinum and/or alkylating agents resistant ovarian cancer cells, and occurs early in the acquisition of resistance of tumour cells to these compounds [27]. Therefore, this mechanism of resistance appears to be most important. However, its previously mentioned complex nature may prohibit adequate evaluation in the clinic.

24.5 CHANGES IN ONCOGENES, TUMOUR SUPPRESSOR GENES AND DRUG RESISTANCE.

Scattered reports can be found in the literature on the relation of changes in oncogenes and tumour suppressor genes and drug resistance. In the next section, only the most appealing literature on this issue will be summarized.

24.5.1 TYROSINE KINASES

The epidermal growth factor receptor (EGFR) and the protein product of the oncogene c-erbB2 are both plasma membrane receptors which function through activation of the tyrosine kinases on the internal domains of the receptor molecules. From most recent studies it appears that c-erbB2 oncogene overexpression *per se* is not a prognostic factor in human ovarian cancer, neither with regard to response to chemotherapy nor survival. At the same time these studies show that c-erbB2 overexpression may have a role in growth regulation in an important proportion (20-40%) of ovarian cancers [74-81]. Moreover, it has been shown that blocking of c-erbB2 overexpression with monoclonal antibodies results in enhanced cytotoxicity of cisplatin in cultured ovarian cancer cells, probably due to blocking of DNA repair by anti-c-erbB2 antibodies [82,83]. The same phenomenon has also been reported for anti-epidermal growth factor receptor (EGFR) antibodies [84].

24.5.2 NUCLEAR TRANSCRIPTION FACTORS

The jun, fos and myc oncoproteins act as nuclear transcription factors that regulate a variety of genes important in normal cellular growth and differentiation processes. C-jun, c-fos and c-myc are immediate early response genes, that can be activated by the exposure of cells to a variety of extracellular stimuli, including growth factors, and chemotherapeutic agents [85,86]. Scanlon *et al.* have provided evidence that fos gene expression may (in part) be responsible for directing the cellular response to DNA damage by cytotoxic agents. Higher fos gene expression after exposure of tumour cells to cisplatin results in the upregulation of DNA synthesis and DNA damage repair enzymes, such as thymidylate synthase, DNA polymerase á, and topoisomerase I. Over-expression of these enzymes results in drug resistance by enhanced repair of DNA damage, while downregulation by anti-fos ribozymes results in restored sensitivity to cisplatin [87-89]. Studies on the role of c-jun and c-myc in cisplatin resistance showed

comparable results [90,91].

Data on expression of c-fos, c-jun, and c-myc in human ovarian cancer are scarce. Scanlon *et al.* reported higher c-fos expression in cisplatin-resistant tumours after platinum chemotherapy in comparison to untreated tumours [88]. In a relatively small study Bauknecht *et al.* separated ovarian cancers into tumours that have low and high expression of c-jun and c-myc. Surprisingly, tumours with high expression were found to respond better to platinum based chemotherapy [92]. The role of the nuclear transcription factors in the clinical course of ovarian cancer has to be explored in larger series of patients to obtain conclusive information on their perhaps important role in response to chemotherapy.

24.5.3 TUMOUR SUPPRESSOR GENES

Changes in the p53 tumour suppressor gene, such as mutations or deletions are among the most common genetic alterations found in ovarian cancer [93]. Loss of p53 function by different ways has been found to increase resistance of cultured tumour cells to a variety of cytotoxic drugs [94]. This increased resistance has been linked to the loss of the presumed triggering role of p53 in the process of apoptosis [95].

Cytotoxicity of most chemotherapeutic drugs appears to be mediated by the induction of apoptosis. Other proteins such as p21, Rb, and Bcl-2, involved in cell cycle control or apoptosis, may also prove to be important determinants of a cell's ability to undergo apoptosis [96]. The near future may show that the cytotoxic action of many anticancer drugs is merely determined by the genotype of the cell rather than the genotoxicity of the agent. Recently, we found p53 immunostaining in 20% of stage I/II and 40% of stage III/IV ovarian cancers [12], which is comparable to results of other studies [93]. Positive immunostaining of p53 in ovarian cancer has been found to be strongly associated with the occurrence of missense mutations [97]. In our study, patients with p53 positive ovarian cancer had significantly shorter progression free and overall survival. Positive p53 immunostaining was associated with poorly differentiated tumours, the presence of ascites, and large residual tumour after first laparotomy. However, in this study, where the majority of responses to chemotherapy was verified by second look laparotomy no relation was found of positive p53 immunostaining with response to chemotherapy.

The negative prognostic impact of positive p53 immunostaining in ovarian cancer appears therefore to be due to more aggressive tumour growth, and not to a different sensitivity to cytotoxic drugs. In a multivariate analysis positive p53 immunostaining did not retain its independent prognostic significance. Two other recent studies also reported a negative prognostic role for positive p53 immunostaining in ovarian cancer [98,99].

The presumed negative prognostic significance of positive p53 immunostaining in ovarian and other malignancies, and the possible role of p53 in response to chemotherapy have lead to the design of *in vitro* and clinical studies in which the defective tumour suppressor gene has been replaced by the insertion of the normal tumour suppressor gene.

The major problem of this kind of gene therapy lies in the delivery of actively expressed vectors to every single tumour cell *in vivo* [100]. However, this approach may especially be promising in ovarian cancer, for which the negative prognostic value of positive p53 immunostaining has been confirmed, and in which the spread of the tumour is largely limited to the easily accessible intraperitoneal cavity.

24.6 CONCLUSIONS

Many factors at different cellular levels are involved in drug resistance. Multiple changes occur at the same time in highly resistant tumour cell lines resulting in the hypothesis that drug resistance is multifactorial. The majority of the respective parameters reviewed have been discovered and studied in cultured cells selected for high levels of resistance. Resistance levels in the clinic are probably much lower, which implies that perhaps single mechanisms will be responsible for resistance in individual patients [28]. Since increased repair of DNA damage caused by platinum compounds or other alkylating agents occurs early and consistently during selection of resistant cell lines this mechanism of resistance appears to be activated first [27]. However, the complexity of DNA repair mechanisms hampers the evaluation of the importance of this mechanism in the clinic. Still, DNA repair inhibiting agents that are targeted to rate-limiting enzymes of DNA repair may show efficacy in the clinic.

Increased cytosolic glutathione levels have been linked to resistance to platinum compounds and alkylating agents. Hamaguchi *et al.* showed that in ovarian cancer cell lines primarily resistant to cisplatin, cross-resistance to drugs such as melphalan and doxorubicin is correlated with enhanced intracellular glutathione levels [56]. This phenomenon reflects the broad cross-resistance patterns in patients with refractory ovarian cancer after platinum chemotherapy. Most studies indicate that modulation of glutathione metabolism may be one of the most promising ways of reversing clinical drug resistance. In phase I clinical trials, melphalan is administered in combination with buthionine sulfoximine. Results with regard to efficacy of this combination in phase II trials have to be awaited.

227

Resistance as a result of decreased intracellular levels of drugs mediated by unknown cell membrane proteins (platinum compounds, alkylating agents) or well characterized cell membrane glycoproteins such as P-glycoprotein (doxorubicin, taxol) are frequently encountered in cultured tumour cell lines. The role of these cell membrane (glyco) proteins in ovarian cancer remains to be established in the clinic. Especially in solid tumours one may presume that physiological barriers, *e.g.* in poorly-vascularized regions of the tumour are also critical in obtaining cytotoxic intracellular drug levels [101].

Further elucidation of the possible links between frequently observed genetic changes in ovarian cancer such as c-erbB2 amplification and p53 mutations and parameters of drug resistance is important because it may offer ways to manipulate encountered drug resistance phenotypes.

After the introduction of platinum containing drugs into combination chemotherapy, the last two decades brought no important changes in chemotherapy for patients with advanced ovarian cancer, resulting in a better outlook for these patients. The recent (intended) inclusion of taxol (and taxotere) in first and second line treatment will probably improve the prognosis for patients with advanced-stage ovarian cancer. However, the exponentially developing understanding of underlying (genetic) mechanisms of drug resistance hopefully will result in a new arsenal of drugs with specific antitumour activity.

REFERENCES

1. Cannistra, S.A. (1993) Cancer of the ovary. *N. Engl. J. Med.* **329**, 1550-9.
2. Ling, V. (1992) Charles F. Kettering prize. P-glycoprotein and resistance to anticancer drugs. *Cancer* **69**, 2603-9.
3. Chan, H.S.L., Bradley, G., Thorner, P. *et al.* (1988) A sensitive method for immunocytochemical detection of P-glycoprotein in multidrug-resistant human ovarian cell lines. *Lab. Invest.* **59**, 870-5.
4. Broxterman, H.J., Kuiper, C.M., Schuurhuis, G.J. *et al.* (1988) Increase of daunorubicin and vincristine accumulation in multidrug resistant human ovarian carcinoma cells by a monoclonal antibody reacting with P-glycoprotein. *Biochem. Pharmacol.* **37**, 2389-93.
5. Bradley, G., Naik, M. and Ling, V. (1989) P-glycoprotein expression in multidrug resistant human ovarian carcinoma cell lines. *Cancer Res.* **49**, 2790-6.
6. Maeda, O., Terasawa, M., Ishikawa, T. *et al.* (1993) A newly synthesized bifunctional inhibitor, W-77, enhances adriamycin activity against human ovarian carcinoma cells. *Cancer Res.* **53**, 2051-6.
7. Rubin, S.C., Finstadt, C.L., Hoskins, W.J. *et al.* (1990) Expression of P-glycoprotein in epithelial ovarian cancer: evaluation as a marker of multidrug resistance. *Am. J. Obstet. Gynecol.* **69**, 163-7.
8. Bourhis, H., Goldstein, L.J., Riou, G. *et al.* (1989). Expression of a human multidrug gene in ovarian carcinomas. *Cancer Res.* **49**, 5062-5.
9. Noonan, K.E., Beck, C., Holzmayer, T.A. *et al.* (1990) Quantitative analysis of MDR1 (multidrug resistance) gene expression in human tumors by polymerase chain reaction. *Proc. Natl. Acad. Sci. USA* **87**, 7160-4.
10. Holzmayer, T.A., Hilsenbeck, S., Von Hoff, D.D. *et al.* (1992) Clinical correlates of MDR1 (P-glycoprotein) gene expression in ovarian and small-cell lung carcinomas. *J. Natl. Cancer Inst.* **84**, 1486-91.
11. Arao, S., Suwa, H., Mandai, M. *et al.* (1994) Expression of multidrug resistance

gene and localization of P-glycoprotein in human primary ovarian cancer. *Cancer Res.* **54**, 1355-9.

12. Van der Zee, A.G.J., Hollema, H., Suurmeyer, A.H. *et al.* (1995) The value of P-glycoprotein, glutathione S-transferase, c-erbB-2, and p53 as prognostic factors in ovarian carcinomas. *J. Clin. Oncol.* **13**, 70-8.

13. Izquierdo, M.A., Van der Zee,A.G.J., Vermorken, J.B. *et al.* (1994) Prognostic significance of the drug resistance associated LRP in advanced ovarian carcinoma. *Ann. Oncol.* **8**, 98.

14. Bell, D.R., Gerlach, J.H., Kartner, N. *et al.* (1987) Detection of P-glycoprotein in ovarian cancer: a molecular marker associated with multidrug resistance. *J. Clin. Oncol.* **3**, 311-5.

15. Sikic, B.I. (1993) Modulation of multidrug resistance: at the threshold. *J. Clin. Oncol.* **11**, 1629-35.

16. Ozols, R.F., Cunnion, R.E., Klecker, R.W. *et al.* (1987) Verapamil and adriamycin in the treatment of drug-resistant ovarian cancer patients. *J. Clin. Oncol.* **5**, 641-7.

17. Cole, S.P., Bhardwaj, G., Gerlach, J.H. *et al.* (1992) Overexpression of a transporter gene in a multidrug resistant human lung cancer cell line. *Science* **258**, 1650-4.

18. Scheper, R.J., Broxterman, H.J., Scheffer, G.L. *et al.* (1993) Overexpression of a Mr 110,000 vesicular protein in non-P-glycoprotein-mediated multidrug resistance. *Cancer Res.* **53**, 1475-9.

19. Muller, M., Meijer, C., Zaman, G.J.R. *et al.* (1994) Overexpression of the gene encoding the multidrug resistance-associated protein results in increased ATP-dependent glutathione S-conjugate transport. *Proc. Natl. Acad. Sci. USA* **91**, 13033-7.

20. Izquierdo, M., van der Zee, A.G.J., Vermorken, J.B. *et al.* (1995) Expression of the new drug resistance-associated marker LRP in ovarian carcinoma predicts poor response to chemotherapy and shorter survival. *J. Natl. Cancer Inst* - submitted.

21. Scheffer, G.L., Wijngaard, P.L.J., Flens, M.J. *et al.* (1995) The drug resistance related protein LRP is the human major vault protein. *Nat. Med.* in press.

22. Arrick, B.A. and Nathan, C.F. (1984) Glutathione metabolism as a determinant of therapeutic efficiency, a review. *Cancer Res.* **44**, 4224-32.

23. Hanigan, M.H. and Rickets, W.A. (1993) Extracellular glutathione is a source of cysteine for cells that express gamma-glutamyl transpeptidase. *Biochemistry* **32**, 6302-6.

24. Richman, P.G. and Meister, A. (1975) Regulation of gamma-glutamyl-cysteine synthetase by nonallosteric feedback inhibition by glutathione. *J. Biol. Chem.* **250**, 1422-6.

25. Godwin, A.K., Meister, A., O'Dwyer, P.J. *et al.* (1992) High resistance to cisplatin in hum-an ovarian cancer cell lines is associated with marked increase of glutathione synthesis. *Proc. Natl. Acad. Sci. USA* **89**, 3070-4.

26. Mistry, P., Kelland, L.R., Abel, G. *et al.* (1991) Relationships between glutathione, glutathione S-transferase and cytotoxicity of platinum drugs and melphalan in eight human ovarian carcinoma cell lines. *Br. J. Cancer* **64**, 215-20.

27. Chu, G. (1994) Cellular responses to cisplatin. *J. Biol. Chem.* **269**, 787-90.

28. Borst, P. (1991) Genetic mechanisms of drug resistance. *Rev. Oncol.* **4**, 87-105.

29. Anderson, M.E. (1989) Enzymatic and chemical methods for the determination of glutathione. In *Glutathione: Chemical, biochemical, and medical aspects* (eds. D. Dolphin, R. Poulson, and O. Avranovic), Wiley, New York, pp.339-65.

30. Allalunis-Turner, M.J., Lee, F.Y.F. and

Siemann, D.W. (1989) Comparison of glutathione levels in rodent and human tumor cells grown *in vitro* and *in vivo*. *Cancer Res.* **48**, 3657-60.

31. Lee, F.Y.F., Vessey, A., Rofstad, E. *et al.* (1989) Heterogeneity of glutathione content in human ovarian cancer. *Cancer Res.* **49**, 5244-8.

32. Britten, R.A., Green, J.A. and Warenius, H.M. (1992) Cellular glutathione (GSH) and glutathione S-transferase (GST) activity in human ovarian tumor biopsies following exposure to alkylating agents. *Int. J. Radiat. Oncol. Biol. Phys.* **24**, 527-31.

33. Hanigan, M.H., Frierson, H.F., Brown, J.E. *et al.* (1994) Human ovarian tumors express gamma-glutamyl transpeptidase. *Cancer Res.* **54**, 286-90.

34. Boyer, T.D. (1989) The glutathione S-transferases: an update. *Hepatology* **9**, 486-96.

35. Mannervik, B. (1985) The isoenzymes of glutathione transferase. *Adv. Enzymol. Relat. Areas Mol. Biol.* **57**, 357-417.

36. Meyer, D.J., Coles, B., Pemble, S.E. *et al.* (1991) Theta, a new class of glutathione transferases purified from rat and man. *Biochem. J.* **274**, 409-14.

37. Mannervik, B. and Danielson, U.H. (1988) Glutathione S-transferases-structure and catalytic activity. *CRC Crit. Rev. Biochem.* **23**, 283-337.

38. Meijer, C., Mulder, N.H. and De Vries, E.G.E. (1990) The role of detoxifying systems in resistance of tumor cells to cisplatin and adriamycin. *Cancer Treat. Rev.* **7**, 389-407.

39. Stelmack, G.L. and Goldenberg, G.J. (1993) Increased expression of cytosolic glutathione S-transferases in drug-resistant L5178Y murine lymphoblasts: chemical selectivity and molecular mechanisms. *Cancer Res.* **53**, 3530-5.

40. Van der Zee, A.G.J., van Ommen, B., Meijer, C. *et al.* (1992) Glutathione S-transferase activity and isoenzyme composition in benign ovarian tumours, untreated malignant ovarian tumours, and malignant ovarian tumours after platinum/cyclophosphamide chemotherapy. *Br. J. Cancer* **66**, 229-34.

41. Rahilly, M., Nafussi, A.A. and Harrison, D.J. (1991) Distribution of glutathione S-transferase isoenzymes in primary epithelial tumors of the ovary. *Int. J. Gynecol. Cancer* **1**, 268-74.

42. Murphy, D., McGown, A.T., Hall, A. *et al.* (1992) Glutathione S-transferase activity and isoenzyme distribution in ovarian tumour biopsies taken before or after cytotoxic chemotherapy. *Br. J. Cancer* **66**, 937-42.

43. Green, J.A., Robertson, L.J. and Clark, A.H. (1993) Glutathione S-transferase expressi-on in benign and malignant ovarian tumours. *Br. J. Cancer* **68**, 235-39.

44. Hamer, D. (1986) Metallothionein. *Ann. Rev. Biochem.* **55**, 913-51.

45. Kraker, A.J., Schmidt, J., Krezoski, S. and Petering, D.H. (1985) Binding of cis-dichlorodiammine platinum(II) to metallothionein in Ehrlich cells. *Biochem. Biophys. Res. Commun.* **130**, 786-92.

46. Kelley, S.L., Basu, A., Teicher, M.P. *et al.* (1988) Overexpression of metallothionein confers resistance to anticancer drugs. *Science* **241**, 1813-5.

47. Schilder, R.J., Hall, L., Handel, L.M. *et al.* (1990) Metallothionein gene over-expression in human ovarian cancer cell lines. *Proc. Am. Assoc. Cancer Res.*, **30**, 525.

48. Murphy, D., McGown, A.T., Crowther, D. *et al.* (1991) Metallothionein levels in ovarian tumours before and after chemotherapy. *Br. J. Cancer* **63**, 711-4.

49. Sladek, N.E. (1994) Metabolism and pharmacokinetic behavior of cyclophosphamide and related oxazaphosphorines. In *Anticancer drugs: reactive metabolism and drug interactions* (ed. G. Powis), Pergamon

Press, Oxford, pp. 79-156.

50. Sreerama, L. and Sladek, N.E. (1994) Identification of a methylcholantrene-induced aldehyde dehydrogenase in a human breast adenocarcinoma cell line exhibiting oxazaphosphorine-specific acquired resistance. *Cancer Res.* **54**, 2176-85.

51. Hilton, J. (1984) Role of aldehyde dehydrogenase in cyclophosphamide-resist-ant L1210 leukemia. *Cancer Res.* **44**, 5156-60.

52. Djuric, Z., Malviya, V.K., Deppe, G. *et al.* (1990) Detoxifying enzymes in human ovarian tissues: comparison of normal and tumor tissues and effects of chemotherapy. *J. Cancer Res. Clin. Oncol.* **116**, 379-84.

53. Liu, L.F. (1989) DNA topoisomerase poisons as antitumor drugs. *Ann. Rev. Biochem.* **58**, 351-75.

54. Beck, W.T. and Danks, M.K. (1991) Mechanisms of resistance to drugs that inhibit DNA topoisomerases. *Semin. Cancer Biol.* **2**, 235-44.

55. Kubota, N., Nishio, K., Takeda, Y. *et al.* (1994) Characterization of an etoposide-resistant human ovarian cancer cell line. *Cancer Chemother. Pharmacol.* **34**, 183-9.

56. Hamaguchi, K., Godwin, A.K., Yakushiji, M. *et al.* (1993) Cross-resistance to diverse drugs is associated with primary cisplatin resistance in ovarian cancer cell lines. *Cancer Res.* **53**, 5225-32.

57. Van der Zee, A.G.J, Hollema, H., de Jong, S. *et al.* (1991) P-glycoprotein and DNA topoisomerase I and II activity in benign tumors of the ovary and in malignant tumors of the ovary, before and after platinum/cyclophosphamide chemotherapy. *Cancer Res.* **51**, 5915-20.

58. Van der Zee, A.G.J., de Vries, E.G.E., Hollema, H. *et al.* (1994) Molecular analysis of the topoisomerase IIà gene and its expression in ovarian cancer. *Ann.*

Oncol. **5**, 75-81.

59. van der Zee, A.G.J., de Jong, S., Keith, W.N. *et al.* (1994) Quantitative and qualitative aspects of topoisomerase I and IIà and á in untreated and platinum/cyclophosphamide treated malignant ovarian tumors. *Cancer Res.* **54**, 749-55.

60. Johnson, S.W., Perez, R.P., Godwin, A.K. *et al.* (1994) Role of platinum-DNA adduct formation and removal in cisplatin resistance in human ovarian cancer cell lines. *Biochem. Pharmacol.* **47**, 689-97.

61. Hoeijmakers, J.H.J. (1993) Nucleotide excision repair II: from yeast to mammals. *Trends in Genet.*, **9**, 211-17.

62. Scanlon, K.J., Kashani-Sabet, M. and Sowers, L.C. (1989) Overexpression of DNA replication and repair enzymes in cisplatin-resistant human colon carcinoma HCT8 cells and circumvention by azidothymidine. *Cancer Comm.* **1**, 269-75.

63. Hwang, B.J., Chu, G. (1993) Purification and characterization of a human protein that binds to damaged DNA. *Biochem*istry **32**, 1657-66.

64. Dabholkar, M., Bostick-Bruton, F., Weber, C. *et al.* (1992) ERCC1 and ERCC2 expression in malignant tissues from ovarian cancer. *J. Natl. Cancer Inst.* **84**, 1512-7.

65. Zhen, W., Link, C.J., O'Connor, P.M. *et al.* (1992) Increased gene-specific repair of cisplatin interstrand cross-links in cisplatin-resistant human ovarian cancer cell lines. *Mol. Cell. Biol.* **12**, 3689-98.

66. Dabholkar, M., Vionnet, J., Bostick-Bruton, F. *et al.* (1994) Messenger RNA levels of XPAC and ERCC1 in ovarian cancer tissue correlate with response to platinum-based chemotherapy. *J. Clin. Invest.* **94**, 703-8.

67. Jekunen, A.P., Homm, D.K., Alcaraz, J.E. *et al.* (1994) Cellular pharmacology of dichloro(ethylenediamine)platinum(II) in

cisplatin sensitive and resistant human ovari-an carcinoma cells. *Cancer Res.* **54**, 2680-7.

68. Sessa, C., Zuchetti, M., Davoli, E. *et al.* (1991) Phase I and clinical pharmacological evaluation of aphidicolin glycinate. *J. Natl. Cancer Inst.* **83**, 1160-4.

69. O'Dwyer, P.J., Moyer, J.D., Suffness, M. *et al.* (1994) Antitumor activity and biochemical effects of aphidicolin glycinate (NSC 303812) alone and in combination with cisplatin *in vivo*. *Cancer Res.* **54**, 724-9.

70. Pegg, A.E. (1990) Mammalian O_6-alkylguanine-DNA alkyltransferase: regulation and importance in response to alkylating carcinogenic and therapeutic agents. *Cancer Res.* **50**, 6119-29.

71. Harris, L.C. and Margison, G.P. (1993) Expression in mammalian cells of the Escherichia coli O_6 alkylguanine-DNA-alkyltransferase gene ogt reduces the toxicity of alkylnitrosoureas. *Br. J. Cancer* **67**, 1196-1202.

72. Baer, J.C., Freeman, A.A., Newlands, E.S. *et al.* (1993) Depletion of O6 alkylguanine-DNA-alkyltransferase correlates with potent-iation of temozolomide and CCNU toxicity in human tumour cells. *Br. J. Cancer* **67**, 1299-1302.

73. Lee, S.M., Harris, M., Rennison, J. *et al.* (1993) Expression of O6 alkylguanine-DNA-alkyltransferase *in situ* in ovarian and Hodgkin's tumors. *Eur. J. Cancer* **29A**, 1306-12.

74. Seidman, J.D., Frisman, D.M. and Norris, H.J. (1992) Expression of the HER-2/neu proto-oncogene in serous ovarian neoplasms. *Cancer* **70**, 2857-60.

75. Meden, H., Marx, D., Rath, W. *et al.* (1992) Overexpression of c-erbB-2-oncogene in 243 cases of primary ovarian carcinoma: frequency and prognostic value. *Geburtsh. Frauenheilk.* **52**, 667-73.

76. Hung, M-C., Zhang, X., Yan, D-H. *et al.* (1992) Aberrant expression of the c-erbB-2/neu protooncogene in ovarian cancer. *Cancer Lett.* **61**, 95-103.

77. Rubin, S.C., Finstad, C.L., Wong, G.Y. *et al.* (1993) Prognostic significance of HER-2/neu expression in advanced epithelial ovarian cancer: a multivariate analysis. *Am. J. Obstet. Gynecol.* **168**, 162-9.

78. Scambia, G., Benedetti Panici, P., Ferrandina, G. *et al.* (1993) Expression of HER-2/neu oncoprotein, DNA-ploidy and S-phase fraction in advanced ovarian cancer. *Int. J. Gynecol. Cancer* **3**, 271-8.

79. Makar, A.Ph., Holm, R., Kristensen, G.B. *et al.* (1994) The expression of c-erbB-2 (HER-2/neu) oncogene in invasive ovarian malignancies. *Int. J. Gynecol. Cancer* **4**, 194-9.

80. Rubin, S.C., Finstadt, C.L., Federici, M.G. *et al.* (1994) Prevalence and significance of HER-2/neu expression in early epithelial ovarian cancer. *Cancer* **73**, 1456-9.

81. Singleton, T.P., Perrone, T., Oakley, G. *et al.* (1994) Activation of c-erbB-2 and prognosis in ovarian carcinoma. *Cancer* **73**, 1460-6.

82. Hancock, M.C., Langton, B.C., Chan, P.T. *et al.* (1991) A monoclonal antibody against the c-erbB-2 protein enhances the cytotoxicity of cis-diamminedichloroplatinum against human breast and ovarian tumor cell lines. *Cancer Res.* **51**, 4575-80.

83. Pietras, R.J., Fendly, B.M., Chazin, V.R. *et al.* (1994) Antibody to HER-2/neu receptor blocks DNA repair after cisplatin in human breast and ovarian cancer cells, *Oncogene* **9**, 1829-38.

84. Christen, R.D., Hom, D.K., Porter, D.C. *et al.* (1990) Epidermal growth factor regulates the *in vitro* sensitivity of human ovarian carcinoma cells to cisplatin. *J. Clin. Invest.* **86**, 1632-40.

85. Curran, T. and Franza, B.R. (1988) Fos and jun: The AP-1 connection. *Cell* **55**, 395-7.

86. Lewin, B. (1991) Oncogenic conversion by regulatory changes in transcription factors. *Cell* **64**, 303-12.

87. Kashani-Sabet, M., Lu, Y., Leong, L. *et al.* (1990) Differential oncogene amplification in tumor cells from a patient treated with cisplatin and 5-fluorouracil. *Eur. J. Cancer* **26**, 383-90.

88. Scanlon, K.J., Kashani-Sabet, M. and Sowers, L.C. (1989) Molecular basis of cisplatin resistance in human carcinomas: model systems and patients. *Anticancer Res.* **9**, 1301-12.

89. Funato, T., Yoshida, E., Jiao, L. *et al.* (1992) The utility of an antifos ribozyme in reversing cisplatin resistance in human carcinomas. *Adv. Enz. Reg.* **32**, 195-209.

90. Sklar, M.D. and Prochownik, E.V. (1991) Modulation of cis-platinum resistance in friend erythroleukemia cells by c-myc. *Cancer Res.* **51**, 2118-23.

91. Rubin, E., Kharbandam, S, Gunji, H. *et al.* (1992) Cis-diamminedichloroplatinum(II) induces c-jun expression in human myeloid leukemia cells: potential involvement of a protein kinase C-dependent signaling pathway. *Cancer Res.* **52**, 878-82.

92. Bauknecht, T., Angel, P., Kohler, M. *et al.* (1993) Gene structure and expression analysis of the epidermal growth factor receptor, transforming growth factor-alpha, myc, jun, and metallothionein in human ovarian carcinomas. *Cancer* **71**, 419-29.

93. Mutch, D.G. and Williams, S. (1994) Biology of epithelial ovarian cancer. *Clin. Obstet. Gynecol.* **37**, 406-22.

94. Lowe, S.W., Ruley, H.E., Jacks, T. and Housman, D.E. (1993) p53-dependent apoptosis modulates the cytotoxicity of anticancer agents, *Cell* **74**, 957-67.

95. Symonds, H., Krall, L., Remington, L. *et al.* (1994) p53-Dependent apoptosis suppresses tumor growth and progression *in vivo*, *Cell* **78**, 703-11.

96. Reed, J.C. (1995) BCL-2 and chemoresistance in cancer. *Proc. Am. Assoc. Cancer Res.* **36**, 711.

97. Kohler, M.F., Marks, J.R., Wiseman, R.W. *et al.* (1993) Spectrum of mutation and frequency of allelic deletion of the p53 gene in ovarian cancer. *J. Natl. Cancer Inst.* **85**, 1513-9.

98. Bosari, S., Viale, G., Radaelli, U. *et al.* (1993) P53 accumulation in ovarian carcinomas and its prognostic implications. *Hum. Pathol.* **24**, 1175-9.

99. Hartman, L.C., Podratz, K.C., Keeney, G.L. *et al.* (1994) Prognostic significance of p53 immunostaining in epithelial ovarian cancer. *J. Clin. Oncol.* **12**, 64-9.

100. Sikora, K. (1994) Genes, dreams and cancer. *BMJ* **308**, 1217-21.

101. Jain, R.K. (1994) Delivery of therapeutic agents to solid tumors: role of vascular and interstitial physiology. *Proc. Am. Assoc. Cancer Res.* **35**, 661.

Chapter 25

Molecular mechanisms of platinum drug resistance

Stephen B. HOWELL, Buran KURDI-HAIDAR, Randolph D. CHRISTEN and

Gerrit LOS

25.1 INTRODUCTION

Development of resistance during a course of treatment with either cisplatin (DDP) or carboplatin (CBDCA) is a common problem, and contributes importantly to our inability to reliably cure even those ovarian cancers that are initially sensitive to these drugs. There is now good evidence that such acquired resistance to due to spontaneous somatic mutation [1,2] of tumour cells to a resistant state followed by selection for and overgrowth of the drug-resistant cells [3-5] by the ongoing chemotherapy. The discovery that loss of DNA mismatch repair can destabilize the human genome, and that such loss occurs commonly in sporadic tumours as well has hereditary non-polyposis colon cancer, has yielded new insight into the possible genetic basis for somatic mutation to drug resistance.

Despite the fact that the platinum-containing drugs are now very widely used in cancer chemotherapy, a complete description of the biochemical pharmacological changes that occur in resistant cells is still lacking. An important observation that has emerged from cell biological and molecular studies of cell lines representative of many types of tumour is that the platinum drugs kill cells via an apoptotic mechanism, and that this is an active process that can be modulated by many signal transduction pathways. Molecular studies of the signal transduction pathways activated during the cellular injury response to DDP is identifying strategies for preventing the emergence of resistance or reversing it once it has developed.

25.2 DRUG-RESISTANCE, SOMATIC MUTATION, AND GENOMIC INSTABILITY

25.2.1 SOMATIC MUTATION AND DRUG RESISTANCE

There is now a very large body of evidence indicating that resistance to the cytotoxic or cytostatic effect of chemotherapeutic and hormonal agents can arise through the process of somatic mutation. The data is consistent with a paradigm in which somatic mutation creates resistant variants that are then selected for by subsequent exposure to the therapeutic agent. The best known of such somatic mutations result in the constitutive over-expression of genes coding for proteins that are responsible for exporting drug from the cell (*e.g.* P-glycoprotein and MRP), the amplification of the enzymes that are the targets of the chemo-therapeutic agents (*e.g.* DHFR and CAD), or the alteration of control processes that regulate the triggering of apoptosis (*e.g.* bcl-2 and bax). A basic prediction that emerges from appreciation of the role of somatic mutation is that the rate of generation of drug-resistant variants in a population will be a function of the mutation rate, and that decreased genomic stability will increase the probability of drug resistance. Over the past several years, three other important principles regarding the development of drug resistance have emerged. First, genetic defects that interfere with the ability of a cell to repair damage to its DNA do create genomic instability in human cells [6-11]. Second, certain kinds of genomic instability do in fact foster the generation of drug-resistant variants in human cells [6]. Third, the cellular injury response produced by the therapeutic agent itself can, in the presence of abnormalities of cell cycle control, cause genomic instability and result in the generation of resistant variants [12,13].

25.2.2 DNA MISMATCH REPAIR

Among the types of genetic defects that can cause genomic instability, the loss of DNA mismatch repair is of particular interest both because it occurs commonly in sporadic ovarian cancers, and because it has the potential of markedly predisposing to the development of drug-resistant variants in the tumour cell population [6]. A cell normally makes a number of mistakes during the replication of DNA, and 'methyl-directed' DNA repair systems exist which promptly correct these mistakes shortly after they occur. Misincorporation of a base or 'slippage' of DNA polymerase on the template can create a short segment of mismatch. Two different types of systems appear to be responsible for repairing these types of errors in human cells, one of which is related to the bacterial mutHLS system and the other to DNA polymerase delta [14,15]. In bacteria and yeast, a minimum of ten proteins participate in the mutHLS-related

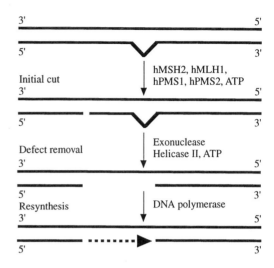

Figure 25.1 Schematic outline of the steps in DNA mismatch repair.

complex that repairs such small loops [7], and of these three are involved in the initiation of excision [16]. Four human homologues of these have now been cloned and their function partially identified. Figure 25.1 shows that the first step involves the binding of hMSH1 to the mismatched segment, and that this is followed by the cutting of the DNA, removal of the segment between the nick and the mismatch, filling of the gap by DNA polymerase delta, and ligation to render the strands whole again.

Loss of DNA mismatch repair can also be due to a defect in DNA polymerase delta function. DNA polymerase delta plays a major role in filling in the gap produced by the mutHLS-related complex and by the nucleotide excision repair system. It has an exonuclease proof-reading function that serves to remove misincorporated bases, and disruption of this function results in loss of DNA mismatch repair in bacteria and yeast [17,18].

Thus far, inactivating mutations in five human genes have been shown to result in the loss of DNA mismatch repair, and these include four genes related to the mutHLS system (hMSH2, hMLH1, hPMS1 and hPMS2) [11,19,20], and one related to DNA polymerase function (pol delta) [14]. Loss of DNA mismatch repair results in the appearance of nucleotide additions or deletions, and transitions and transversions in both repetitive and non-repetitive sequences scattered throughout the genome [6,21]. One consequence of the loss of DNA mismatch repair shows up in DNA sequences called microsatellites [17,22,23]. Microsatellites are stretches of DNA in which the same sequence of two, three or four bases is repeated many times (*e.g.* $(CA)_n$ $(CCA)_n$ or $(GATA)_n$). Microsatellites appear to be sequences where there is a high risk that DNA polymerase will 'slip' during replication creating a mismatched loop that is normally recognized and repaired by the DNA mismatch repair system [24]. If the DNA mismatch repair system is defective, then the loop will persist, and on the next round of DNA replication will generate two chromosomes with different numbers of di-, tri- or tetra-nucleotide repeats in allelic microsatellite sequences. This phenomenon is referred to as microsatellite instability; the term instability indicates that these simple repetitive sequences are prone to alteration by replication errors that are not corrected.

Microsatellite instability can be detected by amplifying the microsatellite sequence using a PCR reaction with primers specific to unique non-repetitive sequences on either side of the microsatellite sequence, and noting that the length of the amplified DNA fragment in the tumour DNA differs from that in the germline DNA. Not all types of microsatellite sequences appear to be at equal risk [6]; studies in many laboratories have documented that some microsatellites have a low probability of reflecting the underlying loss of DNA mismatch repair whereas other micro-satellites are more 'informative'. This variation offers one explanation for why some laboratories have

reported detecting microsatellite instability in only a small fraction of tumours [19], while others, analysing different microsatellite sequences, have found microsatellite instability in a greater percentage of the same histological type of tumour [25].

One might expect that once loss of DNA mismatch repair had occurred in a cell it would result in the appearance of mutations in many genes in the subsequent generations. There is now good evidence that this occurs [6,21]. The genes at greatest risk are likely to be those that contain reiterated short sequences, such as the HGPRT [6,26,27], and p53 [28] genes, or microsatellite sequences within or near their coding regions such as the BRCA1 [29], the androgen receptor [30], c-myc [19], and myotonin protein kinase [31] genes. More importantly, it appears that the genomic instability created by loss of DNA mismatch repair also leads to the mutational activation of oncogenes and/or the inactivation of tumour suppressor genes. Loss of DNA mismatch repair due to mutation of the hMSH2, hMLH1, hPMS1, hPMS2 and the pol delta gene is known to underlie the majority of the cases of hereditary non-polyposis colon cancer (HNPCC) [10,11,14,20]. Subjects who are heterozygous at one of the genes involved with DNA mismatch repair (e.g. hMSH2+/-) have adequate DNA mismatch repair function. However, at some point during the development of the tumour the remaining wild type allele is lost or mutated so that the cell loses all DNA mismatch repair function [20,32]. The resulting genomic instability likely plays a role in causing the series of genetic changes involving inactivation of the p53 gene and activation of ras that are required to create a fully malignant colon cancer [33]. The mutation rate at microsatellite sequences can be extraordinarily high ($0.6–3.8 \times 10^2$ [6]) and it is increased 100–1000-fold at selectable markers such as the HGPRT and ouabain resistance loci [6,7].

25.2.3 MICROSATELLITE INSTABILITY OFTEN OCCURS IN SPORADIC TUMOURS

In addition to HNPCC, microsatellite instability has now been found in sporadic non-familial cases of cancer arising in many different organs [19,22,23,34-37], suggesting that loss of DNA mismatch repair is an important component of the transformation process in many kinds of cancer. Since the simultaneous mutation of both alleles of a DNA mismatch repair gene is likely to occur with low probability, the genetic pathogenesis of sporadic cancers most likely involves a combination of loss of a portion of one chromosome (loss of heterozygosity, LOH) and mutation of the gene on the other chromosome [32]. This is consistent with the observation that clonal loss of heterozygosity occurs quite early in the transformation of the breast epithelium, at least as it can be appreciated histologically.

Loss of heterozygosity can be demonstrated even in hyperplastic breast duct lesions classified by the pathologist as non-malignant when analysed by microdissection and PCR. Recent studies from the Vogelstein group have demonstrated that microsatellite instability in sporadic non-familial colon cancers can be traced directly to loss of DNA mismatch repair resulting from the mutation or loss of both of the wild type alleles of one of the DNA mismatch repair genes [32], and this provides a paradigm for the appearance of microsatellite instability in other types of sporadic tumours. Microsatellite instability has been found in a wide variety of tumours including gastric [34,38,39], breast [19,40-42], pancreatic [34], endometrial [35,43], small cell lung [37], bladder cancers [44], soft tissue sarcomas, primary brain tumours [19] and ovarian carcinomas [19,34,45].

25.2.4 RELATIONSHIP BETWEEN LOSS OF DNA MISMATCH REPAIR, GENOMIC INSTABILITY, AND DRUG RESISTANCE

Loss of DNA mismatch repair can both directly result in drug resistance by knocking out the cells' ability to detect damage, and indirectly foster resistance by increasing the mutation rate. Loss of DNA mismatch repair causes resistance to an alkylating agent in the human lymphoblastoid cell line MT1 [8]. Although one might have expected that loss of DNA mismatch repair would cause the cells to be more sensitive due to the persistence of DNA damage, paradoxically for the methylating agent MNNG it causes the cell to become several hundred-fold more resistant.

A similar effect has been observed when proteins capable of binding to platinated DNA are knocked out in *Saccharomyces cerevisiae* [46]. The best explanation for this relates to the fact that alkylating agents (as well as most other anticancer drugs) cause cell death by apoptosis. Triggering of apoptosis requires that the cell be able to recognize the presence of the alkylation damage in DNA, and it may be lack of detection or lack of attempted repair that causes failure to generate an apoptotic signal [8,46]. The hMSH2 gene product is able to bind to adducts produced in DNA by cisplatin and carboplatin (Fishel, R. - personal communication) and is likely to recognize adducts produced by alkylating agents commonly used in the treatment of breast cancer such as melphalan, cyclophosphamide, and nitrogen mustard.

Loss of DNA mismatch repair could contribute to the generation of drug resistant variants in several ways. First this type of genomic instability could be effective in creating drug-resistant variants through the mutational activation of defence mechanisms such as export pumps (*e.g.* P-glycoprotein in the case of many natural product drugs). Second, it may result in the inactivation of steps required for intracellular metabolic conversion of drugs to their active form, or the activation of detoxification mechanisms.

There is some data suggesting that this type of genomic instability does in fact predispose to the development of drug-resistant mutants.

One colon cancer cell line with defective DNA mismatch repair and a homozygous hMLH1 mutation [10] has been reported to demonstrate microsatellite instability and have a general increase in the rate of spontaneous and drug-selected mutation to a drug-resistant phenotype [7]. The same thing has been observed in another colon carcinoma cell line that demonstrates microsatellite instability [6]. However, the magnitude of this effect for drugs with different mechanisms of action is unknown, and there is no information on whether loss of DNA mismatch repair due to mutations in hMSH2 is more or less devastating than loss of DNA mismatch repair due to mutations in hMLH1, hPMS1, hPMS2, pol delta or other genes whose products are involved in DNA mismatch repair.

Finally, there is evidence consistent with the hypothesis that cells selected for resistance to a drug that produces adducts in DNA that are recognized by hMSH2 show a decrease rather than increase in DNA mismatch repair function. Selection of two different human ovarian carcinoma cell lines (2008 and A2780) for resistance to cisplatin (DDP) results in a situation where 20 to 37-fold more adducts in DNA are required to kill 50% of the cells. In the DDP-resistant A2780/CP70 cells, there is a small increase in the rate of removal of adducts from DNA [47], but this is not seen in the DDP-resistant 2008/C13*5.25 cells [48]. It is clear that DDP adducts can be removed from DNA by nucleotide excision repair [49], and current thinking is that they can also be removed by DNA mismatch repair and that these pathways may share elements in common. Thus, the situation in the A2780/CP70 cells is consistent with a loss of DNA mismatch repair, and some compensatory increase in nucleotide excision repair, whereas in the 2008/C13*5.25 cells the data are consistent with a loss of DNA mismatch repair without any increase in nucleotide excision repair.

25.2.5 MODULATION OF GENOMIC STABILITY BY CELLULAR STRESS AND ENVIRONMENTAL FACTORS

Evidence from several kinds of experiments suggests that the impact of genomic instability on the development of drug-resistant variants can be influenced by the integrity of various types of cell cycle checkpoint controls, and signals arriving at the nucleus from both cell surface and intracellular receptor systems that reflect the effects of growth factors, hormones, and nutrition environment [50].

First, recent studies in *E. coli* have demonstrated that growth under nutrient-limiting conditions favours the outgrowth of genetic variants with base deletions in runs of DNA mononucleotides that resemble those observed in human microsatellite sequences [51,52]. This suggests that metabolite insufficiency may increase the probability of replication errors of the type normally corrected by DNA mismatch repair, and raise the possibility that the nutritional and hormonal environment have an important impact on genomic stability and mutation frequency in cells with loss of DNA mismatch repair function.

Second, cells exposed to various kinds of metabolic stress or injury normally arrest in G_1 (reviewed in [53]). If, due to loss of DNA mismatch repair, mutations have occurred in one or more of the genes involved in G_1 checkpoint control, then cells progress into S phase under circumstances where they should not, and dramatic increases in the generation of drug-resistant variants result. Murine cells that fail to arrest in G_1 due to loss of p53 function have a more than 10^3-fold increase in the number of PALA resistant variants [12,54], and similar results have been observed in human diploid fibroblasts [13]. In this particular situation, one manifestation of the induced genomic instability is chromosome breakage.

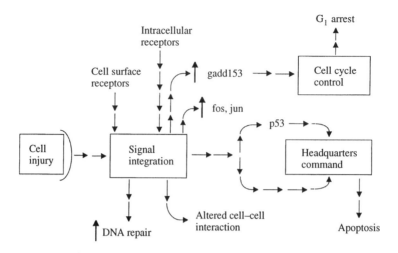

Figure 25.2 Schematic diagram of pathways involved in the DDP-induced cellular injury response.

Thus, pre-existing genomic instability that has resulted in the loss of cell cycle controls can be dramatically amplified by cellular stress.

25.3 CISPLATIN KILLS CELLS BY APOPTOSIS

Treatment of both murine [55] and human [56] cancer cells with clinical relevant exposures to DDP kills them by triggering apoptosis, a process that requires cellular energy, transcription, and translation (reviewed in [57]). Despite the fact that DDP-induced apoptosis has now been shown in many different tumour types, apoptosis is not always readily demonstrable by the appearance of DNA degradation 'ladders' produced by activation of endogenous endonucleases that degrade DNA intranucleosomally. While DDP produces a 'nucleosomal ladder' pattern of DNA degradation in some cell types [55], it fails to do so in many others.

In human ovarian carcinoma cell lines, it is more typical to find a wide spectrum of large fragment sizes. Ormerod *et al.* [56] found a predominance of fragments in the 30–50

kilobase range in one ovarian carcinoma cell line. There is wide variation among ovarian carcinoma cell lines in the ease with apoptosis can be detected by any assay of apoptotic cells death. In our hands, while fragmentation of the DNA can be detected by failure of [^{3}H]dThd-labelled fragments to precipitate in acid [58], this signal is only observed at very high levels of drug exposure.

Flow cytometric quantitation of fragments by has not proven highly reproducible nor quantitative, and the same has been true for detection of apoptosis by the TUNEL assay which is sensitive to broken DNA ends and gaps that can be revealed by incorporation of a labelled nucleotide [59]. This may be related to the fact that even following lethal exposure to the platinum drugs, relatively few adducts are formed per genome such that strand breaks resulting from attempted repair may bequite sparse. A clear distinction between apoptosis and necrosis cannot be made in some cell systems, and there may be a subtle shift from predominance of apoptosis at relatively low levels of drug exposure towards necrosis as very high levels.

25.3.1 SIGNAL TRANSDUCTION PATHWAYS INVOLVED IN CISPLATIN-INDUCED APOPTOSIS

Cellular injury produced by cisplatin provokes a programmed response that results in the activation of some genes, the inactivation of others, major shifts in cellular metabolism and cell cycle progression, and eventually the triggering of apoptosis. At the present time little is known about which signal transduction pathways are involved in this complex cellular injury response, but it is clear that the pathways activated by the platinum drugs are similar in many respects to those activated by other kinds of cellular injury. It is possible at this point to identify some elements of the injury response system that must be present (Figure 25.2).

Successful activation of the cellular injury response requires that the cell have a detector capable of sensing the presence of damage. In the case of the platinum drugs DNA appears to be the primary target, and several proteins have now been identified that can bind with high affinity to platinated DNA and may serve the role of detector. Lippard, Whitehead and their colleagues have demonstrated that several members of the HMG class of proteins contain motifs that permit tight binding to DNA distorted by intrastrand or interstrand adducts [60,61]. Recently, Fox *et al.* [46] have shown that, in *Saccharomyces cerevisiae* photolyase also binds to platinated DNA. Finally, the two molecules (p70 and p80) that together make up the Ku antigen [62] may serve this role. This molecular complex binds avidly to gapped and broken DNA, and serves to attract and activate DNA protein kinase [63]. Once activated, this complex can phosphorylate a number of substrates that might be involved in the repair of DDP adducts including RPA and p53. The actual role of any of these candidates in the process of detecting cisplatin damage remains conjectural at the present time.

A second required component of the cellular

injury response signal transduction pathway is an integration circuit that serves to combine signals arriving from multiple parts of the cell. This conclusion is based on the fact that sensitivity to cisplatin can be altered by a number of different growth factors that bind to receptors on the cell surface [64,65]. For example, a one hour concurrent exposure to EGF is capable of enhancing the cytotoxicity of DDP to human head and neck carcinoma cells in log phase growth by a factor of 3.8 ± 0.2-fold [64,66]. This brief exposure causes neither a mitogenic response, and nor any change in the perturbation of cell cycle phase distribution caused by DDP exposure. In the 2008 human ovarian carcinoma cell system, the EGF effect is not related to any alteration in the biochemical pharmacology of DDP, but the effect does require activation of the EGF receptor, and its magnitude is proportional to the number of receptors present on the cell surface [64].

Sensitization to cisplatin has also been observed when cells were treated with an antibody that can bind to the EGF receptor in an *in vivo* model system [66] presumably by virtue of the ability of the antibody to activate at least some component of the EGF receptor signal transduction pathway. EGF exposure does not change the biochemical pharmacology of cisplatin, therefore the hypothesis is that the signal generated by activation of the EGF receptor amplifies that generated by the damage detector. Antibody that binds to and partially activates the HER2/neu receptor in human breast and ovarian carcinoma cells has also been reported to enhance sensitivity to cisplatin [67]. At what point the receptor signals impinge on those generated by the damage detector is unknown, and is the focus of current research.

Signals originating from intracellular receptors are also capable of modulating those generated by the damage detector. This conclusion devolves from studies showing that activation of protein kinase C with phorbol ester analogues can sensitize many types of human cancer cell lines to cisplatin and several of its analogues [68,69]. Exposure of human ovarian carcinoma 2008 cells to 0.1μM TPA for one hour concurrently with graded concentrations of cisplatin increased the sensitivity of these cells to cisplatin by a factor of 2.5, and to carboplatin by a factor of 2.8 [70]. Activation of protein kinase A, which is another intracellular kinase that plays an important role in signal transduction, also enhances sensitivity to cisplatin in the 2008 system [71].

Yet another component of the signal transduction system must serve to interface cellular injury response signals generated by the DNA damage detector with the motor responsible for driving cell cycle progression. Cells exposed to cisplatin demonstrate both a concentration-dependent slowing of progression through S phase, and a G_2 arrest whose magnitude and duration are related to total drug exposure. Many other kinds of DNA damaging agents produce an arrest in G_1 as well as G_2. However, in 2008 human ovarian cancer cells G_1 arrest following cisplatin injury is dwarfed by the much greater magnitude of the G_2 arrest.

While the issue of how often cisplatin causes a G_1 arrest in human cancer cells remains unanswered, recent reports have identified mechanisms that might account for such an effect in cancer cells [53]. Cisplatin is one of the cytotoxic drugs that cause an increase in the expression and activity of p53 [72]. p53 is a transcription factor that can activate the transcription of p21 which is an effective inhibitor of the cyclin-dependent kinases. The latter are regulators of the phosphorylation of $p107^{Rb}$ which regulates exit from the G_1 phase of the cell cycle [73,74]. Current evidence suggests that if $p107^{Rb}$ cannot be phosphorylated, then it continues to sequester transcription factors, such as E2F-DP, capable of activating genes responsible for S phase function [75].

Finally, the signal transduction pathways involved in the cellular injury response must connect with the trigger for the apoptotic response. How this trigger works is not known, but the activation process is highly regulated as are the individual biochemical reactions that result in nuclear degeneration [76]. Apoptotic activity can now be measured biochemically in cell-free systems, and the generation of such activity is a function of both time and temperature [77,78]. Factors involved in the initiation of the reaction that generates apoptotic activity may be different from those that regulation the rate of its development. The development of apoptotic activity is clearly influenced by proteins of the bcl-2, bcl-X, and Ich-1 family [76,79] and the long list of partners with which these proteins form dimers or multimers [80,81].

25.4 DISCUSSION

The probability of generating a resistant cell is a function of the number of different genes where a mutation can result in drug resistance as well as the mutation rate and the number of cells at risk. The complexity of the cellular injury response triggered by cisplatin, and that fact that there appear to be multiple points where the signal arising from the detector that eventually activates apoptosis can be dampened or amplified, suggests that mutations in many different genes will be capable of altering sensitivity to the platinum-containing drugs. One implication is that, with many different genes at risk, small changes in genomic stability may result in large changes in the probability that a tumour will contain at least one resistant cell at any particular point in its growth [1]. Under these circumstances, interventions directed at controlling the mutation rate may be as important to the development of drug resistance as factors such as dose intensity of treatment, total dose, or the use of combination chemotherapy.

We generally do not think of the mutation rate in a tumour as being susceptible to modulation. However, the discovery of the importance of DNA mismatch repair as a determinant of genomic stability and mutation rate, and the observation that the impact of loss of DNA mismatch repair can be modified by environmental influences, suggests that it may be possible to modify mutation rate. The recent identification of the critical role of hMSH2 and hMLH1 in maintaining DNA mismatch repair makes it easier to understand how mutation rate might be altered through changes in the level of expression of one or both of these genes, or genes coding for other proteins required for successful management of mismatches developing in DNA during normal cellular replication. Although this chapter has emphasized the role of DNA mismatch repair as a determinant of genomic stability, it should be remembered that cisplatin adducts are also removed from the genome by nucleotide excision repair, and that failure of this repair system not only makes cell highly susceptible to cisplatin but can also influence mutation rate by allowing the persistence of adducts that themselves are mutagenic.

REFERENCES

1. Goldie, J.H. and Coldman, A.J. (1979) A mathematic model for relating the drug sensitivity of tumors to their spontaneous mutation rate. *Cancer Treat. Rep.* **63**, 1727-33.
2. DeMars, R. (1974) Resistance of cultured human fibroblasts and other cells to purine analogs in relation to mutagenesis detection. *Mut. Res.* **14**, 335.
3. Prestayko, A.W. (1980) Cisplatin, a preclinical overview. In, *Cisplatin, Current status and new developments* (eds. A.W. Prestayko, S.T. Crooke and S.K. Carter). Academic Press, New York, pp 1-7.
4. Skipper, H.E. (1979) A review and more quantitative analysis of the results of many internally controlled combination chemotherapy trials carried out over the past 15 years (L1210 and leukemia and P388 leukemia). *Southern Res. Inst.* monograph #2
5. Schabel, F.M.,Jr., Skipper, H.E. and Trader, M.W. (1980) Concepts for controlling drug-resistant tumor cells. In, *Breast Cancer, Experimental and Clinical Aspects* , (eds. H.T. Mouridsen and T. Palshof) Pergamon Press, Oxford, pp 199-212.
6. Bhattacharyya, N.P., Skandalis, A., Ganesh, A. *et al.* (1994) Mutator phenotypes in human colorectal carcinoma cell lines. *Proc. Natl. Acad. Sci. USA* **91**, 6319-23.
7. Parsons, R., Li, G.M., Longley, M.J., *et al.* (1993) Hypermutability and mismatch repair deficiency in RER+ tumor cells. *Cell* **5**, 1227-36.
8. Kat, A., Thilly, W.G., Fang, W.-H. *et al.* (1993). An alkylation-tolerant, mutator human cell line is deficient in strand-specific mismatch repair. *Proc. Natl. Acad. Sci. USA* **90**, 6424-8.
9. Murren, J.R., De Rosa, W., Durivage, H.J. *et al.* (1991) High-dose cisplatin plus dacarbazine in the treatment of metastatic melanoma. *Cancer* **67**, 1514-7.
10. Papadopoulos, N., Nicolaides, N.C., Wei, Y.-F. *et al.* (1994) Mutation of a mutL homolog in hereditary colon cancer. *Science* **263**, 1625-9.
11. Fishel, R., Lescoe, M.K., Rao, M.R.S. *et al.* (1993) The human mutator gene homolog MSH2 and its association with hereditary nonplyposis colon cancer. *Cell,* **75**, 1027-38.
12. Livingstone, L.R., White, A., Sprouse, J. *et al.* (1992) Altered cell cycle arrest and gene amplication potential accompany loss of wild-type p53. *Cell* **70**, 923-35.
13. Yin, Y., Tainsky, A., Bischoff, F.Z. *et al.* (1992) Wild-type p53 restores cell cycle control and inhibits gene amplification in cells with mutant p53 alleles. *Cell* **70**, 937-48.
14. da Costa, L.T., Liu, B., El-Deiry, W.S. *et al.* (1995) Polymerase and variants in RER colorectal tumours. *Nat. Genet.* **9**, 10-11.
15. Modrich, P. (1994) Mismatch repair, genetic stability, and cancer. *Science,* **266**, 1959-60.

16. Grilley, M., Griffith, J. and Modrich, P. (1993) Bidirectional excision in methyl-directed mismatch repair. *J. Biol. Chem.* **268**, 11830-7.

17. Strand, M., Prolla, T.A., Liskay, R.M. and Petes, T.D. (1993) Destabilization of tracts of simple repetitive DNA in yeast by mutations affecting DNA mismatch repair. *Nature* **365**, 274-6.

18. Schaaper, R.M. and Radman, M. (1989) The extreme mutatot effect *of Escherichia coli* mutD5 results from saturation of mismatch repair by excessive DNA replication errors. *Embo J.* **8**, 3511-6.

19. Wooster, R., Cleton-Jansen, A.-M., Collins, A. *et al.* (1994) Instability of short tandem repeats (microsatallites) in human cancers. *Nat. Genet.* **6**, 152-6.

20. Leach, F.S., Nicolaides, N.C., Papadopoulos, N. *et al.* (1993) Mutations of a mutS homolog in hereditary nonpolyposis colorectal cancer. *Cell* **75**, 1215-25.

21. Modrich, P. (1991) Mechanisms and biological effects of mismatch repair. *Ann. Rev. Genet.* **25**, 229-53.

22. Ionov, Y. (1993) Ubiquitous somatic mutations in simple repeated sequences reval a new mechanism for colonic carcinogenesis. *Nature* **363**, 558-61.

23. Thibodeau, S.N., Bren, G. and Schaid, D. (1993) Microsatellite instability in cancer of proximal colon. *Science* **260**, 816-8.

24. Kunkel, T.A. (1993) Slippery DNA and diseases. *Nature* **365**, 207-8.

25. Orth, K., Hung, J., Gazdar, A. *et al.* (1994) Genetic instability in human ovarian cancer cell lines. *Proc. Natl. Acad. Sci. USA* **91**, 9495-9.

26. Eshleman, J.R., Lang, E.Z., Bowerfind, G.K. *et al.* (1995) Increased mutation rate at the hprt locus accompanies microsatellite instability in colon cancer. *Oncogene* **10**, 33-7.

27. Groden, J. (1993) Mutational analysis of patients with adenomatous polypoals, identical inactivating mutations in unrelated individuals. *Am. J. Hum. Genet.* **52**, 263-72.

28. Sugarbaker, P.H., Gianola, F.J., Speyer, J.L. *et al.* (1985) Prospective randomized trial of intravenous v intraperitoneal 5-FU in patients with advanced primary colon or rectal cancer. *Semin. Oncol.* **3 Suppl 4**, 101-11.

29. Miki, Y., Swensen, J., Shattuck-Eidens, D. *et al.* (1994) A strong candiate for the breast and ovarian cancer susceptibility gene BRCA1. *Science* **266**, 66-71.

30. La Spada, A.R., Wilson, E.M., Lubahn, D.B. *et al.* (1991) Androgen receptor gene mutations in X-linked spinal and bulbar muscular atrophy. *Nature* **352**, 77-9.

31. Fu, Y.H., Freidman, D.L., Richards, S. *et al.* (1993) Decreased expression of myotonin-protein kinase messenger RNA and protein in adult form of myotonic dystrosphy. *Science* **260**, 235-8.

32. Liu, B., Nicolaides, N.C., Markowitz, S. *et al.* (1995) Mismatch repair gene defects in sporadic colorectal cancers with microsatellite instability. *Nat. Genet.* **9**, 48-55.

33. Fearon, E.R. and Vogelstein B. (1990) A genetic model for colorectal tumorigenesis. *Cell* **51**, 759-67.

34. Han, H.-J., Yanagisawa, A., Kato, Y. *et al.* (1993) Genetic instability in pancreatic cancer and poorly differentiated type of gastric cancer. *Cancer Res.* **53**, 5087-9.

35. Risinger, J.I., Berchuck, A., Kohler, M.F. *et al.* (1993) Genetic instability of microsatellites in endometrial carcinoma. *Cancer Res.* **53**, 5100-3.

36. Lothe, R.A., Peltomaki, P., Meling, G.I. *et al.* (1993) Genomic instability in colorectal cancer, relationship to clinicopathological variable and family history. *Cancer Res.* **53**, 5849-52.

37. Merlo, A., Mabry, M., Gabrielson, E. *et al.* (1994) Frequent microsatellite instability in primary small cell lung cancer. *Cancer Res.* **54**, 2098-101.

38. Rhyu, M.G., Park, W.S. and Meltzer, S.J.

(1994) Microsatellite instability occurs frequently in human gastric carcinoma. *Oncogene* 1, 29-32.

39. Mironov, N.M., Aguelon, M.A., Potapova, G.I. *et al.* (1994) Alterations of (CA)n DNA repeats and tumor suppressor genes in human gastric cancer. *Cancer Res.* 54, 41-4.

40. Yee, C.J., Roodi, N., Verrier, C.S. and Parl F.F. (1994) Microsatellite instability and loss of heterozygosite in breast cancer. *Cancer Res.* 54, 1641-4.

41. Glebov, O.K., McKensie, K.E., White, C.A. and Sukumar, S. (1994) Frequent p53 gene mutations and novel alleles in familial breast cancer. *Cancer Res.* 54, 3703-9.

42. Peltomaki, P., Lothe R.A., Aaltonen, L.A *et al.* (1993) Microsatellite instability is associated with tumors that characterize the hereditary non-polyposis colorectal carcinoma syndrome. *Cancer Res.* 53, 5853-5.

43. Burks, R.T., Kessis, T.D., Cho, K.R and Hedrick, L. (1994) Microsatellite instability in endometrial carcinoma. *Oncogene* 9, 1163-6.

44. Gonzalez-Zulueta, M., Ruppert, J.M., Tokino, K. *et al.* (1993) Microsatellite instability in bladder cancer. *Cancer Res.* 53, 5620-3.

45. Osborne, R.J. and Leech, V. (1994) Polymerase chain reaction allelotyping of human ovarian cancer. *Br. J. Cancer* 69, 429-38.

46. Fox, M.E., Feldman, B.J. and Chu, G. (1994) A novel role for DNA photolyase, binding to DNA damaged by drugs is associated with enhanced cytotoxicity in *Saccharomyces cerevisiae*. *Mol. Cell. Biol.* 14, 8071-7.

47. Johnson, S.W., Swiggard, P.A., Handel, L.M.,*et al.* (1994) Relationship between platinum-DNA adduct formation and removal and cisplatin cytotoxicity in cisplatin-sensitive and -resistant human ovarian cancer cells. *Cancer Res.* 54, 5911-6.

48. Mamenta, E.L., Poma, E.E., Kaufmann, W.K. *et al.* (1994) Enhanced replicative bypass of platinum-DNA adducts in cisplatin-resistant human ovarian carcinoma cell lines. *Cancer Res.* 54, 3500-5.

49. Chao, C.C. (1994). Enhanced excision repair of DNA damage due to cis-diamminedichloroplatinum (II) in resistant cervix carcinoma HeLa cells. *Eur. J. Pharmacol.* 268, 347-55.

50. White, A.E., Livanos, E.M. and Tlsty, T.D. (1994) Differential disruption of genomic integrity and cell cycle regulation in normal human fibroblasts by the HPV oncoproteins. *Genes Dev.* 8, 666-77.

51. Harris, R.S., Longerich, S. and Rosenberg, S.M. (1994) Recombination in adaptive mutation. *Science* 264, 258-260.

52. Cairns, J. and Foster, P.L. (1991) Adaptive reversion of a frameshift mutation in Escherichia coli. *Genetics* 128, 695-701.

53. Hartwell, L.H. and Kastan, M.B. (1994) Cell cycle control and cancer. *Science* 266, 1821-8.

54. Livingstone, L.R., White, A., Sprouse, J. *et al.* (1992) Altered cell cycle arrest and gene amplification potential accompany loss of wild-type p53. *Cell* 70, 923-35.

55. Barry, M.A., Behnke, C.A. and Eastman, A. (1990) Activation of programmed cell death (apoptosis) by cisplatin, other anticancer drugs, toxins and hyperthermia. *Biochem. Pharmacol.* 40, 2353-61.

56. Ormerod, M.G., O'Neill, C.F., Robertson, D. and Harrap, K.R. (1994) Cisplatin induces apoptosis in a human ovarian carcinoma cell line without concomitant internucleosomal degradation of DNA. *Exp. Cell Res.* 211, 231-7.

57. Kerr, J.F.R., Winterford, C.M. and Harmon, B.V. (1994) Apoptosis, its significance in cancer and cancer therapy. *Cancer* 73, 2013-26.

58. Matzinger, P. (1991) The JAM test. A simple assay for DNA fragmentation and cell death. *J. Immunol. Meth.* 145, 185-92.

59. Gorczyca, W., Gong, J. and Darzynkiewicz, Z. (1993) Detection of DNA strand breaks in

individual apoptotic cells by the *in situ* terminal deoxynucleotidyl transferase and nick translation assays. *Cancer Res.* **53**, 1945-51.

60. Toney, J.H., Donahue, B.A., Kellett, P.J. *et al.* (1989) Isolation of cDNAs encoding a human protein that binds selectively to DNA modified by the anticancer drug cis-diamminedichloroplatinum(II). *Proc Natl Acad Sci USA* **86**, 8328-32.

61. Donahue, B.A., Augot, M., Bellon, S.F. *et al.* (1990) Characterization of a DNA damage-recognition protein from mammalian cells that binds to intrastrand d(GpG) and d(ApG) DNA adducts of the anticancer drug cisplatin. *Biochemistry* **29**, 5872-80.

62. Gottlieb, T.M. and Jackson, S.P. (1993) The DNA-dependent protein kinase, requirement for DNA ends and association with Ku antigen. *Cell* **72**, 131-42.

63. Anderson, C.W. (1993) DNA damage and the DNA-activated protein kinase. *TIBS* **18**, 433-437.

64. Christen, R.D., Hom, D.K., Porter, D.C. *et al.* (1990) Epidermal growth factor regulates the *in vitro* sensitivity of human ovarian carcinoma cells to cisplatin. *J. Clin. Invest.* **86**, 1632-40.

65. Isonishi, S., Jekunen, A.P., Hom, D.K. *et al.* (1992) Modulation of cisplatin sensitivity and growth rate of an ovarian carcinoma cell line by bombesin and tumor necrosis factor alpha. *J. Clin. Invest.* **90**, 1436-42.

66. Fan, Z., Baselga, J., Masui, H. and Mendelsohn, J. (1993) Antitumor effect of anti-epidermal growth factor receptor monoclonal antibodies plus cis-diamminedichloroplatinum on well established A431 cell xenografts. *Cancer Res.* **53**, 4637-42.

67. Pietras, R.J., Fendly, B.M., Chazin, V.R. *et al.* (1994) Antibody to HER-2/neu receptor blocks DNA repair after cisplatin in human breast and ovarian cancer cells. *Oncogene* **9**,
1829-38.

68. Isonishi, S., Andrews, P.A. and Howell, S.B. (1990) Increased sensitivity to cis-diamminedichloroplatinum(II) in human ovarian carcinoma cells in response to treatment with 12-0-tetradecanoylphorbol-13-acetate. *J. Biol. Chem.* **265**, 3623-7.

69. Basu, A., Teicher, B.A. and Lazo, J.S. (1990) Involvement of protein kinase C in phorbol ester-induced sensitization of HeLa cells to cis-diamminedichloroplatinum (II). *J. Biol. Chem.* **265**, 8451-7.

70. Isonishi, S., Hom, D.K., Eastman, A. and Howell, S.B. (1994) Enhancement of sensitivity of platinum(II)-containing drugs by activation of protein kinase C in a human ovarianc carcinoma cell line. *Br. J. Cancer* **69**, 217-21.

71. Mann, S.C., Andrews, P.A. and Howell, S.B. (1991) Modulation of cis-diamminedichloroplatinum(II) accumulation and sensitivity by forskolin and 3-isobutyl-1-methylxanthine in sensitive and resistant human ovarian carcinoma cells. *Int. J. Cancer* **48**, 866-72.

72. Fritsche, M., Haessler, C. and Brandner, G. (1993) Induction of nuclear accumulation of the tumor--uppressor protein p53 by DNA-damaging agents. *Oncogene* **8**, 307-18.

73. Xiong, Y., Hannon, G.J., Zhang, H. *et al.* (1994) P21 is a universal inhibitor of cyclin kinases. *Nature* **366**, 701-3.

74. Peter, M. and Herskowitz, I. (1994) Joining the complex, cyclin-dependent kinase inhibitory proteins and the cell cycle. *Cell* **79**, 181-4.

75. Nevins, J.R. (1992) E2F, a link between the Rb tumor suppressor protein and viral oncoproteins. *Science* **258**, 424-9.

76. Reed, J.C. (1994) Bcl-2 and the regulation of programmed cell death. Mini review, cellular mechanisms of disease series. *J. Cell Biol.* **124**, 1-6.

77. Newmeyer, D.D., Farschon, D.M. and Reed, J.C. (1994) Cell-free apoptosis in xenopus

egg extracts, inhibition by Bcl-2 and requirement for an organelle fraction enriched in mitochondria. *Cell* **79**, 353-64.

78. Lazebnik, Y.A., Cole, S., Cooke, C.A. *et al.* (1993) Nuclear events of apoptosis *in vitro* in cell-free mitotic extracts, a model system for analysis of the active phase of apoptosis. *J. Cell. Biol.* **123**, 7-22.

79. Oltvai, Z.N. and Korsmeyer, S.J. (1994) Checkpoints of dueling dimers foil death wishes. *Cell* **79**, 189-92.

80. Yang, E., Zha, J., Jockel, J. *et al.* (1995) Bad, a Heterodimeric Partner for Bcl-XL and Bcl-2, displaces Bax and promotes cell death. *Cell* **80**, 285-91.

81. Miyashita, T. and Reed, J.C. (1995) Tumor suppressor p53 is a direct transcriptional activator of the human bax gene. *Cell* **80**, 293-9.

Chapter 26

Prospects for improved cisplatin analogues

Lloyd R. KELLAND

26.1 INTRODUCTION

Cisplatin is one of the most active and widely used anticancer drugs currently available [1]. Nonetheless, the search for a better cisplatin analogue has been actively pursued ever since the drug's introduction into clinical practice almost 25 years ago and has, to date, resulted in thousands of analogues being synthesized and over 20 having entered phase I clinical evaluation. Two broad strategies have been adopted to analogue development in accordance with the two major limitations of cisplatin, viz. severe toxicities (especially nephro- and neurotoxicity, nausea and vomiting) and the propensity of many tumours to exhibit resistance to the drug. Notably, resistance may occur both at the onset of treatment (intrinsic resistance), e.g. in colorectal and non-small cell lung cancer, or be acquired after an initial promising response, e.g. in ovarian cancer.

This article describes the current status of cisplatin analogue development especially in terms of the amelioration of the severe toxicities of the parent drug and regarding the circumvention of tumour resistance.

26.2 CARBOPLATIN

At present, carboplatin (paraplatin, cis-diammine, 1,1-cyclobutane dicarboxylato-platinum (II)) is the only cisplatin analogue to be both widely used clinically and to have received world-wide registration and acceptance. While the introduction of carboplatin has undoubtedly made a substantial impact on reducing the toxicities associated with cisplatin-based chemotherapy, the results of many randomized and cross-over trials indicate that the two drugs are essentially equiactive but also share cross-resistance [2]. For example, the recently published results from the long-term follow up (median time of nine years) of the first randomized trial of cisplatin ($100mg/m^2$ every four weeks for five courses and $30mg/m^2$ for a further five courses) versus carboplatin ($400mg/m^2$ every four weeks for ten courses) showed that five-year survival rates were not significantly different for the two agents (15% for cisplatin and 19% for carboplatin) while those patients allowed to cross-over between the two arms due to progressive or non-responding disease exhibited a low (14.3%) response rate to the other compound [3]. Thus, the toxicity profile of platinum-based chemotherapy has shifted (myelosuppression, especially thrombo-cytopaenia, is dose-limiting with carboplatin [4]) but the important issue of overcoming tumour resistance remains.

Today, the main area of contention regarding carboplatin concerns whether it should be used in preference to the more toxic parent drug in disease types (such as ovarian

249

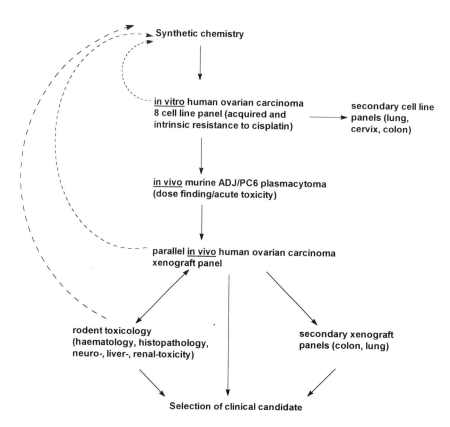

Figure 26.1 CRC Centre for Cancer Therapeutics preclinical evaluation cascade for the discovery of better cisplatin analogues.

and testicular cancer) where platinum-based drugs have demonstrable efficacy and whether it might be better suited to studies of dose intensity (*e.g.* with haematological support by growth factors) [5].

26.3 A STRATEGY FOR THE DISCOVERY OF A BETTER CISPLATIN ANALOGUE

Following our collaborative research programme with the Johnson Matthey Company which led to the discovery of carboplatin [6], we have continued our collaborative efforts to discover and develop new platinum analogues which focus on the central issue of tumour resistance. This has involved a critical re-appraisal of the preclinical tumour models traditionally used in the discovery of anticancer drugs, including platinum drugs, which has predominantly relied upon rapidly growing murine lines (such as the L1210 and P388 leukaemias and, in our own studies, the ADJ/PC6 plasmacytoma). Our re-appraisal has culminated in a preclinical evaluation cascade (Figure 26.1) involving a mechanism - directed, disease - orientated approach focusing largely on human ovarian carcinoma (a disease where intrinsic and acquired resistance to cisplatin/carboplatin severely limits patient survival) which conceptually might offer better predictiveness,

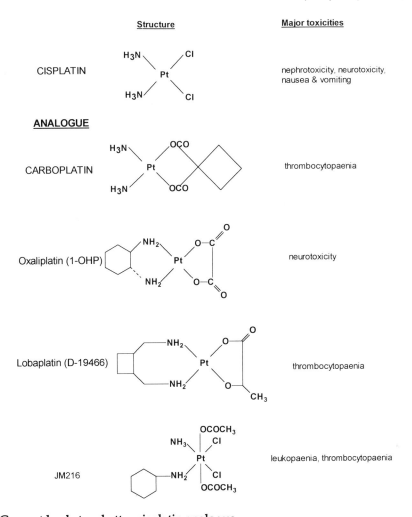

Structure   **Major toxicities**

Figure 26.2 Current leads to a better cisplatin analogue.

of the target disease in man. Similarly to the approach to preclinical anticancer drug screening adopted at the National Cancer Institute [7] and keeping in mind the need to establish an early indicator of therapeutic index for novel complexes, we have utilized *in vitro* cell line and parallel xenograft panels of human ovarian carcinoma [8,9]. All compounds are initially evaluated against an eight cell line panel comprising five 'parent' cell lines (which differ in intrinsic sensitivity to cisplatin by over 100-fold) and three examples of sublines

possessing acquired cisplatin resistance where the major mechanism(s) underlying resistance has been determined (41McisR, resistance predominantly due to reduced drug accumulation [10]; CH1cisRresistance due to enhanced DNA repair and/or increased tolerance to platinum-DNA adducts [11]; and A2780cisR, resistance being due to a combination of decreased drug accumulation, increased glutathione levels and increased DNA repair [12]).

Compounds exhibiting *in vitro* potency

against either the cell lines possessing 'mechanism-directed' acquired resistance to cisplatin and/or the SKOV-3 or HX/62 cell lines representative of intrinsic drug resistance are then selected for further *in vitro* evaluation against panels of other human tumour types (colon, lung and cervix) and *in vivo* antitumour testing (using appropriate parallel xenograft lines following an initial dose-finding/acute toxicity study in mice bearing the ADJ/PC6 plasmacytoma). Notably, the cascade includes an early investigation of the potential toxic side effects of novel compounds (*e.g.* effects on the haematopoietic system, kidney, liver and including the use of a recently described rat nerve conduction velocity model to determine possible neurotoxic effects [13]). At several stages of the cascade, feedback to synthetic chemistry allows appropriate structure-activity refinement to be achieved.

26.4 CURRENT LEADS TO A BETTER CISPLATIN ANALOGUE

While a substantial reduction in the toxic side-effects of cisplatin has been achieved through the introduction of carboplatin, there has been markedly less success, to date, in the circumvention of tumour resistance to cisplatin. Figure 26.2 shows the structures of three analogues which may be considered as the only major leads at present to a platinum-based drug possessing a broader spectrum of clinical activity; namely, oxaliplatin, lobaplatin and, emerging from the above described cascade, the orally administrable JM216 (*bis*-acetato amminedichloro cyclohexyl-amine platinum (IV)).

26.5 OXALIPLATIN

Oxaliplatin(1-OHP) (Figure 26.2) represents the current lead compound from the 1,2-diaminocyclohexane (DACH) class of platinum complex whose promising preclinical antitumour properties were described by Burchenal and colleagues almost 20 years ago

[14]. These complexes were shown to circumvent acquired cisplatin resistance in murine L1210 leukaemia models both *in vitro* and *in vivo*. However, studies in other preclinical models of acquired cisplatin resistance (including the ADJ/PC6 plasmacytoma and human ovarian carcinoma xenografts) have shown that circumvention of resistance by DACH platinum complexes is not universal [9,15] and has cast doubt on the predictive utility of the L1210 mouse leukaemia for human malignancies. Furthermore, clinical trials with DACH platinum complexes were initially plagued by formulation difficulties (*e.g.* with DACCP; DACH 4-carboxyphthalato platinum II) [16] and latterly by dose-limiting neurotoxicity (*e.g.* with the more water soluble tetraplatin, Ormaplatin; tetrachloro DACH platinum IV) [17]. While the dose-limiting toxicity of oxaliplatin is also neurotoxicity [18] and results from single agent phase II trials have not been reported, oxaliplatin did exhibit some evidence of activity in phase I trial (four partial responses) [18] and was part of a complex treatment protocol involving chrono-modulated 5-fluorouracil, leucovorin in patients with metastatic colorectal cancer, which showed an encouraging objective response rate of 53% [19]. However, the contribution of the platinum drug to this response rate is difficult to ascertain.

While the troublesome neurotoxicity observed with the recently clinically evaluated DACH complexes tetraplatin and oxaliplatin may be attributable to the DACH carrier ligand itself (and has led to the withdrawal of tetraplatin), further clinical evaluation of DACH platinum complexes would be of interest if the neurotoxic effects could be reduced by chemical refinement or concomitant usage of neuroprotective agents. Because of these toxicity limitations the important issue as to whether DACH platinum complexes might offer clinical utility against cisplatin-resistant disease remains unanswered.

26.6 LOBAPLATIN

Lobaplatin (D-19466; 1,2-diaminomethyl cyclobutane-platinum II lactate) has recently completed phase I clinical trials in Germany and the Netherlands; as with carboplatin, thrombocytopaenia being the dose-limiting toxicity [20,21]. As for the DACH complexes, preclinical data suggested a lack of cross-resistance of lobaplatin in at least some tumour models [22]. In four acquired cisplatin resistant human tumour cell lines, lobaplatin was non-cross resistant in one testicular carcinoma cell line, partially cross-resistant in the A2780 human ovarian carcinoma cell line and fully cross-resistant in two gastric carcinoma cell lines [22]. Some evidence of *in vivo* activity against two parallel acquired cisplatin resistant testicular and ovarian xenografts was also observed. Although some responses (two partial, one complete, all in patients with ovarian cancer) were observed in the phase I trials [21,22], at present it is too early to predict whether lobaplatin will offer clinical utility in platinum refractory disease. Disappointingly however, no objective responses were observed in a recently reported phase II trial of lobaplatin in 17 patients with cisplatin-resistant ovarian cancer [23].

26.7 JM216

JM216 was selected for clinical trial from a collaborative programme between the Institute of Cancer Research, The Johnson Matthey Company and Bristol Myers Squibb, primarily set up to discover a cisplatin analogue capable of oral administration. Such a drug should further facilitate patient comfort and convenience during platinum-based chemotherapy and allow the possibility of treatment on an out-patient basis (and thereby reducing hospitalization costs). Synthetic efforts concentrated on a novel class of platinum complex, the ammine/amine (or 'mixed amine') platinum (IV) dicarboxylates

possessing lipophilic axial ligands and asymmetric carrier ligands. Parallel studies utilizing the *in vitro* human ovarian carcinoma cell line panel forming part of the above described drug evaluation cascade (Figure 26.1) revealed that these complexes might also offer utility against cisplatin-resistant tumours [24].

Preclinically, JM216 has been shown to possess several encouraging properties:
1. In toxicology terms, JM216 resembled carboplatin rather than cisplatin with myelosuppression being dose-limiting in mice [25]. Moreover, JM216 in rodents showed no nephrotoxicity [26] nor neurotoxicity in head-to-head experiments where both cisplatin and tetraplatin were neurotoxic [13]. JM216 was also less emetic in ferrets than cisplatin (unpublished observations).
2. Orally administered JM216 exhibited broadly comparable antitumour activity to that observed for intravenously administered cisplatin or carboplatin against our panel of human ovarian carcinoma xenografts and showed greater antitumour selectivity in mice bearing the murine ADJ/PC6 plasmacytoma [27].
3. JM216 exhibited greater antitumour activity against a human ovarian carcinoma xenograft when administered orally on a daily for five days schedule (every 21 days) (growth delay of 91 days) compared to administering the same total dose as a bolus every 21 days (growth delay of only 52 days) [28].
4. *In vitro*, JM216 showed circumvention of acquired cisplatin resistance in three of six human tumour cell lines (whereas tetraplatin exhibited partial or full cross-resistance in all six pairs) [27]. Companion mechanistic data has shown that JM216 is capable of circumventing cisplatin resistance due to reduced drug accumulation [10,27,29].

JM216 entered phase I clinical trial in August 1992, initially on a single dose every 21 days schedule [30], and also using daily administration for five days every 21 days. In accordance with the rodent toxicology data, myelosuppression (including both leukopaenia and thrombocytopaenia) was the dose-limiting toxicity; no nephro- or neurotoxicity has been observed and emesis has been controllable. A partial response and a reduction in the ovarian tumour marker CA125 was observed in a patient with ovarian cancer which had recurred following treatment with cisplatin [30]. In the single dose study (involving 31 patients) a maximum tolerated dose was not reached due to non linear pharmacokinetics (possibly due to the drug's poor aqueous solubility limiting its dissolution and availability for gastrointestinal

absorption) [30]. JM216 has also been shown to be a prodrug, being rapidly biotransformed following oral administration to six platinum-containing peaks, a major metabolite being the platinum II species cis-ammine dichloro (cyclohexylamine) platinum (JM118) [31]. JM216 has now entered phase II trials (in ovarian and lung carcinomas) in both Europe and America.

26.8 ADDITIONAL CLINICALLY-EVALUATED CISPLATIN ANALOGUES

Figure 26.3 shows the chemical structures of a further eight cisplatin analogues which have

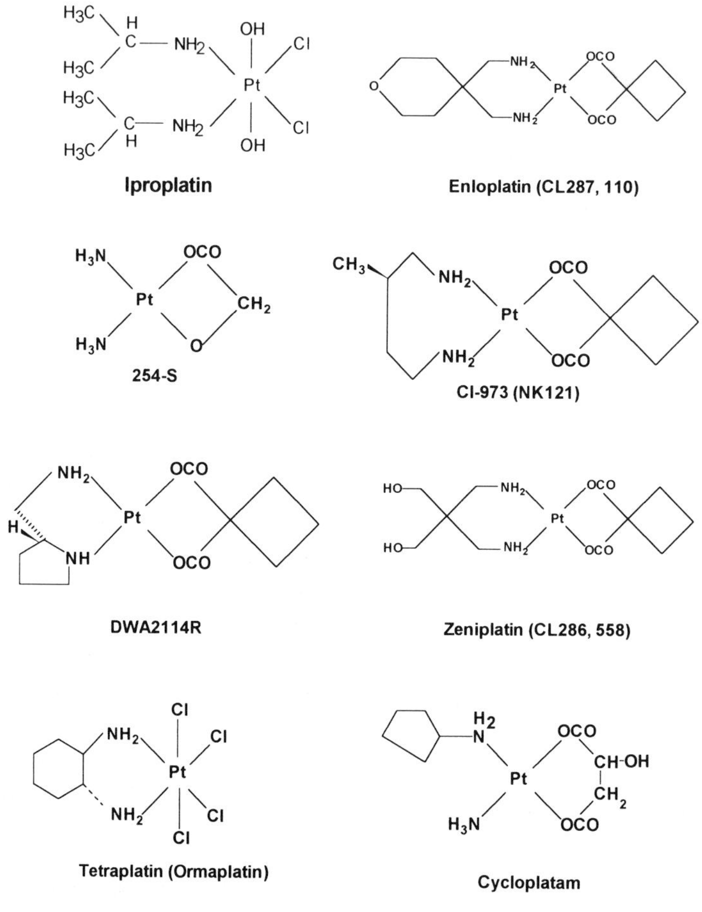

Figure 26.3 Some additional cisplatin analogues recently having undergone or currently undergoing trials.

254

recently undergone or are currently undergoing clinical trial. Iproplatin (CHIP) represents the most extensively used of these analogues, and, as with carboplatin, was selected for clinical trial on the basis of possessing a favourable preclinical toxicity profile to that of cisplatin with accompanying retention of efficacy. However, the results of randomized trials of iproplatin versus carboplatin in ovarian [32] and cervical [33] cancer showed that iproplatin was more toxic than carboplatin (especially to the gastrointestinal tract) and, moreover, less active. In the ovarian trial, median survival was significantly shorter for the iproplatin arm (68 weeks *versus* 114 weeks; p=0.008) [32]. As with carboplatin, iproplatin also shares cross-resistance with cisplatin [32]. Taken together, these clinical data indicate that iproplatin does not offer any advantage over carboplatin.

Many of the other cisplatin analogues which have entered clinical trial share identical or similar leaving group chemistry to carboplatin (*e.g.* zeniplatin, enloplatin, CI-973, DWA2114R) and would be predicted to possess similar toxicological properties. Surprisingly however, both zeniplatin and enloplatin produced some nephrotoxicity in patients and have now been withdrawn. While the Japanese-based complexes CI-973, DWA2114R and 254-S continue to be studied in Japan, based on presently available information none appear likely to make a significant impact in treating cisplatin-resistant disease. Cycloplatam is currently undergoing clinical evaluation in Russia although little information concerning its efficacy is currently available. Further details of the clinical and preclinical properties of these cisplatin analogues have recently been summarized [34].

26.9 SUMMARY AND FUTURE PROSPECTS

While much has been achieved in making platinum-based chemotherapy more acceptable to the cancer patient (largely through the introduction of carboplatin), disappointingly, there has been little clinical success to date in overcoming resistance. Although much more is now known from *in vitro* cell line studies concerning how tumour cells develop resistance to cisplatin, these findings have not yet been translatable to improving platinum-induced response rates in the clinic. Unfortunately, one of the few preclinical leads to an improved cisplatin analogue, the DACH-containing complexes such as tetraplatin and oxaliplatin, have not been thoroughly studied due to dose-limiting neurotoxicity. Two other possible leads, lobaplatin and the orally active complex, JM216, are at too early a stage of clinical evaluation to be confident about their possible utility in cisplatin-resistant disease. However, JM216 may also further enhance patient comfort during platinum-based chemotherapy, possibly including treatment on an out-patient basis.

Our establishment of a preclinical evaluation cascade for the discovery of better cisplatin analogues focuses on *in vitro* and parallel *in vivo* models of cisplatin-sensitive and -resistant human ovarian carcinoma and has, to date, aided in the identification of two lead structural classes of complex; the ammine/amine platinum(IV) dicarboxylates (from which JM216 emerged) and, more recently, two independent series of active *trans* platinum complexes [35,36]. A lead *trans* platinum complex, JM335 (*trans*-ammine (cyclohexylamine) dichloro-dihydroxo platinum (IV)) has been shown to be as cytotoxic as cisplatin against our panel of human ovarian carcinoma cell lines and, moreover, to overcome acquired cisplatin resistance in six of seven pairs of lines. JM335 is the first *trans*-platinum complex to possess marked *in vivo* activity against both murine (ADJ/PC6) and four of six human ovarian carcinoma xenografts [36]. These complexes are of particular interest since they contravene the original structure-activity rules for platinum complexes (based on the observation that the *trans* isomer of cisplatin is inactive as an antitumour agent) and possess DNA-binding properties which differ from that of cisplatin (and carboplatin) [36]. It is hoped that the established preclinical drug evaluation cascade will also provide further novel leads.

It is apparent from almost 25 years of analogue development that overcoming clinical resistance to cisplatin is a demanding challenge. The available clinical data from the current analogues suggests that more needs to be done if this challenge is to be fully met. Complementary strategies to circumvent clinical cisplatin resistance such as pharmacological modulation of platinum resistance mechanisms (see [37] for a recent review), dose-intensification of existing platinum drugs (especially carboplatin) [5] and combination with other active anticancer drugs with generally non-overlapping toxicities and mechanisms of resistance (such as paclitaxel) [38] are also being actively pursued. Together with further elucidation of the molecular mechanisms involved in determining tumour sensitivity and resistance to cisplatin, there are encouraging indications that significant improvements in platinum-based chemotherapy are achievable.

ACKNOWLEDGEMENTS.

Studies described from the CRC Centre for Cancer Therapeutics at the Institute of Cancer Research were supported by grants from the UK Cancer Research Campaign, the Medical Research Council, the Johnson Matthey Technology Centre (JMTC) and Bristol Myers Squibb Oncology. Thanks are due to Dr Barry Murrer (JMTC) and my colleagues Professor Ken Harrap, Drs Mark McKeage, Ian Judson, Florence Raynaud, Kirste Mellish and Swee Sharp for many helpful discussions.

REFERENCES

1. Loehrer, P.J. and Einhorn, L.H. (1984) Cisplatin. *Ann. Intern. Med.* **100**, 704-13.

2. Williams, C.J., Stewart, L., Parmar, M. and Guthrie, D. (1992) Meta-analysis of the role of platinum compounds in advanced ovarian carcinoma. *Semin. Oncol.* **19**, 120-8.

3. Taylor, A.E., Wiltshaw, E., Gore, M.E. *et al.*, (1994) Long term follow up of the first randomised study of cisplatin versus carboplatin for advanced epithelial ovarian cancer. *J. Clin. Oncol.* **12**, 2066-70.

4. Calvert, A.H., Harland, S.J., Newell, D.R. *et al.* (1985) Phase I studies with carboplatin at the Royal Marsden Hospital. *Cancer Treat. Rev.* **12**, 51-7.

5. Calvert, A.H., Newell, D.R. and Gore, M.E. (1992) Future directions with carboplatin, Can therapeutic monitoring, high-dose administration, and hematologic support with growth factors expand the spectrum compared with cisplatin? *Semin. Oncol.* **19**, 155-3.

6. Harrap, K.R. (1985) Preclinical studies identifying carboplatin as a viable cisplatin alternative. *Cancer Treat. Rev.* **12**, 21-33.

7. Skehan, P., Storeng, R., Scudiero, D. *et al.* (1990) New colorimetric cytotoxicity assay for anticancer drug screening. *J. Natl. Cancer Inst.* **82**, 1107-12.

8. Hills, C,A., Kelland, L.R., Abel, G. *et al.* (1989) Biological properties of ten human ovarian carcinoma cell lines, calibration *in vitro* against platinum complexes. *Br. J. Cancer* **59**, 527-34.

9. Harrap, K.R., Jones, M., Siracky, J. *et al.* (1990) The establishment, characterization and calibration of human ovarian carcinoma xenografts for the evaluation of novel platinum anticancer drugs. *Ann. Oncol.* **1**, 65-76.

10. Loh, S.Y., Mistry, P., Kelland, L.R. *et al.* (1992) Reduced drug accumulation as a major mechanism of acquired resistance to cisplatin in a human ovarian carcinoma cell line, circumvention studies using novel platinum(II) and (IV) ammine/amine complexes. *Br. J. Cancer* **66**, 1109-15.

11. Kelland, L.R., Mistry, P., Abel, G. *et al.* (1992) Mechanism-related circumvention of acquired cis-diamminedichloroplatinum(II) resistance using two pairs of human ovarian carcinoma cell lines by ammine/amine platinum(IV) dicarboxylates. *Cancer Res.* **52,** 3857-64.

12. Behrens, B.C., Hamilton, T.C., Masuda, H. *et al.* (1987) Characterization of a cis-diamminedichloroplatinum(II)-resistant human ovarian carcinoma cell line and its use in evaluation of platinum analogs. *Cancer Res.* **47,** 414-8.

13. McKeage, M.J., Boxall, F.E., Jones, M. and Harrap, K.R. (1994) Lack of neurotoxicity of oral bis-acetatoamminedichloro cyclohexy-lamine platinum (IV) in comparison to cisplatin and tetraplatin in the rat. *Cancer Res.* **54,** 629-31.

14. Burchenal, J.H., Kalaher, K., Dew, K. and Lokys, L. (1979) Rationale for development of platinum analogs. *Cancer Treat. Rep.* **63,** 1493-8.

15. Goddard, P.M., Valenti, M.R. and Harrap, K.R. (1991) The role of murine tumour models and their acquired platinum-resistant counterparts in the evaluation of novel platinum antitumour agents, a cautionary note. *Ann. Oncol.* **2,** 535-40.

16. Scher, H.I., Kelsen, D., Kalman, L. *et al.* (1984) Phase II trial of 1,2-diamino-cyclohexane (4-carboxyphthalato) platinum (II) (DACCP) in non small cell lung cancer. *Cancer Chemother. Pharmacol.* **12,** 101-3.

17. Schilder, R.J., LaCreta, F.P., Perez, R.P. *et al.* (1994) Phase I and pharmacokinetic study of Ormaplatin (Tetraplatin, NSC 363812) administered on a day 1 and day 8 schedule. *Cancer Res.* **54,** 709-17.

18. Extra, J.M., Espie, M., Calvo, F. *et al.* (1990) Phase I study of oxaliplatin in patients with advanced cancer. *Cancer Chemother. Pharmacol.* **25,** 299-303.

19. Levi, F.A., Zidani, R., Vannetzel, J-M. *et al.* (1994) Chronomodulated versus fixed infusion-rate delivery of ambulatory chemotherapy with oxaliplatin, fluorouracil, and folinic acid (leucovorin) in patients with colorectal cancer metastases, a randomized multi-institutional trial. *J. Natl. Cancer Inst.* **86,** 1608-17.

20. Gietema, J.A., de Vries, E.G.E., Sleijfer, D.th. *et al.* (1993) A phase I study of 1,2-diamminomethyl -cyclobutane-platinum (II) lactate (D-19466, lobaplatin) administered daily for 5 days. *Br. J. Cancer* **67,** 396-401.

21. Gietema, J.A., Guchelaar, H-J., de Vries, E.G.E. *et al.* (1993) A phase I study of lobaplatin (D-19466) administered by 72h continuous infusion. *Anticancer Drugs* **4,** 51-5.

22. Harstrick, A., Bokemeyer, C., Scharnofkse, M. *et al.* (1993) Preclinical activity of a new platinum analogue, lobaplatin, in cisplatin-sensitive and -resistant human testicular, ovarian, and gastric carcinoma cell lines. *Cancer Chemother. Pharmacol.* **33,** 43-7.

23. Kavanagh, J.J., Finnegan, M.B., Edwards, C.L. *et al.* (1995) A trial of lobaplatin (D-19466) in platin resistant epithelial ovarian cancer. *Proc. Am. Assoc. Cancer Res.* **36,** 2393 (Abstract).

24. Kelland, L.R., Murrer, B.A., Abel, G. *et al.* (1992) Ammine/amine platinum (IV) dicarboxylates, a novel class of platinum complex exhibiting selective cytotoxicity to intrinsically cisplatin-resistant human ovarian carcinoma cell lines. *Cancer Res.* **52,** 822-8.

25. McKeage, M.J., Morgan, S.E., Boxall, F.E. *et al.* (1994) Preclinical toxicology and tissue distribution of novel oral antitumour platinum complexes, ammine/amine platinum(IV) dicarboxylates. *Cancer Chemother. Pharmacol.* **33,** 497-503.

26. McKeage, M.J., Morgan, S.E., Boxall, F.E. *et al.* (1993) Lack of nephrotoxicity of oral ammine/amine platinum (IV) dicarboxylate complexes in rodents. *Br. J. Cancer* **67,** 996-1000.

27. Kelland, L.R., Abel, G., McKeage, M.J. *et al.* (1993) Preclinical antitumor evaluation of bis-acetato-ammine-dichloro-cyclohexylamine platinum(IV), an orally active platinum drug. *Cancer Res.* 53, 2581-6.

28. McKeage, M.J., Kelland, L.R., Boxall, F.E. *et al.* (1994) Schedule dependency of orally administered bis-acetato-ammine-dichloro cyclohexylamine-platinum (IV) (JM216) *in vivo. Cancer Res.* 54, 4118-22.

29. Mellish, K.J., Kelland, L.R. and Harrap, K.R. (1993) *In vitro* platinum drug chemosensitivity of intrinsic and acquired cisplatin-resistant human cervical carcinoma cell lines. *Br. J. Cancer* 68, 240-50.

30. McKeage, M.J., Mistry, P., Ward, J. *et al.* (1995) A phase I and pharmacological study of an oral platinum complex (JM216), dose-dependent pharmacokinetics with single dose administration. *Cancer Chemother. Pharmacol.* In Press

31. Raynaud, F., Odell, D., Boxall, F.E. *et al.* (1995) Metabolism of the oral platinum drug JM216 in ultrafiltrates of patients plasma, mouse plasma, ovarian carcinoma cell lines and plasma incubation medium. *Proc. Am. Assoc. Cancer Res.* 36, 2374 (abstract).

32. Trask, C., Silverstone, A., Ash, C.M. *et al.* (1991) A randomized trial of carboplatin versus iproplatin in untreated advanced ovarian cancer. *J. Clin. Oncol.* 9, 1131-7.

33. McGuire, W.P., Arseneau, J., Blessing, J.A. *et al.* (1989) A randomized comparative trial of carboplatin and iproplatin in advanced squamous carcinoma of the uterine cervix, A Gynecologic Oncology Group Study. *J. Clin. Oncol.* 7, 1462-8.

34. Kelland, L.R. (1993) New Platinum antitumor complexes. *Crit. Rev. Oncol./Hematol.* 15, 191-219.

35. Farrell, N., Kelland, L.R., Roberts, J.D. and van Beusichem, M. (1992) Activation of the *trans* geometry in platinum antitumor complexes, a survey of the cytotoxicity of *trans* compounds containing planar ligands in murine L1210 and human tumor panels and studies on their mechanism of action. *Cancer Res.* 52, 5065-72.

36. Kelland, L.R., Barnard, C.F.J., Mellish, K.J. *et al.* (1994) A novel *trans*-platinum coordination complex possessing *in vitro* and *in vivo* antitumour activity. *Cancer Res.* 54, 5618-22.

37. Timmer Bosscha, H., Mulder, N.H. and de Vries, E.G. (1992) Modulation of cis-diamminedichloroplatinum(II) resistance, a review. *Br. J. Cancer* 66, 227-38.

38. Trimble, E.L., Adams, J.D., Vena, D. *et al.* (1993) Paclitaxel for platinum-refractory ovarian cancer, Results from the first 1,000 patients registered to National Cancer Institute Treatment Referral Center 9103. *J. Clin. Oncol.* 11, 2405-10.

Part Five

Strategies for Gene Therapy

Chapter 27

Gene therapy: general principles and pre-clinical models

Anne P. SHAPTER and Jonathan S. BEREK

27.1 INTRODUCTION

Despite many recent advances in treatment modalities for ovarian cancer, including the advent of platinum based chemotherapy, this cancer remains a significant cause of morbidity and mortality with very little improvement in survival being demonstrated over the years. The optimal treatment for this disease has not yet been determined and alternative therapeutic options must therefore be evaluated. Gene therapy has become an important therapeutic treatment approach in many cancers including renal carcinoma and malignant melanoma [1-4] and may prove to make a significant contribution to the reduction of the morbidity and mortality associated with cancer of the ovary.

The term gene therapy applies to a broad range of techniques directed at modifying gene expression and function and has been studied in non-cancerous genetic diseases such as sickle cell anaemia [5,6] and adenosine deaminase deficiency [7-9] as well as malignant diseases. Gene therapy may be used to introduce exogenous genes into a host in order to correct a genetic defect or alternatively it may involve activation or suppression of an endogenous gene.

Theoretically, gene modification may be directed at germline cells in which the genetic changes would potentially be inherited by future generations, or alternatively it may be targeted at somatic cells in which case only the host would be affected by the specific modification.

In recent years, much cancer therapy research has been conducted in the field of immunotherapy. In broad terms, immunotherapy is aimed at stimulating the various components of the immune system in such a manner as to elicit an anti-tumour response. Many studies in the area of gene therapy of cancer have incorporated the principles of immunotherapy in that target cells are genetically modified to produce immune substances such as cytokines and lymphokines in attempts to alter tumourigenicity.

As cancer is most definitely a disease in which genetic factors play a key role, it is appropriate that gene therapy research be targeted at this disease. Many gene therapy trials are in progress and the first clinical gene therapy trial for ovarian cancer is soon to begin [10,11]. There are many ways in which to genetically modify tumour cells and research is being conducted to find the optimal gene therapy approach to ovarian cancer.

261

27.2 METHODS OF INTRODUCING GENES INTO CELLS

There have been many techniques used to transfer DNA into mammalian cells. These techniques can be divided into two broad categories which include:

1. physical and chemical methods.
2. biological methods.

In order for a gene transfer technique to be considered successful, a given gene must be taken up by a significant number of cells of a particular type and must then be expressed by that cell type.

27.2.1 PHYSICAL AND CHEMICAL METHODS OF GENE TRANSFER

There are a variety of physical and chemical techniques which have been used to introduce DNA into cells and the most important methods are discussed below. In the chemical methods of DNA transfer, a significant portion of cells will take up and transiently express the DNA but only a small percentage of cells will permanently incorporate it into their chromosomes. The physical methods of DNA transfer have traditionally demonstrated variable to poor efficiency.

Microinjection

Direct injection of DNA into the nucleus of a cell can be accomplished via glass micropipettes.

The process is tedious and its usefulness is limited by the fact that only several hundred cells can be injected at a given time [12]. In addition, the genes are integrated into the host genome at random sites and may therefore activate or inactivate host cell genes via insertion [13]. However, the process is efficient in that a large portion of the injected cells actually stably integrate the injected DNA. Microinjection is used today in the generation of transgenic animals [14].

Electroporation

In the technique of electroporation, a cell is briefly exposed to an electrical impulse which causes transient breakdown of the cell membranes and renders the cell temporarily permeable to DNA molecules. The efficiency of this method varies with the type of medium used and is more efficient when applied to actively growing cells.

Calcium phosphate facilitated transfection

It has been shown that a number of insoluble salts including calcium phosphate contribute to an increased rate of DNA uptake by cells. Under proper conditions, calcium phosphate forms a precipitate with DNA and certain cells will incorporate DNA when exposed to this precipitate.

This method of DNA transfer is advantageous because of its simplicity but has the major disadvantage of being an inefficient way to transfer genetic material.

Liposome fusion

Liposomes are artificial phospholipid vesicles which have the capability of encapsulating DNA molecules and have therefore proven to be useful as vectors for DNA transfer [15,16]. The phospholipid vesicles containing DNA fuse spontaneously with cell membranes and subsequently deposit DNA into the cytoplasm of the cell. Liposomes show promise in the gene therapy of cancer in that they can be directly injected into tumour sites [17].

Ballistic particles

One of the most recently developed and novel methods of gene transfer involves the use of spherical gold particles which are coated with the DNA molecules to be transferred. The particles are then fired at the cell in such a manner as to penetrate the cell membrane. More research is needed to determine the clinical usefulness of this approach but initial results are promising [18].

27.2.2 BIOLOGICAL METHODS OF GENE TRANSFER

Retroviral vector transfer

Many of the problems involving inefficient gene transfer, integration, and expression which have been encountered with the physical and chemical techniques have been solved by the use of biological methods of transfer and especially by the use of retroviral vectors. A murine retrovirus known as Moloney murine leukemia virus (MoMuLV) [19-21] was one of the first retroviruses to be used in human gene therapy and can accommodate a gene of 7–8 kb size. In general, retroviral vectors are characterized by their ability to transfer foreign genes into host cells and their inability to replicate their own viral genome.

The retroviral genome consists of single-stranded RNA which is converted to a DNA form by the enzyme reverse transcriptase upon infection of a cell. The advantage of a retroviral vector is that foreign DNA which has been integrated into the retroviral genome can be efficiently incorporated into the genome of a host cell where it can be permanently expressed. When a retroviral vector is constructed, the genes required for replication of the viral genome are removed and replaced with a foreign gene. A packaging cell line is then used to provide the necessary machinery for viral particle assembly. The replication incompetent retroviral vector can therefore enter a target cell and introduce the new gene; however, once inside the cell, the virus itself is unable to replicate.

One limitation of the retroviral vector system is that the target cells must be actively replicating in order for transfer to occur. In addition, a particular retroviral vector may have a limit to the size of the gene that it can accommodate as noted above

with regard to MoMuLV. Despite these disadvantages, the use of retroviruses as vectors for gene therapy has allowed significant advances in this area.

Adenoviral vectors

Much research in the gene therapy of cancer has recently focused on the use of adenoviral vectors as an alternative to retroviruses in gene transfer [22]. Adenoviral vectors differ from retroviral vectors in their ability to introduce genes into non-replicating cells and they also differ in that they do not generally integrate into the host genome. However, it has been demonstrated that genes introduced into cells via adenoviral vectors may be expressed for at least several weeks. Adenoviral vectors are capable of transferring genes as large as 7 to 8 kb. These vectors are further characterized by their affinity for lung tissue [23].

Adeno-associated viral vectors

A third biological method of gene transfer which has received much attention recently involves the use of an adeno-associated viral vector which has no known pathogenicity for humans [24]. Adeno-associated viral vectors are advantageous in that they demonstrate stable integration of genetic material into the host genome and have not been shown to alter expression of host genes. They are capable of transferring genes no greater than 4 kb in size.

27.3 CLINICAL APPROACHES TO CANCER GENE THERAPY

There are several general clinical approaches to cancer gene therapy in humans. These include *ex vivo* gene therapy, *in vivo* gene therapy, and *in situ* gene therapy [25]. The *ex vivo* approach was the first to be used and has since been applied to several different cell types. The other two approaches have thus far been used less frequently.

27.3.1 *EX VIVO* GENE THERAPY

In the *ex vivo* gene therapy approach, target cells are removed from the patient's body and gene transfer is conducted in the laboratory. The modified cells are then tested for successful transduction and are subsequently returned to the patient. This approach to gene therapy was initially developed in bone marrow [25] but has been applied to other tissue types such as hepatocytes and lymphocytes.

27.3.2 *IN VIVO* GENE THERAPY

The *in vivo* approach to cancer gene therapy involves the introduction of a vector directly into the body where gene transfer subsequently takes place. One major limitation of this approach is that it requires the target cell to have a mechanism whereby the vector can recognize this particular cell type. This approach may be utilized in the future to treat non-small-cell lung cancer by retrovirally mediated transduction of the p53 tumour suppressor gene [26,27]. As the tumour cells are likely to be the only replicating cells in the vicinity, they are likely to be the only cells which will be targeted by the vector.

27.3.3 *IN SITU* GENE THERAPY

Several studies have demonstrated the utility of an *in situ* approach to gene therapy in animal models [28-30]. In this approach, cells capable of producing a retroviral vector containing the gene of interest are implanted in the vicinity of the tumour and transfection subsequently takes place. The studies which have demonstrated this method have used genes which confer drug sensitivity on successfully transduced cells. The *in situ* approach has been proposed in the treatment of glioblastoma of the brain [28-30].

27.4 GENE THERAPY OF OVARIAN CANCER

Despite the fact that much cancer therapy research in the last decade has been directed towards gene therapy, the majority of this research thus far has not involved cancer of the ovary. Cancer of the ovary is thought to be an ideal target for gene therapy as tumour cells are easily accessible via malignant ascites. In addition, as it has been demonstrated that immune mechanisms may contribute significantly to the pathogenesis of this disease [31], the alteration of the immune response through gene therapy offers a potential treatment.

One clinical protocol which has been approved but has not yet begun [11] involves the use of the herpes simplex virus thymidine kinase gene (HSV-TK) in a retroviral vector. Freeman and colleagues [10] previously demonstrated that combining tumour cells which have been modified by this gene (HSV-TK positive cells) with unmodified tumour cells in a murine intraperitoneal tumour model yields tumour regression in the presence of gancyclovir. A clinical protocol for ovarian cancer based on this study was subsequently developed and approved.

Another clinical protocol for ovarian cancer which is a form of gene therapy was developed by Deisseroth and colleagues [32]. This protocol involves the transfer of the multiple drug resistance (MDR) gene via a retroviral vector into the stem cells of the bone marrow by an *ex vivo* approach [33,34]. These bone marrow cells are removed from the patient prior to chemotherapy, transduced in the laboratory, and are subsequently returned to the patient. The purpose of modifying these bone marrow cells is to make them more resistant to the toxic effects of such chemotherapeutic agents as paclitaxel (Taxol) so that the patient can continue to receive and benefit from such agents. As ovarian cancer does not typically metastasize to bone marrow, it is unlikely that this approach will cause resistance of tumour cells to chemotherapy.

As noted previously, much of the research in gene therapy to date has been conducted with cancers other than cancer of the ovary. For example, one recent proposal involves the introduction of the tumour suppressor gene p53 via a retroviral vector directly into the tumour site in patients with non-small-cell cancer of the lung [35] as p53 has been shown to be mutated in greater than 50% of these cases [36]. Another interesting approach to this particular cancer involves the transduction of tumour cells in a similar fashion with an anti-sense transcript RNA to the *Ki-ras* protein [37] as this oncogene is mutated in approximately one-third of cases [38]. One recently approved protocol for patients with metastatic melanoma and renal carcinoma involves subcutaneous vaccination with irradiated tumour cells engineered to secrete interleukin-2 (IL-2) [39].

As research continues in attempts to find the optimal gene therapy approach to ovarian cancer, the various principles developed for the treatment of other forms of cancer may be applied to cancer of the ovary. One recent study [40] demonstrated that tumour-infiltrating lymphocytes from the ascites of patients with ovarian or pancreatic cancers demonstrated increased cytotoxicity when retrovirally transduced with the gene for tumour necrosis factor (TNF) alpha. Another interesting study [41] demonstrated that liposome-plasmid DNA complexes used for transfection inhibited proliferation of human ovarian cancer cells *in vitro* and *in vivo* and this effect did not vary with different plasmids.

We are in the process of conducting gene therapy experiments using a murine ovarian teratocarcinoma (MOT) cell line which arose spontaneously in female C3HeB/FeJ mice [42,43]. The MOT cell line behaves similarly to human ovarian cancer in that animals who receive an intra-peritoneal inoculation of tumour cells develop ascites and intra-abdominal implants. Despite the fact that this tumour line has been previously used in various studies, it has not been well characterized. We have demonstrated that the tumour line has inherent immunogenicity as animals who receive serial intraperitoneal inoculations with irradiated cells do not develop tumour on re-challenge with fresh non-irradiated cells (unpublished data).

The inherent immunogenicity of the MOT cells make this tumour line a good candidate for gene therapy and immunotherapy experiments as anti-tumour responses may potentially be elicited by the enhancement of this immunogenicity. We have demonstrated that MOT cells grown in culture can be engineered to secrete IL-2 (unpublished data) and are currently exploring the use of several different vector systems including retroviral and adenoviral vectors to determine the best way to induce an anti-tumour response. As the MOT cells can be genetically modified *ex vivo* and as this tumour line behaves so similarly to human ovarian cancer, it provides an excellent animal model for gene therapy experiments. New treatment modalities discovered through this model may eventually be applied to human ovarian cancer in the hopes of improving the outcome of this disease.

27.5 CONCLUSIONS

In recent years, gene therapy has become a very important aspect of cancer therapy research and clinical trials for various types of cancers using a variety of gene therapy approaches are in progress. As the morbidity and mortality associated with ovarian cancer remains significant despite the development of newer chemotherapeutic agents, it is imperative that research continue in order to evaluate alternative therapeutic options. Gene therapy provides such an alternative to traditional treatment approaches and as research continues and more clinical trials are developed, it may prove to contribute significantly to the overall prognosis of this disease.

REFERENCES

1. Rosenberg, S.A., Lotze, M.T., Yang, J.C. *et al.* . (1989) Experience with the use of high-dose interleukin-2 in the treatment of 652 cancer patients. *Ann. Surg.* **210**, 474-84.
2. Economou, J.S., Figlin, R.A., Jacobs, E. *et al.* (1992) Clinical Protocol: The treatment of patients with metastatic melanoma and renal cell cancer using in vitro expanded and genetically-engineered (neomycin phospho-transferase) bulk, CD8(+) and/or CD4(+) tumour infiltrating lymphocytes and bulk, CD8(+) and/or CD4(+) peripheral blood leukocytes in combination with recombinant interleukin-2 alone, or with recombinant interleukin-2 and recombinant alpha interferon. *Hum. Gene Ther.* **3**, 411-30.
3. Rosenberg, S.A., Aebersold, P., Cornetta, K. *et al.* (1990) Gene transfer into humans-Immunotherapy of patients with advanced melanoma, using tumour-infiltrating lymphocytes modified by retroviral gene transduction. *N. Engl. J. Med.* **323**, 570-8.
4. Lotze, M.T., Rubin, J.T., Edington, H.D. *et al.* (1992) Clinical Protocol: The treatment of patients with melanoma using interleukin-2, interleukin-4 and tumour infiltrating lymphocytes. *Hum. Gene Ther.* **3**, 167-77.
5. Palmer, T., Thompson, A. and Miller, A.D. (1989) Production of human factor IX in animals by genetically modified skin fibroblasts: potential therapy for hemophilia B. *Blood* **73**, 438-45.
6. Hsueh, J.L., Qiu, X., Zhou, J. *et al.* (1992) Clinical protocol for human gene transfer for hemophilia B. *Hum. Gene Ther.* **3**, 543-6.
7. Palmer, T., Hock, R., Osborne, W. *et al.* (1987) Efficient retrovirus-mediated transfer and expression of a human adenosine deaminase gene in diploid skin fibroblasts from an adenosine deaminase-deficient human. *Proc. Natl. Acad. Sci. USA* **84**, 1055-9.
8. Williams, D.A., Orkin, S. and Mulligan, R.C. (1986) Retrovirus-mediated transfer of human adenosine deaminase gene sequences into cells in culture and into murine hematopoietic cells *in vivo*. *Proc. Natl. Acad. Sci. USA* **83**, 2566-70.
9. Blaese, R.M., Anderson, W.F., Culver, K.W. *et al.* (1990) Clinical Protocol: The ADA human gene therapy protocol. *Hum. Gene Ther.* **1**, 327-62.
10. Freeman, S.M., Whartenby K.A., Koeplin, D.S. *et al.* (1992) Tumour regression when a fraction of the tumour mass contains the HSV-TK gene. *J. Cell. Biochem. Suppl.* **16F**, 47.
11. Freeman, S.M., McCune, C., Angel, C. *et al.* (1992) Treatment of ovarian cancer using HSV-TK gene vaccine-regulatory issues. *Hum. Gene Ther.* **3**, 341-6.
12. Tolstoshev,P. and Anderson, W.F. (1995) Gene Therapy. In *The Molecular Basis of Cancer* (eds J. Mendelsohn, P.M. Howley, M.A. Israel and L.A. Liotta), W.B. Saunders, Philadelphia, pp.534-57.
13. Larrick, J.W. and Burck, K.L. (1991) Gene transfer: introduction of DNA into cells using physical and biological methods. In *Gene Therapy*, Elsevier, New York, pp.71-104.
14. Larrick, J.W. and Burck, K.L. (1991) Germline gene manipulation and transgenic animals. In *Gene Therapy*,

Elsevier, New York, pp.161-87.

15. Staubinger, R.M. and Papahadjopoulos, D. (1983) Liposomes as carriers for intracellular delivery of nucleic acids. *Meth. Enzymol.* **101**, 512-27.

16. Felgner, P.L., Gadek, T.G., Holm, M. *et al.* (1987) Lipofection: a highly efficient lipid-mediated DNA-transfection procedure. *Proc. Natl. Acad. Sci. USA* **84**, 7413-7.

17. Nabel, G.J., Chang, A., Nabel, E. *et al.* (1992) Clinical Protocol: Immunotherapy of malignancy by *in vivo* gene transfer into tumours. *Hum. Gene Ther.* **3**, 399-410.

18. Yang, N.S., Burkholder, J., Roberts, B. *et al.* (1990) *In vivo* and *in vitro* gene transfer to mammalian somatic cells by particle bombardment. *Proc. Natl. Acad. Sci. USA* **87**, 5968-72.

19. Gilboa, E., Eglitis, M.A., Kantoff, P.N. *et al.* (1986) Transfer and expression of cloned genes using retroviral vectors. *BioTechniques* **4**, 504-12.

20. Eglitis, M.A. and Anderson, W.F. (1988) Retroviral vectors for introduction of genes into mammalian cells. *BioTechniques* **6**, 608-14.

21. Tolstoshev, P. and Anderson, W.F. (1990) Gene expression using retroviral vectors. *Curr. Opin. Biotechnol.* **1**, 55.

22. Berkner, K.L. (1988) Development of adenovirus vectors for the expression of heterologous genes. *BioTechniques* **6**, 616-29.

23. Miller, A.D. (1992) Human gene therapy comes of age. *Nature* **357**, 455-60.

24. McLaughlin, S.K., Collis, P., Hermonat, P. *et al.* (1988) Adeno-associated virus general transduction vector: analysis of proviral structures. *J. Virol.* **63**, 1963-73.

25. Parkman, R. (1986) The application of bone marrow transplantation to the treatment of genetic diseases. *Science* **232**, 1373-8.

26. Mukhopadhyay, T., Cavender, A., Branch, C.D. *et al.* (1991) Expression and regulation of wild type p53 gene (wtp53) in human non-small cell lung cancer (NSCLC) cell lines carrying normal or mutated p53 gene. *J. Cell. Biochem.* **15F**, 22.

27. Chen, P.L., Chen, Y., Bookstein, R. *et al.* (1990) Genetic mechanisms of tumour suppression by the human p53 gene. *Science* **250**, 1576-80.

28. Short, M.P., Choi, B.C., Lee, J.K. *et al.* (1990) Gene delivery to glioma cells in rat brain by grafting of a retrovirus packaging cell line. *J. Neurosci. Res.* **27**, 427-39.

29. Ezzeddine, Z.D., Maruza, R.L., Platika, D. *et al.* (1991) Selective killing of glioma cells in culture and *in vivo* by retrovirus transfer of the herpes simplex virus thymidine kinase gene. *New Biol.* **3**, 608-14.

30. Culver, K.W., Ishii, H., Blaese, R.M. *et al.* (1992) *In vivo* gene transfer with retroviral vector producer cells for treatment of experimental brain tumours. *Science* **256**, 1550-2.

31. Berek, J.S. and Martinez-Maza, O. (1994) Molecular and Biologic Factors in the Pathogenesis of Ovarian Cancer. *J. Repro. Med.* **39**, 241-8.

32. Deisseroth, A.B (1994) Clinical Protocols. Use of safety-modified retroviruses to introduce chemotherapy resistance sequences into normal hematopoietic stem cells for chemoprotection during the therapy of ovarian cancer: a pilot trial. *Cancer Gene Ther.* **1**, 291.

33. McLachlin, J.R., Eglitis, M.A., Veda, K. *et al.* (1990) Expression of a human complementary DNA for the multidrug resistance gene in urine hematopoietic precursor cells with the use of retroviral gene transfer. *J. Natl. Cancer Inst.* **82**, 1260-3.

34. Sorrentino, B.P., Brandt, S.J., Bodine, D. *et al.* (1992) Selection of drug-resistant bone marrow cells in vitro after retroviral

transfer of human MDR1. *Science* **257**, 99-103.

35. Roth, J.A (1994) Clinical Protocols. Clinical protocol for modification of tumour suppressor gene expression and induction of apoptosis in non-small fell lung cancer with an adenovirus vector expressing wild type p53 and cisplatin. *Cancer Gene Ther.* **1**, 291.

36. Hollstein, M., Sidransky, D., Vogelstein, B. *et al.* (1991) p53 mutation in human cancers. *Science* **253**, 49-53.

37. Mukhopadhyay, T., Cavender, A., Branch, C.D. *et al.* (1990) Expression of antisense K-ras message in a human lung cancer cell line with a spontaneous activated k-ras oncogene alters the transformed phenotype. *Proc. Am. Assoc. Cancer Res.* **32**, 304.

38. Rodenhuis, S., Slebos, R.J.C., Boot, A.J.M. *et al.* (1988) Incidence and possible clinical significance of K-ras oncogene activation in adenocarcinoma of the human lung. *Cancer Res.* **48**, 5738-41.

39. Rosenberg, S.A., Anderson, W.F., Blaese, M.R. *et al.* (1992) Initial proposal of clinical research project: immunization of cancer patients using autologous cancer cells modified by the insertion of the gene for interleukin-2. *Hum. Gene Ther.* **3**, 75-91.

40. Itoh, Y., Koshita, Y., Takahashi, M. *et al.* (1995) Characterization of tumour-necrosis-factor-gene-transduced tumour-infiltrating lymohocytes from ascitic fluid of cancer patients: analysis of cytolytic activity, growth rate, adhesion molecule expression and cytokine production. *Cancer Immunol. Ther.* **40**, 95-102.

41. Hofland, H. and Huang, L. (1995) Inhibition of human ovarian carcinoma cell proliferation by liposome-plasmid DNA complex. *Biochem. Biophys, Res. Commun.* **207**,492-6.

42. Feldman, G.B., Knapp, R.C., Order, S.E. *et al.* (1972) The role of lymphatic obstruction in the formation of ascites in a murine ovarian carcinoma. *Cancer Res.* **32**, 1663-6.

43. Fekete, E. and Ferringno, M.A. (1972) Studies on a transplantable teratoma of the mouse. *Cancer Res.* **12**, 438-40.

Chapter 28

Approaches to gene therapy

Ian R. HART

28.1 INTRODUCTION

Chemotherapy has not cured the majority of patients with advanced stage neoplastic disease and this has encouraged the search for novel approaches to cancer treatment. Gene therapy is one modality which currently is being studied.

Gene therapy for cancer may be based upon two general approaches. Cells are either removed from the patient for genetic modification *ex vivo*, followed by their subsequent readministration to the patient, or attempts are made to modify the cells *in situ*. In both situations the transfected cells could either be the neoplastic cells themselves or potential immune-effector cells.

The *in vitro* transduction protocols are laborious, time-consuming and potentially liable to technical failure which has led us to focus our efforts on the conceptually simpler approach of trying to modify cells *in situ*. We studied neoplastic cells as targets for transduction by introducing exogenous cDNAs and explored how this might modify the subsequent behaviour of successfully manipulated neoplasia.

28.2 NATURE OF GENES TO BE INTRODUCED FOR CANCER THERAPY

In situ modification of tumour cells probably requires the introduction of genes which belong to one of three broad categories:

(a) those which are capable of reversing the neoplastic phenotype by reversing or correcting the underlying genetic lesion,
(b) those which are able to stimulate or enhance a cytotoxic immune response to the modified cells, and
(c) those which encode for an enzyme capable of converting an inert prodrug to an active cytotoxic compound so that only the modified cells which express this enzyme are susceptible to its toxic effects.

28.2.1 GENES WHICH REVERSE THE NEOPLASTIC PHENOTYPE

This corrective approach, which is the way that gene therapy is likely to be utilized for monogenic dysfunctions, appears to have many potential drawbacks for anti-tumour therapy. In many advanced stage cancers the number of genetic aberrations which have accumulated by the time of presentation may be considerable and it may not be evident as to which is the underlying genetic lesion. Therefore, the choice of gene to be introduced may not be apparent. A further potential drawback with this approach is that the requirement appears to be to introduce either a normal copy of a tumour suppressor gene or anti-sense to a dominant acting oncogene into each and every individual neoplastic stem cell. Omission or failure to transduce even a few such stem cells would lead to the overgrowth of the uncorrected

269

cells. Thus, if for example mutations in the BRCA1 gene do contribute to the development of spontaneous ovarian tumours, restoration of normal BRCA1 function may require the transduction of the whole population of neoplastic cells. This is because in this type of approach there is no amplification of effector activity, but a single-hit, single-response mechanism.

Despite these theoretical considerations, this approach has been shown to work in at least one animal model system [1]. Here, introduction of anti-sense to an activated Kirsten-ras gene prevented the growth of human lung tumours transplanted ortho-topically into the lungs of athymic mice [1]. Notwithstanding this apparent success, it has been our feeling that initial positive results in the use of gene therapy in the cancer field are more likely to result from the use of genes which fall into categories (b) and (c) as outlined above.

28.2.2 IMMUNITY STIMULATING GENES

Our understanding of the molecules involved in regulating the immune response to tumours and how they may be manipulated therapeutically has advanced rapidly in recent years. Accordingly interest has been generated in the possible introduction of requisite cDNAs for these molecules to elicit a sustained and dramatic immune response. Such genes might include those encoding for identified tumour antigens, major histocompatibility complex antigens (MHC), co-stimulatory molecules, like B7, or cytokines such as interleukin-2 or interleukin-12 [2].

The obvious theoretical advantage of this approach is the potential avoidance of the requirement (*i.e.* to transduce the vast majority of neoplastic cells) that limited the potential application of genes which reverse the neoplastic phenotype. Indeed, in rodent model systems it has been shown that

expression of MHC antigens in less than 1% of cells within a tumour was sufficient to induce significant inhibition of cancer growth [3]. Equally it seems possible that the immune effector cells stimulated to kill tumour cells will be capable of dealing with those cells which already have metastasized to distant sites.

The advantage of this potential response is that the need to target DNA to all sites of tumour growth is obviated, activated effector cells serve as the targeting mechanism.

28.2.3 GENES ENCODING FOR ENZYMES WHICH CONVERT INERT PRODRUGS TO ACTIVE CYTOTOXICS

In this approach to therapy selective susceptibility to drug-mediated killing is a consequence of expression of a specific introduced gene. The two systems best characterized have been the cytosine deaminase gene, capable of converting 5-fluorocytosine to the toxic compound 5-fluorouracil [4] and the Herpes simplex virus thymidine kinase gene, which confers sensitivity to the nucleoside analogue, ganciclovir [5]. Other prodrug activating enzymes are rapidly becoming available and even more effective agents will likely be developed in succeeding years.

Initially this approach would seem to suffer from exactly those limitations raised with regard to the potential reversal of the neoplastic phenotype by corrective genes, that is, the introduction of cDNA into one cell would seem to be unlikely to confer a field effect. Thus, limitation of efficiency of transduction would appear to be a major factor mitigating against the likely success of this potential approach. It is apparent, however, that there is a dramatic bystander effect, with these prodrug activating compounds which leads to greater response levels than would be obtained from the expected 'single hit-single cell death' kinetics.

This bystander effect, which is well recognized but poorly characterized, appears to be dependent upon the transfer of toxic metabolites from one cell to another; presumably via gap junctions [5]. The practical consequence of the existence of this phenomenon is that transduction of approximately only 10% of the cells within a tumour mass is sufficient to achieve substantial anti-tumour efficacy [6].

28.3 CHOICE OF VECTOR DELIVERY SYSTEMS

There are a number of different delivery systems, some of viral origin and some of non-viral origin, which have been assessed for the delivery of DNA to tumours *in situ*. At this time no single delivery system has overwhelming advantages over the others.

28.3.1 PLASMID DNA

Plasmid DNA has been used to introduce genes into mammalian tumour cells. Generally the efficiency of uptake has been increased by complexing the plasmid DNA with cationic liposomes or precipitating with calcium phosphate. *In vitro* the efficiency achieved with this mode of DNA delivery has been low. Surprisingly, however, results obtained *in vivo* look rather more promising than those obtained *in vitro*. It has been shown, for example, that muscle tissue will take up and express plasmid DNA delivered directly by injection [7]. Equally, the inoculation of DNA into small tumour deposits has resulted in up-take and expression by a sufficient number of tumour cells to bring about therapeutic effects [8,9]. The integration frequency of the plasmid into the host genome is low and while levels of expression may be high, they may also be transient.

The recent demonstration that pretreatment of ovarian cancer cells, both *in vitro*

and *in vivo*, with cisplatin enhances the efficacy of uptake and expression of plasmid DNA complexed with cationic lipids offers hope that this integration frequency may be modified and increased [10]. The fact that such modifications were achieved using a common cytotoxic drug raises the possibility that combination gene and chemotherapy may well be the route to be exploited for targeting of ovarian carcinoma.

28.3.2 RETROVIRUSES

Recombinant retroviruses have been employed in several gene therapy protocols. These retroviral vectors are capable of binding to and infecting a variety of replicating cells and also can accept up to 8kb of non-viral sequences so that they tend to be very useful for the delivery of extra DNA to tumour cells.

Amphotropic retroviruses bind to a receptor with homology to a phosphate transporter which is expressed widely in a variety of cells. Thus, though some degree of tumour cell targeting specificity is achieved by the virus' requirement to transduce only dividing cells, these vectors essentially are non-specific in terms of their spectrum of infectivity. Because the virus integrates into the host genome expression of the introduced gene may be relatively permanent, rather than transient, but this does carry the safety risk of insertional mutagenesis. When this potential disadvantage is added to the fact that retroviruses can be produced only at low titres and that they are inactivated by complement it is clear that currently available retroviral vectors probably are not optimal for *in situ* delivery.

28.3.3 ADENOVIRUSES

Adenoviral vectors offer a number of potential advantages over retroviral vectors for the *in vivo* delivery of DNA. They can be produced at high titres (up to 10 pfu/ml).

Lacking an envelope they are more stable than retroviruses and less susceptible to complement inactivation; they can transduce a wide range of cell types, including terminally differentiated cells and cells in G_0 resting phase, and, because they rarely integrate into the genome but generally maintain an extra-chromosomal existence, they are unlikely to give rise to insertional mutagenesis.

The disadvantage, of course, is that genes introduced by adenoviral vectors are expressed only transiently. Although adenoviruses induce an immune response the illnesses they cause generally tend to be mild and self-limiting. Whether repeated administrations, as a consequence of the need to maintain exogenous gene expression beyond the transient, would be detrimental in cancer patients is presently unknown.

28.3.4 OTHER VIRAL VECTORS

Several DNA viruses, apart from adenoviruses, are being investigated as potential vector delivery systems. These viruses, which include parvovirus, herpes simplex virus and adeno-associated virus, presently are in their infancy in terms of development for *in vivo* delivery of DNA [11].

28.4 SPECIFICITY OF GENE EXPRESSION

The major limitation in all these approaches to delivering genes *in vivo* is not only the lack of efficiency but also the lack of specificity. The use of recombinant retroviruses may be sufficient to limit expression of DNA to dividing cells but the occasions when such limitation is sufficient to confer complete anti-tumour specificity are infrequent. Tumours of the central nervous system, where only the neoplastic cells are dividing, probably represent the best example of this phenomenon [12].

Efforts are underway to engineer retroviruses, by incorporating receptor ligands such as erythropoetin into the extracellular portions of the *env* glycoprotein [13], and adenoviruses, by modifying the fibre protein, so that these vectors bind preferentially to selected cell types. While some of these approaches look interesting *in vitro* their efficacy *in vivo* requires greater investigation.

An alternative approach to that of targeting the vector delivery system to the requisite cell type would be to target expression of the inserted gene. This could be achieved by placing the heterologous gene under transcriptional control of a promoter which functions in a tissue-specific manner. In this way delivery to a range of cell types could be tolerated since gene expression would only be achieved in the desired cell types. This approach originally was described by Huber and his colleagues [14] who used the promoter sequence of the alphafetoprotein gene to limit gene expression to liver tumours. Since then this concept has been shown to hold true for a number of other tumour types. Thus the promoter sequences of the tyrosinase gene have limited heterologous gene expression to cells of the melanocytic lineage [15,16], the c-erbB2 promoter has limited gene expression to breast cells [17] and the surfactant protein promoter has limited gene expression to lung tumours [18]. When these transcriptional elements have been incorporated into vectors which have then been delivered systemically the major limitation has been not the specificity of expression conferred by the promoter element, but the efficiency of delivery by the viral construct [19].

In a disease like ovarian cancer, where the disease generally remains limited until very late in development, intracavity administration may be a delivery route which overcomes these problems of systemic delivery. We intend for example to use the promoter of the MUC-1 gene [20] to direct expression of the HSVtk gene to ovarian cancer cells.

The human MUC-1 gene is expressed by normal glandular epithelial cells and has been shown to be up-regulated in many cancer cells where high levels of the gene product, PEM or polymorphic epithelial mucin, are to be found [20]. Recently it was shown that more than 90% of ovarian cancers express high levels of this PEM gene product [21]. Analysis of five sequences of the MUC-1 gene has shown that the capacity to direct expression of reporter genes to PEM-expressing tumour cells can be conferred by as little as 743 base pairs of the five sequence [22]. The use of the MUC-1 promoter to limit expression to epithelial cells should then increase the specificity of gene expression already conferred by direct installation into the abdomen.

The recent demonstration by us [19] and other groups [23] that the cytotoxic effects obtained with the prodrug-activating systems elicit a strong immune response suggests that such a combination of genes may represent the best hope for effective gene therapy.

REFERENCES

1. Georges, R. N., Mukhopadhyay, T., Zhang, Y. *et. al.* (1993) Prevention of orthotopic human lung cancer growth by intratracheal instillation of a retroviral antisense K-ras construct. *Cancer Res.* 53, 1743-6.

2. Tahara, H. and Lotze, M. T. (1995) Antitumour effects of interleukin-12 (IL-12): applications for the immunotherapy and gene therapy of cancer. *Gene Ther.* 2, 96-106.

3. Plautz, G. E., Yang, Z.-Y., Wu, B.-Y. *et. al.* (1993) Immunotherapy of malignancy by *in vivo* gene transfer into tumors. *Proc. Natl. Acad. Sci. USA* 90, 4645-9.

4. Harris, J. D., Gutierrez, A. A., Hurst, H. C. *et. al.* (1994) Gene therapy for cancer using tumour specific prodrug activation. *Gene Ther.* 1, 170-5.

5. Moolten, F. L. (1986) Tumor chemosensitivity conferred by inserted herpes thymidine kinase genes: paradigm for a prospective cancer control strategy. *Cancer Res.* 46, 76-5281.

6. Vile, R. G. and Hart, I. R. (1993) Use of tissue-specific expression of the herpes simplex virus thymidine kinase gene to inhibit growth of established murine melanomas following direct intratumoural injection of DNA. *Cancer Res.* 53, 3860-4.

7. Wolff, J. A., Malone, R. W., Williams, P. *et. al.* (1990) Direct gene transfer into mouse muscle *in vivo*. *Science* 247, 1465-8.

8. Nabel, G. J., Nabel, E. G., Yang, Z. Y. *et. al.* (1993) Direct gene transfer with DNA-liposome complexes in melanoma: expression, biologic activity and lack of toxicity in humans. *Proc. Natl. Acad. Sci. USA* 90, 11307-11.

9. Vile, R. G. and Hart, I. R. (1994) Targeting of cytokine gene expression to malignant melanoma using tissue specific promoter sequences. *Ann. Oncol.* 5, 559-65.

10. Son, K. and Huang, L. (1994) Exposure of human ovarian carcinoma to cisplatin transiently sensitizes the tumor cells for liposome-mediated gene transfer. *Proc. Natl. Acad. Sci. USA* 91, 12669-72.

11. Ali, M., Lemoine, N. R. and Ring, C. J. A. (1994) The use of DNA viruses as vectors for gene therapy. *Gene Ther.* 1, 367-84.

12. Culver, K. W., Ram, Z., Wallbridge, S. *et. al.* (1992) *In vivo* gene transfer with retroviral vector-producer cells for treatment of experimental brain tumors. *Science* 256, 1550-2.

13. Kasahara, N., Dozy, A. M. and Kan, Y. W. (1994) Tissue-specific targeting of retroviral vectors through ligand-receptor

interactions. *Science* 266, 1373-6.

14. Huber, B. E., Richards, C. A. and Krenitsky, T. A. (1991) Retroviral-mediated gene therapy for the treatment of hepatocellular carcinoma: an innovative approach for cancer therapy. *Proc. Natl. Acad. Sci. USA* 88, 8039-43.

15. Vile, R. G. and Hart, I. R. (1993) *In vitro* and *in vivo* gene targeting to melanoma cells. *Cancer Res.* 53, 962-7.

16. Hart, I. R. and Vile, R. G. (1994) Targeted therapy for malignant melanoma. *Curr. Opin. Oncol.* 6, 221-5.

17. Hollywood, D. and Hurst, H. C. (1993) A novel transcription factor, OB2-1, is required for over-expression of the proto-oncogene c-erbB-2 in mammary tumour lines. *EMBO J.* 12, 2369-75.

18. Smith, M. J., Rousculp, M. D., Goldsmith, K. T. *et. al.* (1994) Surfactant protein α-directed toxin gene kills lung-cancer cells in-vitro. *Hum. Gene Ther.* 5, 29-35.

19. Vile, R. G., Nelson, J. A., Castleden, S. *et al.* (1994) Systemic gene therapy of murine melanoma using tissue specific expression of the HSVtk gene involves an immune component. *Cancer Res.* 54, 6228-34.

20. Gendler, S. J., Lancaster, C. A., Taylor-Papadimitrious, J. *et. al.* (1990) Molecular cloning and expression of the human tumour-associated polymorphic epithelial mucin. *J. Biol. Chem.* 265, 15286-93.

21. Granowska, M., Mather, S. J., Jobling, T. *et. al.* (1990) Radiolabelled stripped mucin, SM3, monoclonal antibody for immuno-scintigraphy of ovarian tumours. *Int. J. Biol. Mark.* 5, 89-96.

22. Kovarik, A., Peat, N., Wilson D. *et. al.* (1993) Analysis of the tissue-specific promoter of the MUC 1 gene. *J. Biol. Chem.* 268, 9917-26.

23. Mullen, C. A., Coale, M. M., Lowe, R. and Blaese, R. M. (1994) Tumors expressing the cytosine deaminase suicide gene can be eliminated *in vivo* with 5-fluorocytosine and induce protective immunity to wild-type tumor. *Cancer Res.* 54, 1503-6.

Chapter 29

Angiogenic growth factors as targets for gene therapy

Stephen K. SMITH

29.1 INTRODUCTION

Two thirds of ovarian cancer patients have advanced disease at diagnosis with highly invasive phenotypes and often ascites [1,2]. A key feature of tumour spread from the ovary is the local invasion that occurs within the peritoneal cavity. Whilst mechanisms of proliferative advantage based on aberrant growth factor and/or oncogene expression and loss of cell cycle control are relevant to tumour spread [3–5], it is now also appreciated that angiogenesis plays a critical role in the malignant transformation of tumours [6].

Tumours which switch to an angiogenic phenotype, express growth factors that promote the local growth of new capillaries [7]. This development benefits not only the individual tumour cells that change phenotype but also adjacent cells that do not undergo this transformation [8]. Growth factors and matrix proteins released by the endothelium further support the progression of the tumour.

Tumours promote this vascular development because they express a range of angiogenic growth factors including αFGF, βFGF [9] and VEGF [10]. Growth factors may also be released by tumour cells from extracellular matrix, and macrophages accumulating at the tumour border further release angiogenic growth factors. The stimulus to angiogenesis reflects a shift in favour of pro-angiogenic growth factors over locally released anti-angiogenic agents [11].

Metastases need angiogenesis at two stages in their development. Firstly, cells are only shed from the primary tumour when it becomes vascularized and secondly, the migrating cells or clumps of cells need to develop a new blood supply when they implant, in the case of ovarian cancer usually inside the peritoneal cavity. Tumours like ovarian cancer that often cause ascites produce factors that increase vascular permeability [12,13].

29.2 VASCULAR ENDOTHELIAL CELL GROWTH FACTOR

Vascular endothelial cell growth factor (VEGF) is a heparin-binding growth factor that has potent angiogenic and endothelial cell proliferative properties [14,15]. The protein has a molecular weight of 23kDa and is the product of a single gene. Five alternate splice variants have been identified, arising from conserved expression of the first four exons, and the rest resulting from differential expression of the four 3' exons. This results in five proteins of 121, 145, 165, 189 and 205 amino acids. Exon six has the heparin

275

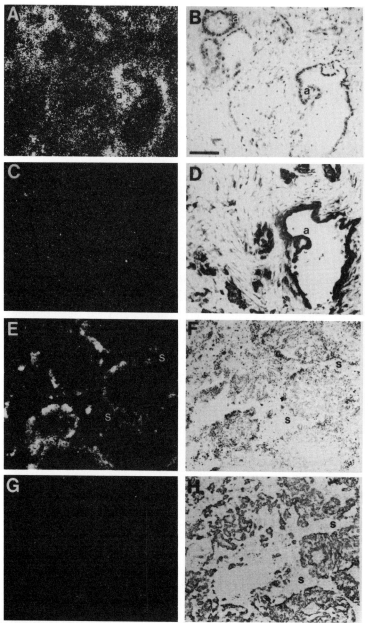

Figure 29.1 Expression of VEGF mRNA by primary and secondary tumour cells.
(a-d) tumour C (moderately differentiated mucinous carcinoma, primary site).
(e-h) tumour 324 (poorly differentiated serous papillary cystadenocarcinoma, secondary site).
(a,b,e,f) *in situ* hybridization with ^{35}S-labelled VEGF antisense cRNA.
(c,g) serial section hybridized with ^{35}S-labelled VEGF sense RNA.
(d,h) immunoperoxidase labelling of the same region with anticytokeratin.
Tumour acini (a) and stroma (s) are indicated. Scale bars = 200 μm.

binding domain and proteins with this exon bind heparin.

Tissue specific expression of VEGF usually includes expression of the 189 variant whilst macrophages only express the 165 and 121 variants. The receptors for VEGF are the fms-like tyrosine kinase, flt, and the kinase domain receptor, KDR [16,17]. These are type III TK receptors and contain a seven immunoglobulin repeat in the extracellular domain.

VEGF was initially thought to be an endothelial cell specific growth factor. Besides its mitogenic effects it also promotes migration and protease release from endothelial cells whilst also increasing vascular permeability [18].

29.3 VEGF AND OVARIAN CANCER

An ^{35}S-labelled VEGF cRNA probe hybridized with serous, mucinous and endometroid primary carcinoma (Figure 29.1). Hybridization was strongest at the margins of papillary tumours and in the glandular structures of both mucinous and endometroid tumours. Similar hybridization was found in secondary deposits of the tumours. Only light hybridization was found to the capsule on non-malignant ovaries. Immunoreactive VEGF was found with the same distribution, suggesting expression of the protein by the primary tumour. Staining in the stromal matrix was also found around malignant epithelial cells suggesting binding of the VEGF to extracellular matrix components. In addition, ovarian cell lines and primary cell cultures obtained from malignant ascitic fluid cells released VEGF into the supernatant as judged by a VEGF Elisa.

Hybridization for flt was not found in any of the tumours, but immunoreactive flt was found in two tumours in blood vessels adjacent to the tumour. Blood vessels in secondary deposits did not express flt.

However, digoxigenin-labelled KDR cRNA probes hybridized not only with blood vessels but also with malignant cells in both mucinous and endometroid carcinomas but not in any of the serous adenocarcinoma sections.

RT-PCR for flt and KDR in both ovarian cell lines and primary cultures from malignant ascitic fluid suggest variable expression amongst invading phenotypes. Thus some cells expressed both receptors whilst others expressed one or other of the receptors. This suggests significant diversity in receptor expression in these cells.

Over-expression of VEGF could arise for a variety of reasons in tumours because several factors known to induce VEGF expression are present. These include oestrogens [19], activators of adenylyl cyclase [20], protein kinase C [21] and hypoxia [22]. Hypoxia has recently been shown to act via the c-src pathway. A further interesting observation is the up-regulation of VEGF in tumours containing mutations of the tumour suppressor gene p53. It is likely that secreted VEGF plays a significant role in inducing ascites. Neutralizing antibodies to VEGF prevent ascitic fluid accumulation.

The finding of KDR but not flt receptor on primary tumour cells raises the prospect of an autocrine role for VEGF in tumour progression. To pursue this question, we cultured malignant cells in the presence of VEGF. No mitogenic activity was found [10]. These findings are consistent with similar observations in Chinese hamster ovarian (CHO) cells [23]. However, other cells that have an invasive phenotype express VEGF receptors and include trophoblast [19], malignant melanoma cell lines [24] and peripheral monocytes [25]. Thus VEGF may not only induce angiogenesis around the tumour, it may also be responsible for the migratory response of invading tumour cells. Studies are underway to address this question.

A second source of VEGF at the tumour site is activated macrophages. These cells present in the peritoneal cavity significantly over-express VEGF only when activated [26]. It is not yet clear if specific macrophage activators induce this response or whether it is just a feature of macrophage activation.

This clear demonstration of the potent angiogenic growth factor expressed by the commonest forms of ovarian cancer without significant expression in the normal ovary suggests a role for VEGF in the progression of malignancy. This role could act through several mechanisms:

1. VEGF secreted by the primary tumour on the outside of the acini promotes the growth of new blood vessels to maintain the primary tumour and provides a conduit for blood born spread.

2. Secreted VEGF in the peritoneal cavity promotes vascular permeability and results in ascites.

3. The presence of KDR receptors (certainly in mucinous and endometroid carcinomas) suggests an autocrine effect of VEGF, though this probably relates more to migration than it does mitosis.

4. VEGF released by the tumour causes the accumulation of activated macrophages at the tumour site that further enhances VEGF secretion.

Ovarian cancer is thus a clear target for the increasing range of anti-angiogenic strategies being developed. Experiments in nude mice show reduction in tumour mass of the order of 80% with intraperitoneal instillation of neutralising VEGF antibodies [27].

A wide range of clinical trials are at present under way to determine the efficacy and toxicology associated with anti-angiogenic strategies. The broad principles that are arising from these studies were reviewed by Folkman [6]. This approach is of low toxicity, does not have any of the side effects associated with chemotherapy and there is no drug resistance [8]. Moreover, there is some suggestions that in combination with cytotoxic therapy it is able to induce cure in animals for which each agent alone is only palliative.

The strategies to promote this therapy in ovarian cancer are several fold:

1. Agents that inhibit angiogenesis such as platelet factor 4 and fumagillin derivatives may be administered systemically. The obvious advantage of this approach is that it may reduce growth of distant metastases. Its disadvantages are the problems of targeting and dosage.

2. Alternatively non-specific anti-angiogenesis agents may be administered after surgery or in combination with cytotoxic agents. This may be particularly important because recent evidence shows increased angiogenic activity in the peritoneal cavity following surgery.

3. Specific gene therapies to inhibit angiogenic growth factor expression may be used with antisense or ribozymes administered in viral or liposomal vectors.

29.4 CONCLUSIONS

In conclusion, ovarian cancer seems particularly susceptible to anti-angiogenic therapies. Careful evaluation of this strategy is now being undertaken in several clinical studies throughout the world.

REFERENCES

1. Young, R.C., Decker, D.G., Wharton, J.T. *et al.* (1983) Staging laparotomy in early ovarian cancer. *JAMA* 250, 3072-6.

2. Plaxe, S.C., Deligdisch, L., Dottino, P.R. *et al.* (1990) Ovarian intraepithelial neoplasia demonstrated in patients with stage I ovarian carcinoma. *Gynecol. Oncol.* 38, 367-72.

3. Fearon, E.R. and Vogelstein, B. (1990) A

genetic model for colorectal tumorigenesis. *Cell* **61**, 759-67.

4. Kacinski, B.M., Carter, D., Mittal, K. *et al.* (1990) Ovarian adenocarcinomas express fms-complementary transcripts and fms antigen, often with coexpression of CSF-1. *Am. J. Pathol.* **137**, 135-47.

5. Wu, S., Boyer, C.M., Whitaker, R.S. *et al.* (1993) Tumor necrosis factor alpha as autocrine and paracrine growth factor for ovarian cancer, monokine induction of tumor cell proliferation and tumor necrosis factor alpha expression. *Cancer Res.,* **53**, 1939-1944.

6. Folkman, J. (1995) Angiogenesis in cancer, vascular, rheumatoid and other disease. *Nat. Med.* **1**, 27-31.

7. Weidner, N., Folkman, J., Pozza, F. *et al.* (1992) Tumor angiogenesis, a new significant and independent prognostic indicator in early-stage breast carcinoma. *J. Nat. Cancer Inst.* **84**, 1875-87.

8. Folkman, J. (1994) Angiogenesis and breast cancer. *J. Clin. Oncol.* **12**, 441-3.

9. Presta, M. (1988) Sex hormones modulate the synthesis of basic fibroblast growth factor in human endometrial adeno-carcinoma cells, implications for the neovascularization of normal and neoplastic endometrium. *J. Cell. Physiol.* **137**, 593-7.

10. Boocock, C.A., Charnock-Jones, D.S., Sharkey, A.M. *et al.* (1995) Expression of vascular endothelial growth factor and its receptors flt and KDR in ovarian carcinoma. *J. Natl. Cancer Inst.* **87**, 506-16.

11. Risau, W. (1990) Angiogenic growth factors. *Prog. Growth Factor Res.* **2**, 71-9.

12. Senger, D.R., Galli, S.J., Dvorak, A.M. *et al.* (1983) Tumor cells secrete a vascular perm-eability factor that promotes accumulation of ascites fluid. *Science* **219**, 983-5.

13. Senger, D.R., Perruzzi, C.A., Feder, J. *et al.* (1986) A highly conserved vascular permeability factor secreted by a variety of human and rodent tumor cell lines. *Cancer Res.* **46**, 5629-32.

14. Ferrara, N. and Henzel, W.J. (1989) Pituitary follicular cells secrete a novel heparin-binding growth factor specific for vascular endothelial cells. *Biochem. Biophys. Res. Comm.* **161**, 851-8.

15. Connolly, D.T., Heuvelman, D.M., Nelson, R. *et al.* (1989) Tumor vascular permeability factor stimulates endothelial cell growth and angiogenesis. *J. Clin. Invest.* **84**, 1470-8.

16. de Vries, C., Escobedo, J.A., Ueno, H. *et al.* (1992) The fms-like tyrosine kinase, a receptor for vascular endothelial growth factor. *Science* **255**, 989-91.

17. Terman, B.I., Dougher-Vermazen, M, Carrion, M.E. *et al.* (1992) Identification of the KDR tyrosine kinase as a receptor for vascular endothelial cell growth factor. *Biochem. Biophys. Res. Comm.* **187**, 1579-86.

18. Pepper, M.S., Ferrara, N., Orci, L. *et al.* (1991) Vascular endothelial growth factor (VEGF) induces plasminogen activators and plasmin-ogen activator inhibitor-1 in microvascular endothelial cells. *Biochem. Biophys. Res. Comm.* **181**, 902-6.

19. Charnock-Jones, D.S., Sharkey, A.M., Boocock, C.A. *et al.* (1994) Vascular endothe-lial growth factor receptor localisation and activation in human trophoblast and chorio-carcinoma cells. *Biol. Reprod.* **51**, 524-30.

20. Garrido, C., Saule, S. and Gospodarowicz, D. (1993) Transcriptional regulation of vascular endothelial growth factor gene expression in ovarian bovine granulosa cells. *Growth Factors* **8**, 109-17.

21. Finkenzeller, G., Marme, D., Weich, H.A. *et al.* (1992) Platelet-derived growth factor-induced transcription of the vascular endo-thelial growth factor gene is mediated by protein kinase C. *Cancer Res.* **52**, 4821-3.

22. Schweiki, D., Itin, A., Soffer, D. *et al.* (1992) Vascular endothelial growth factor induced by hypoxia may mediate hypoxia-initiated angiogenesis. *Nature* **359**, 843-5.

23. Ferrara, N., Winer, J., Burton T. *et al.* (1992) Expression of vascular EGF does not promote transformation but confers a growth advantage *in vivo* to Chinese hamster ovary cells. *J. Clin. Invest.* **91**, 160-70.

24. Gitay-Goren, H., Halaban, R. and Neufeld, G. (1993) Human melanoma cells but not normal melanocytes express vascular endothelial growth factor receptors. *Biochem., Biophys. Res. Comm.* **190**, 702-8.

25. Shen, H., Clauss, M., Ryan, J. *et al.* (1993) Characterization of vascular permeability factor/vascular endothelial growth factor receptors on mononuclear phagocytes. *Blood* **81**, 2767-73.

26. McLaren, J., Prentice, A., Charnock-Jones, D.S. *et al.* (1995) Involvement of vascular endothelial growth factor in endometriosis, pivotal role of peritoneal macrophages. *Nat. Med.*- submitted

27. Kim, K.J., Li, B., Winer, J. *et al.* (1993) Inhibition of vascular endothelial growth factor-induced angiogenesis suppresses tumour growth *in vivo*. *Nature* **372**, 841-4.

Chapter 30

Gene therapy: virus-directed enzyme prodrug

Rachael G. BARTON, Moira G. GILLIGAN, Peter F. SEARLE,

Lawrence S. YOUNG and David J. KERR

30.1 INTRODUCTION

Carcinogenesis is characterized by the aberrant function of cellular genes which control cell division. In the majority of common solid tumours it is the accumulation of several different mutations which eventually leads to the development of a malignant phenotype. Such mutations may include the 'gain of function' of cellular proto-oncogenes and the 'loss of function' of tumour suppressor genes. Advances in recombinant DNA technology have led to the isolation of many relevant genes and provided the means to manipulate these *in vitro*, as well as to reintroduce the manipulated genes into living cells. The success of these techniques *in vitro* has raised the possibility that gene transfer to cancer cells might form the basis for new and powerful clinical therapies.

The poor results of the conventional treatment of ovarian carcinoma and its severe life-threatening nature justify the careful development of gene therapy in advanced disease. Ovarian carcinoma may be an advantageous target for gene therapy as the disease remains localized to the peritoneal cavity for much of its natural history. Surgery can often reduce the bulk of

disease to small metastatic nodules on the peritoneal surface which are in contact with peritoneal fluid and therefore accessible to agents administered via the intraperitoneal route [1].

In principle, faulty genes could be silenced, or their normal function restored by the transfer of a 'corrective gene'. This approach suffers from the inherent improbability that 100% of malignant cells can be successfully corrected and the possibility that 'uncorrected' cells, or those which have undergone further mutations could eventually repopulate the tumour. A more promising option is to destroy malignant cells using genetic manipulation either to target drugs specifically to the cancer or to enhance tumour immunogenicity and induce cytotoxic immune response specifically directed against the cancer cells. It is these two approaches which are the focus of active research in the Gene Therapy Group in the University of Birmingham CRC Institute for Cancer Studies.

30.2 VIRUS DIRECTED ENZYME PRODRUG THERAPY (VDEPT)

Cytotoxic drugs can undoubtedly induce tumour cell death in up to 100% of a given *in*

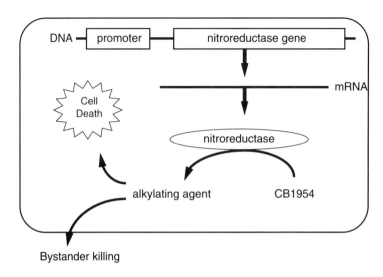

Figure 30.1 Tumour specific expression of the bacterial gene coding nitroreductase which activates CB1954 to an active alkylating species.

vitro population depending on the dose-response curve. The most effective drug concentrations *in vitro* cannot, however, be used clinically because of their systemic toxicity. VDEPT aims to avoid this problem by using a genetically modified virus to express, in tumour cells, an enzyme which converts an inactive prodrug to a short-lived cytotoxic metabolite thus producing maximum local cell kill with minimal systemic toxicity.

Several prodrugs have been proposed for this purpose, including ganciclovir which is activated by herpes simplex virus thymidine kinase, and 5-fluorocytosine, activated by cytosine deaminase [2]. One particularly promising prodrug is CB1954 (5-(aziridin-1-yl)-2,4-dinitrobenzamide), a weak alkylating agent which showed promising curative activity against the rat Walker 256 tumour [3]. It was entered into clinical trials in 1970 but disappointingly, no anti-tumour activity was seen in human subjects. It was subsequently shown that CB1954 is reduced by the rat enzyme DT diaphorase to a

strongly active, difunctional alkylating agent which cross-links DNA but that the human and mouse forms of DT diaphorase are deficient in this reaction [4]. On a dose basis, the active species is up to 100 000 times more cytotoxic than the prodrug [5].

A nitroreductase from *E. coli* was found to perform the same reduction 60 to 100-fold faster than the rat diaphorase [6]. Our VDEPT strategy aims to express this bacterial nitroreductase selectively in tumour cells, making them susceptible to killing by CB1954 (Figure 30.1).

An important feature of VDEPT is the 'bystander effect' which describes the killing of a significant proportion of non-expressing cells when prodrug is administered to a mixed population consisting of cells containing the activating enzyme and those without. This is presumably due to the transfer of activated drug from a cell in which it is produced to others in the vicinity which lack the enzyme [7]. Coculture of cells which activate CB1954 with insensitive cells resulted in killing of both populations in the

282

presence of the prodrug, and DNA interstrand cross-links could be detected in the intrinsically insensitive cells [8]. Thus, expression of nitroreductase in just a fraction of cells within each tumour deposit should allow killing of a much larger proportion of the cancer upon prodrug administration. Repeat cycles of transduction and prodrug administration might allow elimination of larger nodules.

Although retroviral vectors are selective for replicating cells, it is not currently feasible to target gene transfer vectors to enter tumour cells selectively, thus viral vectors introduced into the peritoneal cavity could potentially enter normal cells, making them susceptible to prodrug also. To avoid this, promoters from genes selectively expressed in tumours will be used to control the expression of nitroreductase, so that the enzyme can only be synthesized in cancer cells.

Carcinoembryonic antigen (CEA) has been identified as a tumour-associated protein in ovarian carcinoma and the complete gene has been cloned, including upstream DNA [9]. Identification of the functional promoter regions within the upstream DNA, and their incorporation into gene therapy vectors will ensure that the nitroreductase is only expressed in tumour cells, and not in normal cells incidentally transduced by the vector.

30.3 IMMUNOLOGICAL APPROACH

The majority of spontaneously arising malignant tumours do not induce an effective host immune response and accumulating evidence suggests they are subject to selection pressure to avoid immune detection. The increased risk of tumour development in the immuno-suppressed suggests that T cell responses may be important in preventing the development of certain cancers, particularly

those with a viral aetiology. There are a few well documented cases of regression of advanced tumours, particularly of melanoma and renal carcinoma, where an immune response seems to have played a major role [10,11]. Is it possible that immunotherapeutic strategies could induce curative immune responses against a greater number of tumours?

One approach to tumour immunotherapy is to develop vaccines against specific tumour antigens. The concept of immunization comes from the field of infectious diseases, where ideally vaccination is performed before the pathogen is encountered, using antigens which are predictable and specific. Virally-induced cancers such as human papilloma virus-associated anogenital carcinomas express viral proteins which may be appropriate antigens for vaccination. However for the majority of cancers without a known viral aetiology, including ovarian cancer, the choice of antigen for vaccination is less apparent, although tumour-associated antigens recognized by CTLs have been identified in melanoma [12] and also in ovarian cancer [13], raising the possibility of patient immunization with specific tumour antigens.

An alternative strategy is to modify the cancer cells to enable them to act as efficient antigen presenting cells in their interactions with T cells. This would allow all the tumour antigens to become potential targets of the immune response without requiring any detailed knowledge of the precise antigenic make-up of the cell. A broadly based immune response would decrease the chance that tumour cell variants could escape destruction by loss of just one antigen.

It is well documented that many experimentally induced tumours express antigens that can mediate tumour rejection, largely dependent on cell-mediated

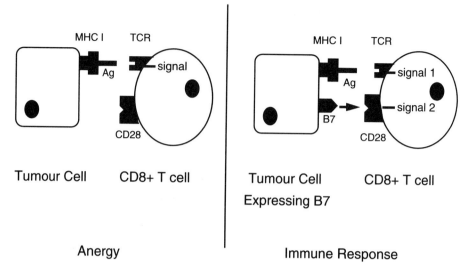

Anergy | Immune Response

Figure 30.2 Transduction of tumour cells with B7 will increase their capacity to elicit an immune response when presented as an autologous tumour cell vaccine.

responses with circulating antibodies playing only a minor role. Both T helper cells (CD3+/CD4+) and cytotoxic T lymphocytes (CD3+/CD8+) are involved in this process. For a tumour antigen to be recognized by CTLs it must be processed within the cell into small peptides. Those which are able to bind in the antigen-binding groove of the major histocompatibility complex (MHC) class I molecules are carried to the cell surface and displayed, where they may be recognized, in combination with the MHC, by the antigen receptor of CD8+ T cells. T helper cells recognize antigen released by tumour cells which has been taken up by antigen presenting cells, processed, and presented at the cell surface on MHC class II molecules. The major effector function of these cells is the secretion of cytokines which act on the same T cells and other cells including CTLs thereby amplifying the immune response.

Although it is accepted that human tumours are less immunogenic than the experimentally induced murine tumours, there is nevertheless reason to believe that tumour specific antigens exist and are presented by MHC proteins on human cancers. So why are the majority of malignant tumours not cured by an immune response?

An explanation has been offered which presents an exciting possibility for gene therapy [14]. Two types of signal are required for T cell activation. One is derived from interaction of the T cell receptor with peptides presented by the MHC class I and II molecules. The second signal is derived from the costimulatory pathway and failure to deliver this may lead to T cell clonal anergy or deletion. The costimulation signal is antigen non-specific and is delivered via T cell surface proteins CD28 or CTLA-4, dependent on interaction with a ligand, B7-1 (or its homologues B7-2 or B7-3) present on specialized antigen presenting cells. The genes for the B7 family of proteins have recently been cloned and encode 44–54kDa

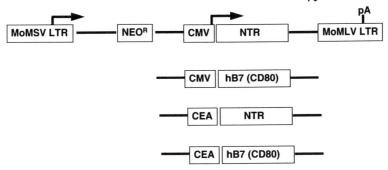

Retroviral vectors

Figure 30.3 Diagramatic representation of retroviral vectors:
CMV = Immediate, early promoter of CMV; CEA = Promoter region of CEA gene;
NTR = Nitroreductase gene; B7 = Gene for B7-1 protein;
NEO = Neomycin phosphotransferase gene; LTR = Retroviral long terminal repeat.

glycoproteins belonging to the immuno-globulin superfamily.

Although carcinomas usually express MHC class I molecules, most lack B7 suggesting that even when a tumour is expressing a potential rejection antigen it is unlikely to activate antitumour T cell responses (Figure 30.2). This hypothesis was tested in a mouse tumour line which expressed a tumour antigen encoded by the E7 gene of HPV 16 but did not express B7 (E7+B7-) [15]. Cells were transfected with the B7 gene (E7+B7+) and these and cells from the parental line were injected separately into immune-competent mice. Whereas the E7+B7- line was able to grow, the E7+B7+ cells were rejected. Mice which had rejected E7+B7+ cells were subsequently able to mount a cell-mediated immune response to E7+B7- cells suggesting that expression of B7 in tumour cells may allow the generation of a tumour specific immune response. Thus, using viral vectors to achieve efficient delivery and expression of B7-1 in tumour cells, they may be enabled to act as efficient antigen-presenting cells and induce a cytotoxic T cell response.

Gene transfer might be achieved most easily using tumour material removed at surgery (*ex vivo*); these could be used to stimulate T cells *ex vivo* which would subsequently be infused to the patient. More simply, the transduced tumour cells could be irradiated then returned to the patient as an autologous vaccine. In some instances it might be possible or desirable to deliver the B7 vector directly to tumour deposits within the patient. Additional local stimulation of immune responses could be achieved by additional modification of the tumour vaccine to express cytokines such as IL2, IL12, and GM-CSF.

30.4 EXPERIMENTAL PROTOCOLS

30.4.1 VDEPT

The nitroreductase coding sequence has been inserted into the LNCX retroviral vector [16], under the transcriptional control of the strong constitutive immediate early promoter of cytomegalovirus (CMV). The construct also contains the prokaryotic neomycin phos-photransferase gene, which confers resistance to G418 in eukaryotic cells (Figure 30.3)

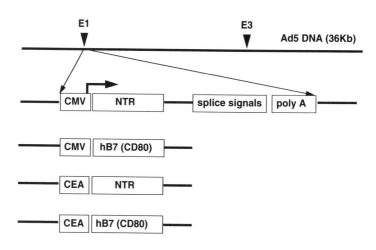

Adenoviral vectors

Figure 30.4 Diagramatic representation of adenoviral vectors:
CMV = Immediate, early promoter of CMV; CEA = Promoter region of CEA gene;
NTR = Nitroreductase gene; B7 = Gene for B7-1 protein;
NEO = Neomycin phosphotransferase gene; polyA = Polyadenylation.

This has been transfected as plasmid DNA into established tumour cell lines in tissue culture. Ovarian, pancreatic and colorectal cells expressing nitroreductase have been shown to be killed upon exposure to low concentrations of CB1954. The construct has been introduced into retroviral packaging cell lines, leading to the generation of retroviral particles, and in cells transduced with the virus, nitroreductase has been detected in the cytoplasm by immuno-fluorescence, and the expressing cells are killed by low concentrations of CB1954. A construct incorporating a short section from the CEA promoter instead of the CMV sequence has been produced and will be similarly tested in CEA-expressing and non-expressing cell lines.

When the system has been fully characterized and optimized *in vitro*, the effectiveness of the therapy will be tested using animal models. Initially, human cell lines transduced *in vitro* will be used to generate tumours in immunodeficient nude or SCID mice, for treatment with prodrug. Cell mixing experiments will be used to characterize bystander cell killing *in vivo*. Subsequently, the efficiency of transduction of tumour cells in established intraperitoneal ovarian tumour xenografts will be examined following intraperitoneal injection of the viral vectors. Localization of nitroreductase enzyme activity will be monitored in the tumour and in normal tissues, and pharmacological assays of the prodrug and its metabolites carried out. The aim of these experiments is to optimize parameters for efficient transduction and maximize prodrug efficacy *in vivo*.

30.4.2 IMMUNOLOGICAL APPROACH

The sequence encoding human B7-1 has similarly been cloned into the LNCX vector, and used to produce retrovirus. Strong expression of B7 has been detected in cell lines transfected with the DNA or transduced with the virus. The virus will be used to transduce freshly isolated ovarian tumour cells, which will be used to stimulate autologous lymphocytes isolated from either peripheral blood, ascitic fluid or solid tumour. Non-transduced tumour cells or cells transduced with the parental vector lacking B7 will also be used in order to compare the effect of B7 on CTL stimulation. *In vivo*, animal studies will require the use of murine tumours in immune competent animals. An attractive possibility is to use tumours which arise in transgenic mice as a model system [17].

Adenoviral vectors are also being developed for both therapeutic approaches, as these can be produced in much higher titre and should allow transduction of virtually 100% of a target cell population irrespective of replication status (Figure 30.4). Although, unlike retroviruses, adenoviral vectors do not integrate in transduced cells and so can give only transient expression lasting for a few days to weeks, this should be sufficient for the intended therapeutic effects to be obtained.

30.5 CLINICAL STUDIES

Following the initial validation of the gene therapy approaches *in vitro* and in mouse models, the most active agents will be moved forward into phase I clinical trials. The nitroreductase expression viruses will necessarily be used directly *in vivo* via the intraperitoneal route. This will allow the homogeneous distribution of virus and prodrug within the compartment harbouring bulk tumour, leading to the generation of high activated drug concentrations locally. Immunotherapy using B7 modulation could involve reinfusion of *in vitro* activated T cells; the use of *in vitro* transduced and irradiated tumour cells as an autologous vaccine; the direct administration of virus to residual tumour; or a combination of these. Phase I

studies will be undertaken involving the administration of each of the planned therapeutic strategies to about 30 patients.

The aim of the studies will be to furnish data on toxicity, dosage and scheduling of the gene therapy and to assess the biological and clinical end points. Biological end points include pharmacokinetic studies of prodrug/active metabolite in the peritoneal fluid and blood; estimation of the expression of therapeutic genes in ovarian cancer cells washed from the peritoneum at intervals and assessment of the cytotoxic T cell response using lymphocytes collected from the peripheral blood and peritoneal cavity. Clinical endpoints comprise bulk of disease and tumour markers. These initial studies will be performed in patients with relatively advanced cancer but once satisfactory endpoints along with dosage, scheduling and toxicity have been established, it will be possible to extend the therapies into an adjuvant setting to follow optimal conventional therapy.

REFERENCES

1. McArdle, C.S., Kerr, D.J., O'Gorman, P. *et al.* (1994). Pharmacokinetic study of 5-fluorouracil in a novel dialysate solution: a long-term intraperitoneal treatment approach for advanced colorectal carcinoma. *Br. J. Cancer* **70**, 762-6.
2. Harris, J.D., Gutierrez, A.A., Hurst, H.C, *et al.* (1994). Gene therapy for cancer using tumour-specific prodrug activation. *Gene Ther.* **1**, 170-5.
3. Cobb, L.M., Connors, T.A., Elson, L.A. *et al.* (1954). 2,4-Dinitro-5-ethylene-iminobenz-amide (CB1954): a potent and selective inhibitor of growth of the Walker carcinoma 256. *Biochem. Pharmacol.* **18**, 1519-27.
4. Boland, M.P., Knox, R.J.and Roberts, J.J. (1991). The differences in kinetics of rat and human DT diaphorase result in a

differential sensitivity of derived cell lines to CB1954 (5-(aziridin-1-yl)-2,4-dinitrobenzamide). *Biochem. Pharmacol.* **41**, 867-75.

5. Roberts, J.J., Friedlos, F. and Knox, R.J. (1986). CB1954 (2,4-dinitro-5-aziridinyl benzamide) becomes an interstrand crosslinking agent in Walker tumour cells. *Biochem. Biophys. Res. Comm.* **140**, 1073-8.

6. Anlezark, G.M., Melton, R.G., Sherwood, R.F. *et al.* (1992). The bioactivation of CB 1954. I. Purification and properties of a nitroreductase enzyme from *Escherichia coli*- a potential enzyme for antibody-directed enzyme prodrug therapy (ADEPT). *Biochem. Pharmacol.* **44**, 2289-95.

7. Harris, J.D., Gutierrez, A.A., Hurst, H.C., *et al.* (1994). Gene therapy for cancer using tumor-specific prodrug activation. *Gene Ther.* **1**, 170-5.

8. Knox, R.J., Friedlos, F., Jarman, M. and Roberts, J.J. (1988). A new cytotoxic, DNA interstrand crosslinking agent, 5-(aziridin-1-yl)-4-hydroxylamino-2-nitrobenzamide, is formed from 5-(aziridin-1-yl)-2,4-dinitro-benzamide (CB 1954) by a nitroreductase enzyme in Walker carcinoma cells. *Biochem. Pharmacol.* **37**, 4661-9.

9. Richards, C.A., Wolberg, A.S. and Huber, B.E. (1993). The transcriptional control region of the human carcinoembryonic antigen gene: DNA sequence and homology studies. *J. DNA Seq. Map.* **4**, 185-96.

10. Knuth, A., Wölfel, T. and Meyer zum Büschenfelde, K.-H. (1992). T-cell responses to human malignant tumours. In *Cancer Surveys. A new look at tumour immunology*. McMichael, A. & Bodmer, W. (ed.). CSHL Press: Cold Spring Harbor, NY. pp 39-52.

11. Oliver, R. and Nouri, A. (1992). T-cell immune response to cancer in humans and its relevance for immunodiagnosis and therapy. In *Cancer Surveys. A new look at tumour immunology*. McMichael, A. & Bodmer, W. (eds.). CSHL Press: Cold Spring Harbor, NY, pp 173-204.

12. Boon, T., De Plaen, E., Lurquin, C. *et al.* (1992). Identification of tumour rejection antigens recognized by T lymphocytes. In *Cancer Surveys. A new look at tumour immunology*. McMichael, A. & Bodmer, W. (eds.). CSHL Press: Cold Spring Harbor, NY. pp 23-37.

13. Ioannides, C.G., Platsoucas, C.D., Rashed, S. *et al.* (1991). Tumor cytolysis by lymphocytes infiltrating ovarian malignant ascites. *Cancer Res.* **51**, 4257-65.

14. Chen, L., Linsley, P.S. and Hellström, K.E. (1993). Costimulation of T cells for tumour immunity. *Immunol. Today* **14**, 483-6.

15. Chen, L., Ashe, S., Brady, W.A., *et al.* (1992). Costimulation of antitumour immunity by the B7 counterreceptor for the T lymphocyte molecules CD28 and CTLA-4. *Cell* **71**, 1093-102.

16. Miller, A.D. and Rosman, G.J. (1989). Improved retroviral vectors for gene transfer and expression. *BioTechniques* **7**, 980-8.

17. Searle, P.F., Thomas, D.P., Faulkner, K.B. and Tinsley, J.M. (1994). Stomach cancer in transgenic mice expressing human papillomavirus type 16 early region genes from a keratin promoter. *J. Gen. Virol.* **75**, 1125-37.

Chapter 31

Immune gene therapy: angiogenesis and apoptosis

William P. COLLINS

31.1 INTRODUCTION

Normal ovaries undergo profound changes in form and function during each ovarian cycle. The crucial events are the expulsion of an egg from a mature follicle (*i.e.* ovulation) and the eventual regression of the corpus luteum. Both processes have many similarities to an inflammatory or immune rejection reaction. In particular there are intense local changes in the production of factors which enhance or inhibit neo-angiogenesis, cell proliferation or cell death (apoptosis), and the type, distribution and concentration of leukocytes [1-3]. Monocytes differentiate into macrophages within the ovary and probably play an important role in the processes of phagocytosis and tissue remodelling, and as antigen presenting cells (APCs). There is at least a five-fold increase in the density of macrophages in the thecal layer of the pre-ovulatory follicle and in the corpus luteum during regression. A large proportion of the cells appear to be immunologically active and express MHC class I and class II molecules. Lymphocytes, especially T-helper cells, are present in relatively low numbers throughout the ovarian cycle [4]. Physiological antigens might be produced by the egg during the resumption of meiosis and by the

programmed death of theca or granulosa cells.

The early development of epithelial cell ovarian cancer has some similarities to the growth of a follicle. Both processes involve a rapid increase in cell numbers (either by mitosis or an inhibition of apoptosis), tissue remodelling and neo-angiogenesis. In contrast, however, established carcinogenesis is often associated with a vast increase in the number of local lymphocytes (particularly CD4+ T-helper (T_H) cells and CD8+ precytotoxic T cells).

An example of such tumour infiltrating lymphocytes (TILs) is shown in Figure 31.1 and is consistent with the hypothesis that the immune system has been selectively, but incompletely activated. There is now compelling evidence for the presence of ovarian tumour antigens and the specific activation of the immune system in human ovarian carcinomas [5].

The immediate aim of immune gene therapy for ovarian cancer is to enhance the tumour specific activation of the immune system and thus destroy the malignantly transformed cells. This approach is likely to complement conventional therapies (including surgery) and new approaches arising from a knowledge of factors affecting neo-angiogenesis and apoptosis. One longer

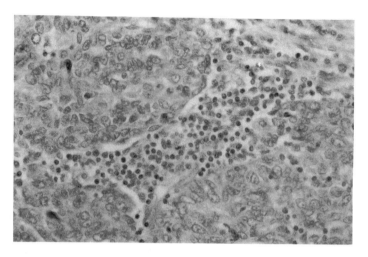

Figure 31.1 An example of lymphocytes infiltrating a serous cystadenocarcinoma.

term aim of immune gene therapy is to produce vaccines which will prevent the development of hereditary forms of the disease.

31.2 IMMUNE GENE THERAPY

Immune gene therapy is a development of immunotherapy and has arisen from the recognition of additional factors that are required to initiate or augment an effective immune response [6].

31.2.1 NORMAL IMMUNE RESPONSE

Activation of the cytotoxic T lymphocytes against foreign proteins requires the processing and expression of appropriate fragments within grooves of the MHC molecules expressed on the surface of professional APCs – notably macrophages and dendritic cells [7]. The APCs display these antigenic peptides in conjunction with molecules of the MHC classes I and II and β_2-microglobulin [8,9]. Co-stimulatory molecules (including B7.1 and B7.2) are also required for the initiation of antigen specific and MHC restricted cell-mediated and

humoral (immunoglobulin based) responses [10-13]. There are also MHC independent natural killer (NK) cells which are able to eliminate some tumour cells [14].

Antigen specific CD4+ T-helper and CD8+ precytotoxic T-cells are activated by binding to the APCs through a complex of receptors including the constitutively expressed CD28 and the inducible CTLA-4 receptor, both of which bind the B7 family of costimulatory molecules.

The combined engagement of the T-cell receptor and activation of the accessory molecules (*e.g.* CD28) results in the increased production of a variety of cytokines including IL-2, IL-4, IL-12, IFNγ, TNFβ and GM-CSF. The nature, level and combination of the cytokines produced by the CD4+ T-helper cells determine the precise consequence of the interaction and whether the activation will result in a cellular or a humoral response. For example the production of IL-2 and IL-4 furthers the activation and proliferation of antigen specific CD8+ cytotoxic T lymphocytes (CTLs) and antibody producing B cells, respectively.

290

The recognition of an MHC bound antigen in the absence of co-stimulating signals results in anergy, that is, an active state of antigen specific T cell dormancy [15,16]. This state can be reversed by the appropriate administration of IL-2 [17]. However, whilst the activation phase of immune stimulation requires the presence of the costimulatory factors, the effector phase destruction of the target antigen, by either cell mediated or humoral responses, is independent of the presence of these accessory factors.

31.2.2 IMMUNE RESPONSE TO OVARIAN CANCER

Ovarian cancer antigens might not evoke a complete immune response due to loss of components in the antigen processing or presentation complex [18,19], defects in the immune activation mechanisms, or the production of immunosuppressive agents by the tumour. In addition, the interaction between T-cell receptors and the MHC/antigen complexes expressed on the tumour cell surface, but in the absence of adequate accessory signals, may have resulted in the establishment of an anergic state. Such anergy could also be the product of T-cell receptor engagement by weak antigens. Therefore, immune gene therapy of ovarian carcinoma should be designed to overcome these potential problems.

31.2.3 APPROACHES TO TREATMENT

One approach to immune gene therapy for cancer involves the use of autologous TILs transfected with a cytokine gene (*e.g.* IL-2 or TNFα) [20]. CD8+ TILs have been directed to ovarian cells expressing the 38kDa folate binding protein by retroviral infection with a chimeric gene construct encoding an antifolate binding protein monoclonal antibody (MOv18 V_H and V_L genes) coupled to the common γ subunit of the IgG/IgE F_c

receptor [21].

The transfer of cytokine genes into tumour cells is another possible way of improving the immune response [22]. The expression of IL-2 or IL-4 by tumour cells has been shown to reduce tumour uptake in experimental animals by enhancing the activity of CD8+ CTLs, or eosinophilic granulocytes and macrophages, respectively [23]. The transfer of genes for immune modulators other than cytokines also results in the activation of the immune system against tumour antigens. A promising group of genes belong to the B7 family (B7.1/CD80 and B7.2/CD86) because their products are essential immune co-stimulatory molecules.

The Immune Gene Therapy Group at King's College Hospital is undertaking a systematic study of the potential efficacy of the co-stimulatory genes in combination with various cytokines for the immune gene therapy of ovarian and other cancers.

31.2.4 MOUSE MODELS

There is no inbred animal model for the study of epithelial ovarian cancer. Consequently it is not possible to study the effects of cytokine or B7 gene transfer on the tumourigenicity of cancer cell lines in syngeneic animals. There has, however, been one report on the inhibited growth of Chinese hamster ovary (CHO) cells transfected with murine IL-4 in nude mice [24].

We initiated our work on immune gene therapy by studying a murine malignant melanoma cell line and demonstrated a progressive increase in the survival rates of mice injected with 10^4 B16F10 cells (which do not express the MHC class I or II complex) infected with Molony murine virus based retroviral vectors encoding mouse B7.1, IL-2, or IL-4. Whilst the expression of B7.1 alone had no detectable effect on the rate of tumour formation, expression of either IL-2 or IL-4 did delay the onset of tumour formation [25]. The expression of any two of these genes further increased the delay in the onset of tumour formation. The combined expression of all three immune modulators totally inhibited tumour formation by the modified cells (unpublished observations).

We have also studied tumour formation in syngeneic mice injected subcutaneously with 10^4 wild type NC breast adeno-carcinoma cells (which express the MHC class I antigens) and in NC cells transduced with the retroviral vector (M_3P) or NC cells expressing murine IL-2, B7.1, or both IL-2 and B7.1. The combination of genes increased the time of disease free survival for a group of 10 animals with from 12 to 50 days. More importantly a distant vaccination (subcutaneous injection in the opposite flank) with irradiated NC cells expressing both B7.1 and IL2 was 80% successful in treating a similar group of animals with established NC tumours [26]. The treatment, however, could not be used as a vaccine to inhibit the uptake of tumours, or prevent the growth of distant metastases after the primary tumour had been removed surgically [26].

31.2.5 NEW VECTORS

We have recently constructed new retroviral vectors containing two different internal ribosome entry sites (IRES) from polio and ECM viruses. One such vector allows the combined expression of B7.1 and IL-2 in target cells which can be selected by their resistance to specific drugs due to expression of the appropriate drug resistance gene placed downstream of the second IRES. The co-ordinated expression of the transduced genes from a single vector has a number of important advantages. These include the simultaneous expression of the transduced genes without interference from internal promoters as well as reliable expression of the upstream genes in the infected target cells

which have been isolated by their expression of the downstream selectable marker gene. This system is being examined for its ability to deliver additional genes, either as single components (by construction of triple IRES vectors), or by the expression of biologically active chimeric immune modulators. Our most immediate aim is the construction of vectors encoding B7.1/IL-2 and herpes simplex virus - thymidine kinase (HSV-*tk*)/zeomycin.

Previous studies with tumour cells expressing HSV-*tk* have shown that the administration of gancyclovir destroys the *tk* expressing cells and the wild type tumour cells – possibly by the bystander effect or appropriate antigen presentation after phagocytosis [27]. We wish to exploit these effects in combination with B7.1/IL-2 vaccination in order to obtain higher levels of immune stimulation (due to the immunogenicity of *tk* and particularly its chimeric constructs), as well as introducing an important safety feature enabling the gancyclovir induced ablation of the transduced cells.

31.2.6 HUMAN OVARIAN CANCER

Human ovarian epithelial cancer cells are difficult to establish in culture. Consequently, attention is being focused on the potential for allogeneic (cells from a different patient(s)) rather than autologous immune gene therapy. Studies have shown that expression of B7.1 by ovarian carcinoma cell lines increases their ability to induce the activation of allogeneic T lymphocytes [28]. Our studies have shown that this action is accompanied by the phosphorylation of tyrosine in specific targets of CD28 activation. Ovarian carcinoma cell lines expressing both B7.1 and IL2 have now been generated and are being analysed in various allogeneic and autologous *in vitro* immune stimulation assays.

31.2.7 POTENTIAL PROBLEMS

There are many potential problems with immune gene therapy for ovarian cancer. For example, some malignant cells might not produce the MHC class I complex or β_2-microglobulin. This limitation may be addressed by the transfer of genes to produce a given MHC molecule (matched or mismatched) or β_2-microglobulin in tumour cells. The expression of a matched MHC molecule by the tumour cells, in the absence of other manipulations is unlikely to result in immune stimulation. By contrast expression of a mismatched MHC is likely to result in inflammatory responses culminating in better immune stimulation. However, this reaction will still leave the problem of tumour recognition by the HLA restricted CTLs unresolved and any therapeutic response will be dependent on the induction of non-HLA restricted immune reactions such as NK activation and humoral responses.

Allogeneic vaccination will be dependent on the induction of inflammatory responses and the indirect presentation of the shared tumour antigens (assuming the presence of such antigens) by the infiltrating APCs. This approach assumes not only the presence of shared tumour antigens, but the active presentation of such an antigen by allogeneic HLA molecules in a manner capable of inducing immune reactions against the autologous tumour. However, the presence of common HLA molecules suggests that presentation of shared antigens by HLA molecules common to the tumour and the vaccinating allogeneic cells could allow such allogeneic cell vaccines to induce antigen specific and HLA restricted, as well as unrestricted, immune responses. All such vaccination strategies remain dependent on two important requirements:
1. The presence of shared tumour antigens.

2. The ability of the immune system to overcome various measures which allow tumour cells to evade immune surveillance. This includes production of immune suppressive cytokines by the cancer.

Finally, adverse reactions may be induced by non-specific immune reactions due to the presence of common antigens in tumour and normal cells. However, these potential, sometimes theoretical, problems must be considered in relation to the lethal nature of the disease and the known adverse effects and limitations of conventional treatments.

31.2.8 COMPLEMENTARY STRATEGIES

Over the last 15 years we have developed and evaluated an ultrasound based screening procedure for early ovarian cancer in asymptomatic women from the community or cancer families [29] and in referred patients from gynaecological outpatient clinics. This core activity enables us to study the biochemical basis of neo-angiogenesis in persistent ovarian tumours and apoptosis in cells (from ovarian cyst and peritoneal fluids) in culture.

We have also noted with concern the number of peritoneal cancers reported at follow-up of women with a family history of ovarian cancer (up to 30%). Consequently, we have initiated a programme to develop complementary cell specific therapies for ovarian and peritoneal cancer based on immune gene therapy or oral pro-drug (or drug) chemotherapy (which have arisen from studies of neo-angiogenic and apoptotic factors). A sonographic image of a serous cystadenocarcinoma illustrating these two processes is shown in Figure 31.2. Active areas of growth (by mitosis or the inhibition of apoptosis) appear dense white, and areas of neo-vascularization are characterized by low resistance, high velocity blood flow.

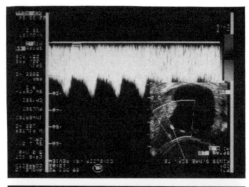

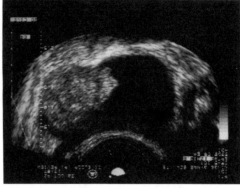

Figure 31.2 Transvaginal sonogram of an ovary containing a serous cystadenocarcinoma. (a - upper print) B-mode imaging showing irregular outline of tumour with dense (white) areas of rapid growth. (b - lower print) colour Doppler imaging with flow velocity waveforms from an area of neo-angiogenesis.

31.3 ANGIOGENESIS AND APOPTOSIS

There is now convincing evidence that neo-angiogenesis and the inhibition of apoptosis are essential components of tumour growth and spread [30].

31.3.1 ANGIOGENIC FACTORS

We have studied the expression of mRNA for known angiogenic factors – including platelet derived endothelial cell growth factor (now known to by thymidine phosphorylase) and vascular endothelial growth factor (VEGF) in benign and malignant ovarian tumours. To date 25 tumours (7 benign, 1 borderline malignancy and 18 malignant) have been examined before surgery for areas of high velocity blood flow by transvaginal ultrasonography with colour Doppler imaging. Ovarian RNA was subsequently extracted from areas of high velocity flow (*i.e.* tissues with a positive scan result) or from solid areas or septa in tissues with a negative scan result.

A ribonuclease protection assay was used to assess the expression of thymidine phosphorylase and VEGF. One benign and 17 malignant tumours (including the borderline malignancy) gave a positive scan result. There was a significant difference

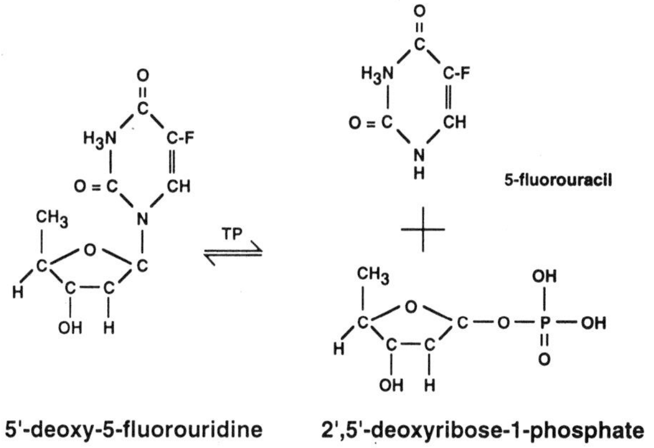

Figure 31.3 Enzymatic activity of thymidine phosphorylase (TP).

between the expression of mRNA for thymidine phosphorylase and VEGF between scan positive and scan negative tissues and between benign and malignant tumours. We conclude that areas of angiogenesis with high blood velocity in ovarian tumours are associated with increased expression of angiogenic factors – particularly thymidine phosphorylase [31].

31.3.2 THYMIDINE PHOSPHORYLASE

Platelet-derived endothelial cell growth factor (PD-ECGF) was originally isolated as the sole endothelial cell mitogenic activity in platelets. The factor was subsequently shown to have a similar structure and activity to thymidine phosphorylase [32]. The enzyme is a non-glycosylated intracellular protein (molecular weight 45kDa) which lacks a secretion signal peptide and has no heparin binding activity. Thymidine phosphorylase (sometimes called uridine or pyrimidine phosphorylase) effects the reversible breakdown of thymidine to thymine and 2'-deoxyribose-1-phosphate. The structure of the substrate and products is shown in Figure 31.3. The thymidine phosphorylase activity of PD-ECGF is involved in the proliferation of endothelial cells [33] and is associated with chemotaxis.

Thymidine has been shown to inhibit neo-angiogenesis *in vitro*, whereas thymine and β-aminobutyric acid (a metabolite of thymine) are stimulatory (unpublished observations).

31.3.3 APOPTOSIS

The rate of cell proliferation has traditionally been perceived as the most important determinant of tumour growth. More recently, however, it has be come apparent that much spontaneous and induced tumour loss occurs by apoptosis [34]. This process is characterized by cell shrinkage, chromatin condensation and systematic DNA cleavage. Apoptotic cells are rapidly engulfed by phagocytes, thus minimizing the inflammatory reaction to degradative cell contents, and possibly enhancing the immune response [35]. Apoptosis is distinct from necrosis which involves the depletion of ATP and metabolic collapse leading to cell swelling, rupture and inflammation.

We have shown that cells derived from cystic and peritoneal fluid from patients with ovarian cancer undergo apoptosis. Of particular interest is the additional finding that up to 2% of cells are binucleate. In some of these cells one of the nuclei exhibits morphological signs of apoptosis. The significance of this finding is being

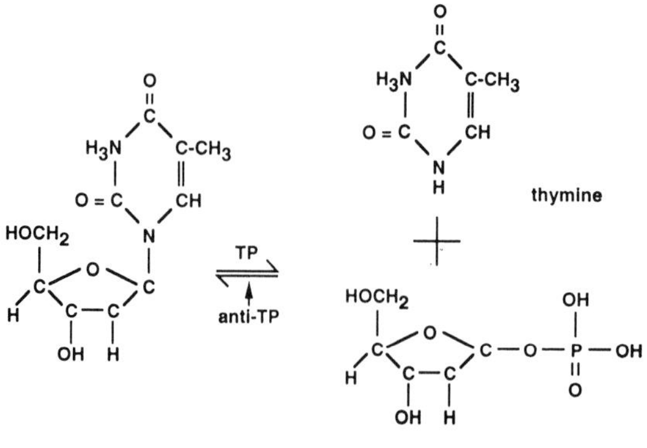

Figure 31.4 An example of prodrug therapy involving thymidine phosphorylase.

investigated. There is also some evidence that thymidine phosphorylase might inhibit apoptosis (unpublished observations) and thereby play a pivotal role in both processes.

31.3.4 THERAPEUTIC POSSIBILITIES

We have used the information that malignant ovarian tumours express relatively large amounts of thymidine phosphorylase to initiate a research program based on the probability that the enzyme can convert a prodrug into an active anti-cancer compound at the target tissue (by analogy with anti-viral treatment which involves the localized production of viral thymidine kinase). Two reports from Japan have indicated that 5'-deoxy-5-fluorouridine can be used in this way [36,37]. The reaction is shown in Figure 31.4. Thus thymidine phosphorylase is thought to release 5-fluorouracil from the prodrug in tumour cells. Another study has shown that 5-fluorouracil can induce apoptosis in cancer of the pancreas, and may also inhibit neo-angiogenesis. This possibility is being explored for ovarian cancer. We also plan to raise monoclonal antibodies against the catalytic site of thymidine phosphorylase, sequence the binding site and synthesize a peptide which would inhibit enzymatic activity. This agent

might also inhibit neo-angiogenesis and enhance apoptosis – thus inhibiting tumour growth and metastases. Current drugs that inhibit angiogenesis have been reviewed [38].

31.4 DISCUSSION

Preliminary data has been obtained from animal models to support the hypothesis that malignant cells transfected with genes for B7.1, IL-2 and IL-4 might complete the activation of the immune system and lead to the destruction of unmodified tumour cells. Human ovarian cancer cells have been transfected with B7.1 and IL-2; the products are expressed, and *in vitro* tests are being used to study T-cell activation and proliferation. The cytotoxic T-lymphocytes are being tested *in vitro* for their ability to lyse syngeneic and allogeneic ovarian cancer.

Concurrently, better vectors for gene transfer are being developed. In particular it is encouraging that various adenoviruses can deliver genes to non-proliferating cells. The use of such vectors would speed up the procedure for reagent preparation and reduce the expense of testing vectors for replication competent viruses. The development of vectors that are cell specific would also enhance the practicability of immune gene therapy [39,40]. There is also some evidence that certain vectors can effect gene transfer after direct injection into the cancerous tissue.

There are, however, some potential problems and limitations to immune gene therapy for ovarian cancer. Consequently, we believe that the systematic use of two complementary procedures may provide the best approach in the short term. Conventional chemotherapy tends to destroy both tumour cells and inactivate the immune system.

We are attempting to develop treatments which either predominantly activate the immune system (immune gene therapy) or destroy tumour cells, but not leukocytes. There is the possibility that the combination of immune gene therapy with prodrug (or drug) therapy (through the activity of thymidine kinase or thymidine phosphorylase) might achieve this objective. There is no doubt that the lack of an inbred animal model for ovarian cancer inhibits the rapid development of alternative and complementary therapeutic procedures. The production of a vaccine against hereditary ovarian cancer remains a long term goal, and awaits the identification of appropriate antigens.

ACKNOWLEDGEMENTS

The Immune Gene Therapy Programme at King's College Hospital and King's College School of Medicine and Dentistry is directed by Dr Farzin Farzaneh (Dept. of Molecular Medicine) and involves the collaboration of many colleagues including: Joop Gäken, David Darling, Marcel Kuiper, Amanda Barnard and Paul Towner, Dept. of Molecular Medicine; Simon Hollingsworth, William Hirst, Andrea Buggins and Guhlam Mufti, Dept. of Haematological Medicine; Mark Peakman and Diego Verani, Dept. of Immunology; Stephen Humphries, Dept. of Histopathology and Juliet McMullen, Karina Reynolds and Darren Stevenson, Department of Obstetrics and Gynaecology. Aspects of the work on ovarian cancer are supported by the Linbury Trust, Wellbeing and the Joint Research Committee of King's College Hospital.

REFERENCES

1. Espey, L.L. (1980) Ovulation as an inflammatory reaction - a hypothesis. *Biol. Reprod.* **22**, 73-106.
2. Espey, L.L. (1994) Current status of the hypothesis that mammalian ovulation is comparable to an inflammatory reaction. *Biol. Reprod.* **50**, 233-8.
3. Brännström, M. and Norman, R.J. (1993) Involvement of leucocytes and cytokines in the ovulatory process and corpus luteum function. *Hum. Reprod.* **8**, 1762-75.
4. Bränström, M., Pascoe, V., Norman, R.J. and McClure, N. (1994) Localization of leucocyte subsets in the follicle wall and in the corpus luteum throughout the human menstrual cycle. *Fertil. Steril.* **61**, 488-95.
5. Kuiper, M., Peakman, M. and Farzaneh, F. (1995) Ovarian tumour antigens as potential targets for immune gene therapy. *Gene Ther.* **2**, 7-15.
6. Schwartz, R.H. (1992) Costimulation of T lymphocytes: the role of CD 28, CTLA-4 and B7/BB1 in interleukin-2 production and immunotherapy. *Cell* **71**, 1065-8.
7. Huang, A.Y.C., Gombek, P., Ahmadzadeh, M. *et al.* (1944) Role of bone marrow-derived cells in presenting MCH class I-restricted tumor antigens. *Science* **264**, 961-5.
8. Goldberg, A.L. and Rock, K.L. (1992) Proteolysis, proteasomes and antigen presentation. *Nature* **357**, 375-9.
9. Clark, E.A. and Ledbetter, J.A. (1994) How B and T cells talk to each other. *Nature* **367**, 425-8.

10. Chen, L., Ashe, S., Brady, W.A., *et al.* (1992) Costimulation of antitumor immunity by the B7 counter receptor for the T lymphocyte molecules CD28 and CTLA-4. *Cell* **71**, 1093-102.

11. Townsend, S.E. and Allison, J.P. (1993) Tumor rejection after direct costimulation of CD8$^+$ T cells by B7-transfected melanoma cells. *Science* **259**, 368-70.

12. Azuma, M., Ito, D., Yagita, H., *et al.* (1993) B7 antigen is a second ligand for CTLA-4 and CD28. *Nature* **366**, 76-9.

13. Freeman, G.J., Gribben, J.G., Boussiotis, V.A., *et al.* (1993) Cloning of B7-2: CTLA-4 counter receptor that costimulates human T cell proliferation. *Science* **262**, 909-11.

14. Möller, P. and Hämmerling, G.J. (1992) The role of surface HLA-A,B,C molecules in tumour immunity. *Cancer Surv.* **13**, 101-27.

15. Schwartz, R.H. (1990) A cell culture model for T lymphocyte clonal anergy. *Science* **248**, 1349-56.

16. Lombardi, G., Sidhu, S., Batchelor, R. and Lechter, R. (1994) Anergic T cells as suppressor cells *in vitro*. *Science* **264**, 1587-9.

17. Beverly, B., Kang, S.M., Lenardo, M.J. and Schwartz, R.H. (1992) Reversal of *in vitro* T cell clonal anergy by IL-2 stimulation. *Int. Immunol.* **4**, 661-71.

18. Restifo, N.P., Esquivel, F., Kawakami, Y. *et al.* (1993) Indentification of cancers deficient in antigen processing. *J. Exp. Med.* **177**, 265-72.

19. Vegh, Z., Wang, P., Vanky, F. and Klein, E. (1933) Selectively down-regulated expression of major histocompatibility complex class I alleles in human solid tumours. *Cancer Res.* **53**, 2416-20.

20. Yannelli, J.R., Hyatt, C., Johnson, S. *et al.* (1993) Characteristics of human tumour cell lines transduced with the cDNA encoding either tumour necrosis factor a (TNF-a) or interleukin -2 (IL-2). *J.*

Immunol. Meth. **161**, 77-90.

21. Hwu, P., Shafer, G.E., Treisman, J. *et al.* (1993) Lysis of ovarian cancer cells by human lymphocytes redirected with a chimeric gene composed of an antibody variable region and the F_c receptor g chain. *J. Exp. Med.* **178**, 361-6.

22. Paul, W.E. and Seder, R.A. (1994) Lymphocyte responses and cytokines. *Cell* **76**, 241-51.

23. Colombo, M.P. and Forni, G. (1994) Cytokine gene transfer in tumor inhibition and tumor therapy: where are we now? *Immunol. Today* **15**, 48-51.

24. Platzer, C., Richter, G., Uberla, K. *et al.* (1992) Interleukin-4-mediated tumor suppression in nude mice involves interferon-g. *Eur. J. Immunol.* **22**, 1729-33.

25. Hollingsworth, S.J., Darling, D., Gäken, J., *et al.* (1995). The therapeutic benefit of interleukin-2 and interleukin-4 transduction of murine B16F10 melanoma cells requires the expression of both cytokines by each cell. *Br. J. Cancer* submitted.

26. Gäken, J., Hollingsworth, S., Darling, D. *et al.* (1995) B7.1/IL-2 induced rejection of NC adenocarcinoma. *J. Exp. Med.* submitted.

27. Freeman, S.M., Abboud, C.N., Whartemby, K.A. *et al.* (1993) The 'bystander effect': tumor regression when a fraction of the tumor mass is genetically modified. *Cancer Res.* **53**, 5274-83.

28. Döhring, C., Angman, L., Spagnoli G. and Lanzavecchia, A. (1994) T-helper-and accessory-cell-independent cytotoxic responses to human tumor cells transfected with a B7 retroviral vector. *Int. J. Cancer* **57**, 754-9.

29. Bourne, T.H., Campbell, S., Reynolds, K.M., *et al.* (1993) Screening for early familial ovarian cancer with transvaginal ultrasonography and colour flow imaging. *BMJ* **306**, 1025-9.

30. Holmgren, L., O'Reilly, M.S. and Folkman, J. (1995) Dormancy of micrometastases: Balanced proliferation and apoptosis in the presence of angiogenesis suppression. *Nat. Med.* **1**, 149-53.

31. Reynolds, K., Farzaneh, F., Collins, W.P. *et al.* (1994) Association of ovarian malignancy with expression of platelet-derived endothelial cell growth factor. *J. Natl. Cancer Inst.*, **86**, 1234-8.

32. Moghaddam, A. and Bicknell, R. (1992) Expression of platelet-derived endomethial cell factor on Escherichia coli and confirmation of thymidine phosphorylase activity. *Biochemistry* **31**, 12141-6.

33. Finnis, C., Dodsworth, N., Pollit, C.E. *et al.* (1993) Thymidine phosphorylase activity of platelet-derived endothelial cell growth factors is responsible for endothelial cell mitogenicity. *Eur. J. Biochem.* **212**, 201-10.

34. Dive, C., Evans, C.A. and Whetton, A.D. (1992) Induction of apoptosis - new targets for cancer chemotherapy. *Cancer Biol.* **3**, 417-27.

35. Savill, J., Fadok, V., Henson, P. and Haslett, C. (1993) Phagocyte recognition of cells undergoing apoptosis. *Immunol. Today* **14**, 131-6.

36. Noda, K., Ikeda, M., Saito, Y. *et al.* (1991) Phase II study of 5'-DFUR in uterine cervical cancer and ovarian cancer. *Gan. To Kagaku Ryoho* **18**, 2557-65.

37. Eda, H., Fujimoto, K., Watanabe, S. *et al.* (1993) Cytokines induce thymidine phosphorylase expression in tumor cells and make them more susceptible to 5'-deoxy-5-fluorouridine. *Cancer Chemother. Pharmacol.* **32**, 338-8.

38. Fan, T-P, D. (1994) Angiosuppressive therapy for cancer. *TIPS* **15**, 33-5.

39. Kasahara, N., Dozy, M. and Kan, Y.W. (1994) Tissue-specific targeting of retroviral vectors through ligand-receptor interactions. *Science* **266**, 1373-5.

40. Sikora, K. (1994) Genetic approaches to cancer therapy. *Gene Ther.* **1**, 149-51.

Part Six

Conclusions and Recommendations

Chapter 32

Conclusions and recommendations

32.1 IS THERE AN IDENTIFIABLE OVARIAN PRE-CANCER?

IMMUNOCYTOCHEMISTRY AND MORPHOLOGY OF OVARIAN SURFACE EPITHELIUM

1.1 Immunofluorescent studies show that cultured surface epithelial cells from apparently normal ovaries from patients with and without a family history of ovarian cancer, show differences in their immunophenotype. In cells from patients with a family history there is persistent expression of cytokeratin but reduced or absent expression of intracellular collagen.

1.2 Expression of the epithelial differentiation marker CA125 is increased in cultured cells from those cases with a family history.

1.3 Cells may be grown in a 3-dimensional collagen sponge matrix, which allows them to reproduce their *in vivo* morphology. Ovarian surface epithelium (OSE) from women without a family history of ovarian cancer, was found to undergo epithelio-mesenchymal conversion in the matrix: OSE cells were dispersed in an abundant extracellular matrix. By contrast, ovarian cancer cells retained their epithelial phenotypes, and were able to form, for example, cysts and papillae. OSE cells from women with family histories of ovarian

cancer also retained their epithelial morphology. In addition, OSE cells from women without family histories were able to contract the sponge matrix. This phenomenon is analogous to wound contraction by fibroblasts *in vivo*. Cells from OSE of women with family histories, as well as cells from ovarian cancers, could not contract the sponges.

1.4 Thus, apparently normal surface epithelium from women with familial ovarian cancer risk appears to have a reduced capacity for epithelio-mesenchymal conversion in response to explantation into culture.

1.5 Reduced responsiveness to environmental signals may represent a very early change in ovarian neoplastic progression. These changes may also reflect a defect or an alteration in the capacity of the cells to undergo repair responses.

1.6 Immunohistochemical studies using a panel of antibodies show that cytokeratins 7,18,19 and 20 but not cytokeratins 10 and 13, are expressed in primary mucinous cystadenocarcinoma of the ovary. This may have practical application in the differentiation between a primary mucinous tumour of the ovary and a colonic metastasis.

1.7 The immunophenotypic diversity of serous papillary adenocarcinoma of the ovary compared to normal surface

303

epithelium has been studied using antibodies to proliferating cell nuclear antigen (PCNA), mib1 and p53. Invasive tumour shows expression with each of these markers, while surface epithelium shows little or no mib1 or p53 expression. Evidence for a transitional stage has been provided. The surface epithelium shows uniform expression of PCNA.

1.8 On the basis of immunohistochemical findings alternative pathways of neoplastic progression have been tentatively suggested:

(a) Normal surface epithelium → Borderline tumour → Invasive tumour

(b) Normal surface epithelium → Invasive tumour (*de novo*)

(c) Normal surface epithelium → Borderline tumour (low malignant potential with no further progression)

Mechanism (c) seems worthy of consideration in view of the relative phenotypic stability of borderline lesions.

P53 AND CANDIDATE OVARIAN CANCER PRECURSOR LESIONS

1.9 An immunohistochemical study of candidate precursor lesions in ovarian cancer shows that p53 expression is more frequent in surface epithelium and epithelial inclusion cysts associated with ovarian serous neoplasia (borderline and malignant) than in normal ovaries. It is likely, therefore, that loss of normal p53 protein function is a key event in ovarian carcinogenesis.

1.10 Ovarian intraepithelial neoplasia (OIN) may be the precursor of ovarian malignancy and, in some cases at least, p53 protein expression may precede overt cytological abnormalities.

RETROVIRAL-LIKE GENOMIC ELEMENTS IN THE OVARY

1.11 A new family of retroviral-like elements have been discovered in the rat genome. Members of this family are specifically transcriptionally active in the adult rat ovary.

1.12 The relationship between potential transcription factor-binding elements in the promoter of the retroviral elements and promoters of the oestrogen receptor, FSH receptor, and LH receptor, as well as the tissue specificity of expression, support promoter-driven activation as the means of induction of transcription of these retroviral elements.

1.13 If promoter-driven activation of these retroviral elements can be proven, the promoter elements may provide a valuable tool to regulate gene expression *in vitro* and *in vivo* including gene therapy strategies.

1.14 The distribution and abundance (in the range of 1 000 copies per genome) of these retroviral genomic elements in the rat genome make them useful tools together with genome scanning to detect genetic abnormalities in transformed rat ovarian surface epithelial cells.

1.15 We recommend that for future studies attempting to identify a precursor lesion for ovarian cancer investigators should consider comparisons of macroscopically normal contralateral ovary and apparently normal peritoneum, in cases of sporadic early stage ovarian cancer.

1.16 We recommend that in p53 studies sequencing should ideally be combined with immunohistochemical approaches.

1.17 We recommend that microdissection techniques should be explored further when comparing phenotypically normal ovarian surface epithelium adjacent to the neoplastic lesion.

1.18 There is presently some concern over the relationship between the use of drugs to stimulate ovulation in infertile women, and the subsequent risk for ovarian neoplasia. **We recommend** further studies to clarify this possible relationship.

32.2 IS OVARIAN CANCER PREVENTABLE?

OVARIAN CANCER INCIDENCE AND RISK FACTORS

2.1 The incidence of ovarian cancer differs by about 5-fold between countries with high and low incidence. This absolute variation is very small when compared with other common solid cancers. There are no obvious geographical clues to aetiology. There has been a slight overall increase in incidence with time. Five year population-based survival in Denmark and Scotland has improved from 25% to 30% between 1970 and 1985. Using three year survival figures, the results are more encouraging (for patients under 55 years the figures have improved from 38% to 55%).

2.2 The strongest risk factor is family history. Others are low parity, older age at first birth, younger menarche and older menopause. There are no identified strong dietary effects. Oral contraceptive use reduces risk. The risk of ovarian cancer appears to be halved among women who use oral contraceptives for 5 years. The effect persists for at least 10 years after use stops. It is not clear whether this extends through the menopause. To date, epidemiological studies of ovarian cancer have been unsatisfactory.

MOLECULAR BASIS OF OVARIAN GROWTH AND DEVELOPMENT

2.3 Allowing for unrestricted pregnancy and lactation there will be about 20 to 40 ovulations in a woman's life time. However in the modern woman there is the potential for about 480 ovulations in a life time. Components of the growth control of ovarian epithelial cells are beginning to be identified. They include: TGF-α, TGF-β, EGFR and gonadotrophins which may achieve effects via growth factor release or via effects on androgen or oestrogen biosynthesis. Detailed mechanisms of growth control and of stromal-epithelial interaction may differ between rodent and human ovary. Caution is needed in extrapolating from animal models.

2.4 It is unclear whether the protective effect of oral contraceptives is due only to prevention of ovulation or also to other factors. There is currently no evidence that tamoxifen alters ovarian cancer risk.

2.5 The role of life-style factors in ovarian cancer risk is poorly understood. Of all risk factors identified, oral contraceptive use is the only consistently found risk determinant, in that alteration of exposure will directly change the risk of developing the disease. A clearer understanding of the mechanism of action of oral contraceptives on ovarian cancer risk could serve to accelerate prospects for prevention.

2.6 We recommend that better epidemiological and biological studies be established to answer the following questions:

(a) Is combined steroid oral contraceptive use protective against post-menopausal ovarian cancer?

(b) Can epidemiological and biological studies elucidate the mechanism of protection by oral contraceptives, and is this apparent protective effect similar in sporadic and familial ovarian cancer?

(c) Can final conclusions be made on the role of diet, including the suggested link with galactose intake?

(d) Is there a link between infertility (plus or minus fertility drugs) and ovarian cancer?

(e) Is there a role for the interaction of stroma and/or blood cells with endocrine mediated responses of ovarian epithelial cells? Is there a difference in sensitivities to exogenous factors between the normal and neoplastic epithelial cells?

32.3 FAMILIAL OVARIAN CANCER

3.1 The recently identified familial breast and ovarian cancer gene BRCA1 was described. Epidemiological studies indicate that:

(a) Female BRCA1 carriers have an 85% risk of breast cancer and a 63% risk of ovarian cancer by age 70 years.

(b) There may be two classes of ovarian cancer susceptibility mutations: type 1 (the more frequent) conferring a relatively low risk of 26% by age 70 years, and type 2 a risk of 85% by age 70 years.

(c) BRCA1 carriers also have a 3-fold increased risk of colon cancer and male carriers have a 4-fold increased risk of prostate cancer.

3.2 High penetrance predisposing mutations have been found in approximately 100 families. These appear to be loss of function mutations, indicating that BRCA1 is a tumour suppressor gene.

3.3 There is a statistically significant association between mutations in the 5' region of the gene and increased risk of ovarian cancer, in BRCA1 carriers.

3.4 There is still some dispute about the frequency of high penetrance BRCA1 mutations in the general population but there is general agreement that it is somewhere between 1:500 and 1:2000.

3.5 BRCA1 is a large gene, spanning approximately 100 kilobases, with 22 coding exons, making mutation screening costly. The BRCA1 gene encodes a protein of 1863 amino acids of unknown function.

3.6 One particular BRCA1 mutation, which is called 1294 Del40, appears to confer an extremely high risk of ovarian cancer.

3.7 While there are examples of large families in which a defined BRCA1 mutation is associated exclusively with breast or ovarian cancer, there are also instances of the same BRCA1 mutation accompanied by breast cancer in one family but ovarian cancer in another. The contribution of modifying genes or of environmental factors in determining the phenotype associated with a given BRCA1 mutation are, at present, unclear.

3.8 There is now evidence of BRCA1 involvement in sporadic ovarian cancer but as yet no evidence for involvement in sporadic breast cancer.

3.9 The *BRCA2* gene, which has been mapped to chromosome 13q12–q13 also confers a susceptibility to ovarian cancer. Preliminary estimates suggest that female carriers have a 17 times relative risk of ovarian cancer although this number is based on only two families.

3.10 In the UKCCCR Familial Ovarian Cancer Registry, Lynch type 2 families appear to be uncommon.

3.11 Site specific ovarian cancer families show evidence of linkage to BRCA1 and BRCA1 predisposing mutations have been identified in a number of such families. However attention is drawn to a recent abstract suggesting linkage of site specific ovarian cancer to chromosome 9q. This has not been confirmed.

3.12 There is no difference in the frequencies of three BRCA1 sequence variants between cancer patients and controls, indicating that these are neutral polymorphisms.

3.13 The UKCCCR Familial Ovarian Cancer Registry of high risk women has been set up, and to date there have been three ovarian cancers and eight breast cancers detected on follow-up in women at risk. This represents an ovarian cancer rate of 0.5 cancers per 100 woman years and a cumulative risk of 1 in 8 of developing ovarian cancer by 70 years of age.

3.14 In a survey of 240 women in the UKCCCR Familial Ovarian Cancer Registry at high risk of ovarian cancer, only 61 received vaginal ultrasonography which was the recommended screening test.

3.15 Approximately 100 000 women in the UK between the ages of 25 and 60 years have a significant family history of either breast or ovarian cancer. When BRCA1 and other relevant gene testing becomes more generally available many of these women may want the test.

3.16 BRCA1 germline mutations are thought to account for 2–5% of all ovarian cancer cases and about 80% of all families with breast and ovarian cancer.

3.17 Women from cancer families appear to have a greater than average knowledge of genetics. There is variance between their actual and perceived risk and there is some misunderstanding as to the significance of family history. At the moment there are very few people in the UK with the skills to run familial ovarian cancer clinics. **We recommend** that the training of cancer geneticists must be addressed. The long term funding of such clinics needs to be determined in some countries. Through the media attention given to the identification of the BRCA1 gene it was felt that the public are demanding information. Proper counselling must be available to women before they are screened for BRCA1 mutations.

3.18 We recommend that cancer genetic training courses for gynaecologists, oncologists and specialist nurses be established.

3.19 Cancer genetic clinics are the means by which research into both the clinical and genetic aspects of familial ovarian cancer may be taken forward. **We recommend** that in the UK the service components of these clinics, including the adequate provision for recording and evaluating the work undertaken, must be funded by the National Health Service.

3.20 There should be a consensus on criteria for referral of women for currently available screening tests. **We recommend** that only women with two first or second degree affected relatives be screened. Until the role of ovarian cancer screening has been defined, all information should be collected within research-orientated registries.

3.21 We recommend that in screening high risk women, serum CA125 level and vaginal ultrasonography should be carried out and serum stored for future analysis.

3.22 A satisfactory answer to the question 'Does prophylactic oophorectomy for women with a strong family history of ovarian cancer, perceived to be at increased risk, actually offer prophylaxis?', is required. **We recommend** that all such women who undergo prophylactic oophorectomy (or hysterectomy with bilateral salpingo-oophorectomy) should be registered nationally. In the UK they should be entered on to the UKCCCR Familial Ovarian Cancer Register.

32.4 MOLECULAR GENETICS

4.1 Somatic losses in ovarian cancers were described. Aggregated results of studies on chromosomes 11 and 17 were described. Loss of heterozygosity near the 11q telomere and both 17 telomeres correlated with a very poor prognosis.

4.2 Losses on chromosome 13 covered both the RB1 and BRCA2 loci and it is therefore unknown which one, if either, of these genes is the target of loss.

4.3 In both mucinous and serous tumours one copy of chromosome 17 is often lost. Xq losses are also common.

4.4 Although allelic imbalance studies are helpful they are not the only way to find novel genes involved in ovarian cancer progression. **We recommend** that other techniques such as comparative genome hybridization (CGH) and differential display are complementary, and so should be adopted.

4.5 **We recommend** that a centralized data register, localizing molecular lesions in sporadic ovarian cancer should be set up, facilitating adequate data collection on different tumour subtypes. This should be done in conjunction with data on response to treatment and analysis of mechanisms of drug resistance.

32.5 OPTIMIZING TREATMENT

ADEQUATE PRIMARY SURGERY

5.1 The incidence of random mutations increases with tumour bulk and these mutations may include the appearance of chemoresistant clones. Therefore cytoreduction of a tumour may contribute to the effectiveness of chemotherapy.

5.2 It has been known for some time that survival is related to the amount of residual disease after cytoreductive surgery. This year a randomized study of interventional cytoreductive surgery mounted by the EORTC has given us randomized data that shows the important contribution that surgery makes to survival. A confirmatory GOG study is currently underway.

5.3 There is now little doubt that surgery is mandatory as part of management of advanced epithelial ovarian cancer although the following questions still remain to be answered:

(a) Timing of cytoreductive surgery: pre-chemotherapy, after the first 2–3 cycles or at a given individualized point as defined by histological markers or response assessment.

(b) The extent of surgery with particular regard to lymphadenectomy.

(c) The timing of chemotherapy after initial cytoreduction.

(d) The role of cytoreductive surgery in selected patients with stage IV disease.

IMMEDIATE POST-SURGICAL TUMOUR GROWTH

5.4 There is now an increasing amount of data to suggest that surgery enhances the proliferation rate of residual disease, possibly mediated via the release of cytokines and growth factors into the peritoneal cavity. These adverse effects may be exacerbated by the immunosuppressive consequences associated with surgery, such as a decrease in NK cells and certain T-lymphocyte subsets.

DOSE INTENSITY

5.5 One possible strategy to improve the results of chemotherapy is to intensify the dose. There have been a number of studies performed and from these it can be concluded that below a particular dose of cisplatin (approximately 50mg/m^2) the efficacy of treatment is impaired.

5.6 However, how much benefit can be gained by relatively small increases (less than 2-fold) above the standard dose remains uncertain, although the total dose given may be important. Carboplatin dosing should only be calculated according to the renal clearance of the drug, preferably using a suitable formula, such as the Calvert Formula. This allows the drug to be administered at a dose that achieves a consistent 'area under the curve' (AUC) and accurately predicts the drug's main side effect, myelosuppression. It is not known whether higher doses of carboplatin are more effective than lower doses when administered in this way, or what is the optimum target AUC to give the best therapeutic ratio. Existing data indicate that a substantial (greater than 2-fold) increase in AUC will be required to impact upon efficacy. In the case of paclitaxel, since the pharmacokinetics are non-linear, more

modest increases in dose may be associated with significant improvements in efficacy. Future trials should compare significantly different doses and take into account drug pharmacokinetics.

THE ROLE OF TAXANES IN RELAPSED/REFRACTORY DISEASE

5.7 Taxanes are undoubtedly an important new development in the treatment of ovarian cancer. In patients with resistant disease and disease that recurs rapidly after the end of first-line chemotherapy, taxanes currently provide the only realistic treatment option. However, the duration of response is short and any possible benefit needs to be weighed against potential side effects, notably alopecia. In late relapsing disease a number of alternative drugs are also active and the role of taxanes in this situation remains to be assessed.

NEW STANDARDS OF CARE IN FIRST-LINE CHEMOTHERAPY

5.8 The GOG have reported that the survival of patients treated with a cisplatin-paclitaxel combination is significantly superior to standard cisplatin-cyclophosphamide in patients who have had suboptimal cytoreduction. In the US this regimen is now considered to be the gold standard therapy and it is no longer possible to mount randomized studies of first line chemotherapy in that country unless all treatment arms contain a taxane. A confirmatory study, albeit using a slightly different dose and schedule of paclitaxel, is being performed by the EORTC/NCI-Canada/Scottish group.

5.9 Current pilot studies with paclitaxel have been focusing on dose and schedule of the compound when given either as a single agent or in combination with carboplatin.

The apparent amelioration of carboplatin-induced thrombocytopenia in this combination is of particular interest.

NEW APPROACHES TO PREVENTION AND THERAPY

5.10 An understanding of the biology of ovarian cancer is vital to allow a more rational approach to the development of new strategies for prevention and treatment.

5.11 A number of alterations in growth factors, oncogenes and tumour suppressor genes have been identified as ovarian epithelium undergoes malignant transformation. Among the factors that regulate growth of normal ovarian epithelium, most stimulate proliferation but TGF-β inhibits it. Ovarian cancer cells have lost autocrine, but not paracrine growth inhibition by TGF-β in at least 40% of cases.

5.12 Synergistic inhibition of ovarian cancer cell growth has been obtained with all-trans retinoic acid and TGF-β, suggesting new approaches to chemoprevention of the disease.

5.13 For therapy of established ovarian cancer, inhibition of tyrosine kinases, inhibition of ras, upregulation of tyrosine phosphatases, replacement of p53 function and inhibition of metalloproteinases provide attractive approaches. Monoclonal antibodies against HER-2/neu can inhibit growth of ovarian tumour cells that over-express the receptor. Use of immunotoxins in combination with radionuclide conjugates reactive with HER-2/neu protein may permit more effective therapy in the near future.

SURVIVAL ANALYSIS USING NEURAL NET TECHNOLOGY

5.14 Neural network design is based on a number of simplified model neurones linked together. If the network is large enough it is able to function as a computer and solve any precisely specified mathematical problem. Artificial neural networks differ from conventional databases in that they have the ability to learn, reorganize data and recognize patterns. These networks may have advantages over more traditional statistical methods such as Cox's regression analysis because they function in a non-time dependent manner. New prognostic factors may be identified using this method and the survival of an individual new patient predicted.

RELAPSE OR RECURRENT DISEASE

5.15 We recommend that the following major areas be addressed:

(a) What is appropriate role of surgery for patients who develop clinical relapse, progressive disease or who require palliation for intestinal obstruction and how do we reselect appropriate candidates for surgery?

(b) What are the appropriate means by which we should measure response to chemotherapy?

(c) Where should treatment be given and by whom?

(d) How do we best palliate symptoms of progressive disease in the context of maximizing the quality of life?

DEFINITIONS OF OPERATIONS FOR OVARIAN CANCER AND SELECTION OF SURGICAL CANDIDATES IN RELAPSING OR RECURRENT DISEASE

5.16 It is important to establish clear definitions of the operative procedures used for ovarian cancer. **We recommend** the adoption of the following definitions:

Primary cytoreductive surgery:
an operation performed prior to the initiation of treatment for advanced ovarian cancer used to remove as much primary and metastatic disease as possible in order to facilitate response to treatment and to improve survival.

Interval cytoreductive surgery:
an operation performed after a short course of induction chemotherapy, *e.g.* 2-3 cycles of chemotherapy, to remove as much primary and metastatic disease as possible to facilitate response to subsequent chemotherapy and to improve survival.

Secondary cytoreductive surgery:
an operation performed in patients who either have persistent disease at the completion of a complete course of chemotherapy or who subsequently develop clinical relapse.

5.17 We recommend that secondary cytoreductive operations and operations to palliate intestinal obstruction should be done only in selected patients as guided by the individual circumstance of the patient and the best judgement of the clinicians to whom her care is entrusted. It was felt in general that secondary cytoreductive operations should be confined to patients who have tumours that exhibit indolent growth, as manifest by disease progression through intervals of one year or greater from the time of complete of primary chemotherapy, or from the time of negative second-look surgery.

5.18 We recommend that biological and molecular markers be studied to predict time to relapse. This might help to categorize patients who are most likely to benefit from secondary cytoreductive surgery.

5.19 Consensus agreement was not achieved on how a rising serum CA125 measurement

could be appropriately integrated into clinical management of patients being followed after achieving clinical remission with primary chemotherapy. **We recommend** that this be studied in a prospective manner in randomized trials.

MEASUREMENT OF RESPONSE TO PRIMARY AND SECOND-LINE CHEMOTHERAPY

5.20 It was agreed that serum CA125 measurement is a more cost-effective as well as a sensitive and specific method for assessing response to second-line chemotherapy compared with computed tomography scans (CT). Serial CA125 measurements have the comparative advantage of being simpler, cheaper and are as reliable as the latter.

5.21 We recommend that response assessment using serial serum CA125 measurement should be incorporated into accepted methods of new drug approval, when it could often replace CT scanning as the primary method of measuring response. The WHO standards should be revised accordingly. CT scans should be used more sparingly. They should not be a substitute for careful serial physical examinations, including pelvic examinations, of the patient during her chemotherapy.

5.22 We recommend the use of specific serum CA125 response criteria that have been developed by retrospective analysis of large cohorts of patients treated with chemotherapy. These criteria are, for example, a 50% response (defined as a 50% fall of CA125 by serial measurement of three to four levels), and a 75% response (defined by a 75% fall of CA125 levels over 3 serial measurements), both over a specified amount of time.

WHERE AND BY WHOM SHOULD PATIENTS WITH OVARIAN CANCER BE TREATED?

5.23 Data from a population based study in Scotland strongly suggest that optimal outcome of management of ovarian cancer patients as measured by survival is best achieved when patients are initially operated on by gynaecologists rather than general surgeons, and are managed in a multidisciplinary clinic. Patients who undergo optimal primary cytoreductive surgery and whose initial treatment includes a platinum compound have a better survival. A correlation has been established between the number of procedures performed by the individual gynaecologist and survival. On a population basis, five year survival could be expected to improve from 24% to 38% if all patients received currently available treatment in such optimal circumstances.

5.24 We recommend that international studies be conducted to confirm the importance of these factors. Such studies should include central histopathology review.

PALLIATION OF SYMPTOMS AND QUALITY OF LIFE

5.25 We recommend that intestinal obstruction is best palliated by a combination of medical and surgical interventions in a strategy designed to maximize the quality of life. Optimal medical management is based on a strategy which uses effective medications but has the fewest side effects.

5.26 We recommend that surgical intervention should be performed only on patients whose subsequent survival is likely to be longer than several weeks.

32.6 OBSTACLES TO SUCCESSFUL TREATMENT

6.1 Regarding clinical drug resistance the following have to be considered:

(a) What are the fundamental cellular mechanisms which underlie the development of clinical drug resistance in ovarian cancer? In particular can resistance be explained on the basis of one or two major factors or is the process multifactorial?

(b) What are the most promising avenues for resistance modulation?

6.2 Mechanisms which underlie resistance to the most important agents in ovarian cancer, namely the platinum compounds, include defective transport, increased intracellular inactivation and enhanced DNA repair. Research in this field is now building on this wealth of data to explore new factors which may explain resistance development clinically.

6.3 There is a general consensus that the failure of cells to engage the process of apoptosis could be an important factor underlying the development of clinical drug resistance. Indeed this could be a common pathway for 'multi drug resistance' as well as platinum resistance. The genetic triggers involved are probably multiple, but a key one is likely to be functional inactivation of the TP53 gene. Mutations in the TP53 gene are common in ovarian cancer, and correlations with response to carboplatin have been established in one study.

6.4 At present there are relatively few other clinical data to support the wealth of preclinical information relating p53 status to drug resistance. Accordingly it was agreed that it was important to develop assays to assess p53 *function* in clinical material from patients before and after chemotherapy.

Sequential tumour biopsies from patients given single agent therapy would be most informative in this respect.

6.5 Over the last few months information has been accruing on the potential importance of the phenomenon of microsatellite instability (MI). Preclinical *in vitro* data suggest a correlation between MI and cytotoxic drug resistance. Cells which have evidence of MI are presumably able to by-pass potentially lethal DNA adducts resulting from a number of cytotoxic drugs thus evading the apoptotic response following DNA damage. The genes which control this process of mismatch repair are currently being analysed. Microsatellite instability is a relatively simple phenomenon to assess in paraffin embedded tumour biopsies, although there are no data as yet relating it to clinical drug resistance.

MULTI-DRUG RESISTANCE

6.6 Multi-drug resistance is an experimental phenomenon which involves cross-resistance to a number of agents. The classical form is mediated by P-glycoprotein which has been detected in clinical material in ovarian cancer at varying levels. In one study increased expression was seen following doxorubicin-containing chemotherapy. Its overall significance is however unclear, but recent data on first-line therapy with taxol or doxorubicin indicate the potential importance of this resistance mechanism.

6.7 Proteins which underlie other forms of multi-drug resistance include the so-called multi-drug resistance-related protein (MRP) whose function includes a role in glutathione conjugate transport. Although this could be relevant in ovarian cancer, clinical studies have not so far shown a correlation between MRP expression and outcome.

6.8 In contrast another protein, lung resistance protein (LRP) has been measured in clinical material and interestingly expression correlates strongly with outcome to cisplatin containing chemotherapy. **We recommend** further studies in this area.

6.9 Data on clinical material and other potential markers for resistance mechanisms, including glutathione-S transferase and metallothionene, are conflicting, and the significance of isolated measurements is doubtful.

6.10 The potential means for circumventing drug resistance include the use of novel cisplatin analogues. These include drugs bearing the DACH complex (*e.g.* oxaliplatin), the lipophilic oral analogue JM216, as well as new trans-platinum compounds. A range of *in vitro* and *in vivo* models have demonstrated the potential for JM216 and this is now in Phase II clinical trial. The models used vary in the extent to which different mechanisms are predominant in determining resistance. This makes it possible to make a rational interpretation of the results of clinical trial.

6.11 Attempts to modulate drug resistance include the use of the gamma glutamyl cysteine synthetase (GGCS) inhibitor, buthionine sulphoximine (BSO). Phase II trials are now planned since in Phase I trials satisfactory glutathione depletion in tumour cells was noted. Such trials should incorporate drugs such as carboplatin as well as melphalan.

6.12 A number of candidate agents for cisplatin modulation, including tamoxifen, have been identified although their mechanisms, which are ER-independent, remain elusive. In respect of Taxol, Phase I trials using the MDR modulator SDZPSC833, have demonstrated a significant pharma-cokinetic interaction, as predicted from trials

313

involving agents such as doxorubicin and etoposide.

6.13 The collection of clinical material from patients with ovarian cancer should be co-ordinated. In particular samples taken prior to chemotherapy and on relapse should be available for study in a number of centres. **We recommend** that a central registry for such material should be considered for Europe, incorporating full clinical data.

6.14 New avenues to explore in assessing mechanisms underlying resistance in this clinical material include the failure of the apoptotic process and the presence of MI (indeed these may be connected). Accordingly **we recommend** a coordinated approach to developing assays for both these features is recommended.

6.15 While it is recognized that modulation based on a single mechanism may not be successful in the majority of cases, **we recommend** such trials. An important feature of these is the incorporation of a biological end point measure to facilitate a rational interpretation of results.

6.16 Ovarian germ cell tumours represent a rare but curable form of ovarian tumour in which cisplatin resistance generally does not occur. Molecular explanations for this are unclear, and **we recommend** further investigations in this area.

32.7 APPROACHES TO GENE THERAPY

7.1 Gene therapy has its origins in attempts to correct genetic deficiencies by replacing defective genes in affected cells. Its applications in cancer lie not in this direction but by using DNA as a drug to render the tumour cells susceptible to chemotherapy, as a means of inducing a therapeutic immune response, or to decrease the undesired toxicity to normal tissues, such as bone marrow, by introducing resistance genes. In this sense perhaps it would better be called *DNA therapy* rather than *gene therapy*.

7.2 One approach depends upon introducing into cancer cells DNA that renders them susceptible to a drug treatment. For example a widely used model system involves the herpes simplex virus thymidine kinase (tk) gene which when expressed renders it susceptible to the drug ganciclovir.

7.3 A second major approach is to try and achieve immune therapy. This could be by modifying the tumour cell or, once targets for cytotoxic T-cell attack have been identified, introducing the appropriate DNA coding for these antigens into professional antigen presenting cells.

7.4 The means of delivery of DNA vary. Direct injection, physical methods or recombinant viruses all have been used. While viruses are efficient vectors they suffer from a number of limitations, such as the possibility of insertional mutagenesis with retroviruses, or the induction of an undesirable immune response with adenoviruses.

7.5 The drug treatment approach involves a 'bystander' effect in which there is killing of adjacent untransduced cells, presumably via transfer across gap junctions. This is important because the ability to target cells efficiently is not yet sufficient to achieve transduction of all cells within the tumour mass. The advantage of the immunotherapy approach is that it involves an amplification event in which the activated immune cells may deal with a number of tumour target cells. Equally the immune treatments are most likely to produce a systemic protection.

7.6 The currently available DNA delivery systems have little if any tissue specificity. One way to overcome this is to target expression of the DNA by using tissue specific promoters. One example is to use a tyrosinase promoter to target expression to melanocytes for the treatment of melanomas. While this approach is not entirely selective for the tumour the specificity achieved may be sufficient for therapeutic purposes. The product of the MUC1 gene is over-expressed in epithelial ovarian carcinomas, and its 5′ flanking promoter sequences could be used to target this tumour type. Promising results have been obtained in murine melanoma model which indicate that cell death as a consequence of the HSV tk/ganciclovir combination may stimulate a strong immune response. These results encourage an approach that combines drug targeted killing with immunotherapy.

7.7 Three model systems were discussed in more detail:

(a) The first involves attacking a tumour through its vasculature. Vascular endothelial growth factor (VEGF) is critical for the growth of vascular endothelial cells. Soluble versions of the extracellular portion of VEGF receptors have been shown to block VEGF activity and provide a promising approach to the inhibition of angiogenesis.

(b) Virus directed enzyme prodrug therapy (VDEPT) can be combined with the introduction of molecules such as B7 or ICAM-1 into tumour cells to enhance the immune response. A particular promising model involves the enzyme nitro imidazole reductase together with the inactive drug CB1954 resulting in a highly active bifunctional alkylating agent. *In vitro* mixtures of transfected and untransfected cells reveal an impressive bystander effect. These responses suggest that intraperitoneal therapy may be possible in ovarian cancer using these reagents.

(c) Alternatively B7.1, IL2, IL4 or other genes may be introduced into removed tumour cells to mimic the action of antigen presenting cells. The transfected cells can then be returned as an irradiated vaccine to the patients.

7.8 Technology for DNA therapy approaches is well ahead of clinical exploitation, and it is likely that only clinical studies will move the field forward significantly.

7.9 **We recommend** that at this stage the emphasis should be on phase I studies that are accompanied by well designed investigations to monitor the response to treatment and in particular the immune response at the cellular level.

7.10 There is no consensus as to the preferred approach to gene therapy and **we recommend** the employment of a range of alternative techniques.

7.11 Approval is more likely to be obtained for DNA-based studies using plasmids rather than viral vectors.

7.12 *In vitro* and *in vivo* models remain inadequate and need further development.

7.13 We recommend that regulatory issues be addressed continuously.

Index